MECHANICAL LOW BACK PAIN

Perspectives in Functional Anatomy

JAMES A. PORTERFIELD, P.T., M.A., A.T.C.

President, Rehabilitation and Health Center, Crystal Clinic
Akron, Ohio
Assistant Professor, Cleveland State University
Cleveland, Ohio

CARL DeROSA, P.T., Ph.D.

Professor and Chairman, Physical Therapy Program
Northern Arizona University
Flagstaff, Arizona

SECOND EDITION

W.B. SAUNDERS COMPANY
A Division of Harcourt Brace & Company

PHILADELPHIA, LONDON, TORONTO, MONTREAL, SYDNEY, TOKYO

W. B. SAUNDERS COMPANY
A Division of Harcourt Brace & Company

The Curtis Center
Independence Square West
Philadelphia, PA 19106

Library of Congress Cataloging-in-Publication Data

Porterfield, James A.
    Mechanical low back pain : perspectives in functional anatomy /
James A. Porterfield, Carl DeRosa. — 2nd ed.
        p.   cm.
    Includes bibliographical references and index.
    ISBN 0-7216-6837-2
    1. Backache—Pathophysiology. 2. Backache—Patients—
Rehabilitation.   I. DeRosa, Carl.   II. Title.
    [DNLM: 1. Low Back Pain.   2. Biomechanics.   3. Lumbosacral Region—
physiology.   WE 755 P849m 1998]
RD771.B217P67   1998
617.5'64—dc21
DNLM/DLC
                                                                    97-14398

MECHANICAL LOW BACK PAIN   ISBN   0-7216-6837-2

Printed in the United States of America.

Last digit is the print number: 9   8   7   6   5   4   3   2   1

To our children Alison, Jeffrey, Sara, Patrick, and Christopher.

PREFACE

One of the basic tenets outlined in the first edition of *Mechanical Low Back Pain: Perspectives in Functional Anatomy* was that treatment philosophies for low back pain needed to change from passive therapeutic interventions to those strategies encouraging a more active rehabilitation approach, i.e., those emphasizing restoration of function. We believe that the concepts outlined in that first edition have rapidly become the accepted standard for today's treatment approach in the management of patients with mechanical low back pain.

Since the first edition, precipitous changes have occurred in the delivery of all health care services. Although the phrase "managed care" is used, it is really costs that increasingly have been managed. These changes in health care mandate the analysis and development of more efficient patient care models. In this second edition we revisit the original treatment philosophies and reorganize, enhance, and direct them toward patient care guidelines designed to comply with present medical and economic criteria. The new challenge raises these central questions: If the patient wants anything more than information and treatment geared toward improving their ability to help themselves, can we as health professionals help them, and is treatment indicated? These questions represent the current medical, therapeutic, and economic realities that serve as the basis for clinical practice.

Rehabilitation of mechanical low back pain thus can be defined as the process through which the patient begins to restore function and at the same time gain valuable information required to improve their ability for self-management. To effectively teach the patient, it is essential that the clinician have a comprehensive understanding of the functional anatomy of the lumbopelvic region, the response of tissues to injury, and the effects that age-related changes have on the specialized connective tissues. The emphasis of this second edition is to integrate this scientific information into a format that can be understood easily by the patient so that successful management can take place with efficient intervention. From this starting point, the steps can then be taken to implement rehabilitation strategies that direct the management—not the "cure"—of their low back pain problem toward optimizing their musculoskeletal health. It is our hope that the information in this textbook provides the clinician with the scientific and clinical knowledge required to maintain a viable clinical practice in an emerging health care system.

ACKNOWLEDGMENTS

As in the first edition of *Mechanical Low Back Pain: Perspectives in Functional Anatomy*, we are grateful for the willingness of numerous friends and colleagues who knowingly, and sometimes unknowingly, assisted us in completion of this second edition. The artwork and photography, which adjoin visual images to thoughts, were provided by an outstanding artist, Tina Cauller, and a very talented photographer, Kurt Lundquist, P.T. Their illustrations and photographs have enhanced the quality and teaching potential of this text.

Our colleagues and friends, John McCulloch, M.D., Phil Sauer, P.T., Vert Mooney, M.D., Jonathan Cooperman, P.T., and Stanley Paris, P.T., Ph.D., continue to be sources of academic and clinical inspiration. We are also indebted to Paul Larsen, P.T., Mike Barry, P.T., Dave Hartwig, P.T., and Greg Redfern, P.T., who assisted us in the preparation of many of the dissections seen in this text, and Troy Gerspacher for his assistance with the photos. A special thanks is also extended to Margaret Biblis and the production teams at W.B. Saunders for their continued help and support.

Most importantly, we thank our wives and best friends, Marlene DeRosa, P.T., and Bonnie Porterfield, who not only offer unequivocal support of our efforts and projects, but who also lovingly tolerate our many moments of "out of the box" thinking. Their encouragement is the source of our energies.

CONTENTS

CHAPTER 1

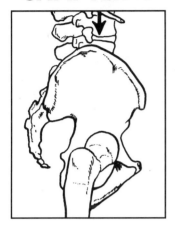

PRINCIPLES OF MECHANICAL LOW BACK DISORDERS

Low back pain has been, and continues to be, one of the enigmas of modern medicine. The problem transcends the typical approach used with other disease processes: determine the cause and implement a treatment strategy to directly impact the cause. On the contrary, the epidemic of low back pain and the disability associated with it has appeared to escalate at the same time that the greatest technological advances related to diagnosis, treatment, and rehabilitation have been made. Back pain has now become not only a medical problem, but a social, legal, and political one as well.

This chapter provides an overview of several topics germane to the concepts presented in this textbook. First, a discussion of costs is presented so that the reader can relate this information to the philosophy of evaluation and treatment presented in Chapters 5 and 6. Following this discussion, a brief review of the natural history of low back disorders and the influence of age, injury, and adaptive changes to the different neuro–musculo–skeletal tissues is presented. The information is then applied to the detailed functional anatomy presented in Chapter 2 (neurosciences), Chapter 3 (muscles of the lumbopelvic region), and Chapter 4 (articulations of the lumbopelvic region).

The goal of this textbook is to provide the reader with a comprehensive understanding of the function-

al anatomy of the lumbopelvic region, on which a practical evaluation scheme can be based, and on which management of the problem can be focused on restoration of function. The overriding assumption, however, is that, through education for self management, the responsibility of rehabilitation is ultimately directed *back* to the patient.

LOW BACK PAIN COSTS

Cost effectiveness has fast become one of the necessary requirements for sound and successful clinical practice and it is essential that any textbook dealing with the topic of low back disorders take this into account. Evaluation and treatment strategies suggested for managing patients with low back pain that fail to recognize the necessity for cost effectiveness are no longer practical in the emerging health care system. The challenge to the clinician is not only to provide quality care, but to do so in a cost-effective manner. In recognition of this responsibility, health care professionals dealing with spinal disorders need to be prepared to justify their treatment based on outcomes that can withstand evaluation not only by medical criteria but by economic criteria as well.[22]

Brief descriptions of costs relative to health care in general and back pain specifically help to illustrate the importance of cost awareness. Aaron and associates have noted that by the year 2000, at the current rate of spending, approximately 15 percent of the gross national product in the United States will be utilized for health care.[1] This rate of health care spending actually exceeds the rate of inflation. However, the precise understanding of the total costs for health care are never fully appreciated because such numbers typically reflect only the *direct costs* of health care— those dollars allocated to medical expenditures such as hospitalization, emergency room visits, visits to health care professionals, outpatient costs, home health visits, rehabilitation costs, and laboratory procedures. Direct costs also include nonmedical costs such as legal expenditures and litigation.

In addition to direct costs, *indirect* and *psychosocial costs* must be considered so that a more comprehensive picture of the total costs to society emerges. *Indirect costs* refer to those costs that are related to lost work output due to a reduced capacity for activity. Such a reduced work capacity obviously impacts productivity in the workplace and is a primary concern with the low back pain problem.[43] Examples of indirect costs are wage loss due to work absence, wage decrease due to job change, work time lost by family members in caring for or transporting an injured family member for health care or rehabilitation, and loss of professional opportunities. Of the many factors that can be considered indirect costs, the inability to work and the time lost from work are the two major indirect costs. These two significant indirect costs are especially relevant in any discussion of disorders of the low back because episodes of back pain are responsible for 25 percent of all lost workdays in the United States, and represent 25 percent of all workers' compensation claims.[35] Further impact of the effect workers' compensation has on the low back problem is addressed below. It has been estimated that chronic low back pain annually results in 225,000 to 300,000 lumbar surgeries and an estimated direct and indirect medical cost of $75 to 100 billion.[35]

Psychosocial costs are more difficult to translate into monetary value because they are associated with pain and suffering and consequently are difficult to accurately measure. Psychosocial costs not only affect the patient, but also family members, co-workers, and other members of society dependent on such human interaction. Increased psychological stress such as job stress, economic stress, self-inflicted stress, and family stress are all potential consequences of disease or injury and are part of the accrued psychosocial costs. It is difficult to measure their cost in terms of actual dollars, but there is no doubt that such psychosocial costs adversely affect the individual's quality of life.

As a result of understanding that psychosocial factors play as important a role as pathology regarding the patient outcome, quality-of-life measures have now assumed paramount importance in determining relevant outcomes for treatment of patients with low back pain. As a result of the increased recognition of the impact of psychosocial costs, outcome and efficacy studies are now being directed toward quality-of-life measures.[20] Because low back pain often prevents or limits work and activities of daily living, one's quality of life is markedly affected. New expectations of the clinician treating patients with low back pain have emerged: outcome measures that ultimately assess the spectrum of health-related quality of life measures. These measures include symptoms, functional status, perception of well-being, and opportunity (Table 1–1).[62] Health-related quality of life measures are the new paradigm for assessing treatment effectiveness and in the further development of policies related to health, injury, and disability. The clinician dealing with spine disorders is now being asked to measure efficacy by assessing quality of life measures and utilize these measure for outcome studies. Physiologic measures are no longer adequate outcome measures. The relationship between changes in such diverse physiologic measures as strength, range of motion, and surgical fusion show little evidence of correlating with changes

---

Table 1–1. Health Related Quality of Life Issues

Symptoms
Pain
Functional Status
Physical
Psychological
Social
Perceptions of Well Being
General Health
Satisfaction with Health
Reported Improvement
Opportunity
Return to Work
Disability Status

in quality of life. If improved physiologic measures indicated that one's quality of life improved, these measures would be adequate. Unfortunately, they do not. Furthermore, sophisticated testing such as electromyography, myelography, discography, and advanced imaging studies are expensive and have a reported 20 to 50 percent rate of error.[12] Hence, quality-of-life measures are assuming a greater weight in judging the efficacy of treatment.

IMPAIRMENT AND DISABILITY

When the costs for diseases of the musculoskeletal system are scrutinized, spine and back injuries are seen to represent the largest component. To fully interpret the costs relative to spine problems, however, one must understand the differences between, and the consequences of, impairment and disability. *Impairment* refers to an anatomic or pathologic abnormality that leads to a loss of bodily ability. In contrast, *disability* refers to a diminished capacity for everyday activities or employment, or the limitation of a person's performance when compared with a fit person of the same age and gender.[50] While impairment is primarily medically determined and based on objective tests and measures of structural limitation, disability is primarily determined from the patient's subjective description. Most often, disability related to the low back is assessed by asking for the patient's impression of how activities of daily living are currently being affected by low back pain. Several reliable and valid tools have been developed for this purpose.[25, 82, 64] Activities of daily living that are often assessed include such functions as sitting, walking, sleeping, dressing, sex life, use of pain medications, etc. Disability relates to the patient's perception of how their particular problem is affecting their activities of daily living and their quality of life.

The significance of understanding the important differences between impairment and disability as they relate to back pain is illustrated by the fact that, for the most part, impairment rates have largely remained stable while disability rates have grown exponentially.[3, 6, 61, 70] Disability-related costs for spinal disorders have been estimated to be $43 billion.[8] In the United States, disorders of the low back are currently the leading cause of disability in people under age 45, the second leading cause of absenteeism from work, the second leading reason for visits to primary care physicians, the fifth most frequent reason for hospi-

talization, and the third ranking reason for surgical procedures.[19, 21, 52, 63] In Europe, the number of patients claiming long-term or permanent disability as a result of chronic low back pain threatens the financial solvency of the welfare system in many countries.[58]

When costs are closely analyzed, however, it is apparent that relatively few patients are responsible for the majority of the costs. Spengler et al. noted that only 10 percent of the claimants for low back injury accounted for nearly 70 percent of the total costs.[70] Leavitt et al., who pioneered the analysis of these skewed costs noted that only 25 percent of workers' compensation claimants accounted for 87 percent of medical and disability claims.[47] The relatively low costs for the remaining 75 percent of claimants are understood when the favorable natural history of low back pain is taken into account.

Therefore, the new clinical challenge has been to identify those factors that may assist the clinician in predicting those patients who have a propensity toward disability, to provide an appropriate treatment strategy and potentially minimize disability costs. Accounting for factors other than spine pathology becomes crucial in attempting to make such a prediction. Factors recognized as having predictive value include (among others) work status at the time of injury, past work history, worker's perception as to whether the injury is compensable, job satisfaction, whether a lawyer had been contacted, and past hospitalizations.[36] Obviously, such a predictive index would be the result of many complex variables. Perhaps one of the best clusters of predictors for identifying which acute low back pain episodes are likely to become chronic disability cases is when it is the perception of the patient that the low back pain episode is work-related plus the absence from work for more than 2 weeks.[48] This is important for the clinician to consider because the 2-week return-to-work "window" suggests a much more active approach to managing the back problem and encouraging early return to work. The treatment approach is highly dependent on the ability to educate the injured person regarding their particular problem and how they can self-manage it, tied to an understanding that a *completely* pain-free state is an unrealistic goal.

Because of the staggering statistics associated with costs, novel evaluation and treatment methods for low back disorders have continually been sought. Attempts to manage the problem have led to research resulting in new knowledge in anatomy, biomechanics, exercise physiology, and neurosciences. This expanding knowledge base has in turn resulted in the modification of some practice habits, the discarding of others, and the addition of new and innovative forms of treatment. Low back pain is especially challenging because of the wide variety of evaluation measurements used, and the lack of standardization in diagnosis or treatment.

Clinical practice has also been continually reshaped by the political, socioeconomic, and legal climate. The rising cost of care for mechanical low back disorders has forced a reexamination of the payment schedules by various third party payers. This change in reimbursement attitudes for services that are provided has mandated new directions for treatment. Additionally, some clinicians have become hesitant to be involved with the industrial low back injury for reasons other than a dwindling reimbursement dollar: This hesitancy can be attributed in part to the perceived low success rate in attempting to manage these patients, as well as to the concern of being drawn into disputes that have resulted in litigation. Since the work-related origin of many industrial back injuries is difficult to prove conclusively, and since the evidence of physical injury is often obscure, back injury claims between employee and employer tend to be more adversarial than other types of claims. The major sources of dispute between the employer and injured worker are the cause of injury, the determination of when the worker is ready to go back to work, and the extent of the impairment and disability.[16] Hadler has noted that psychological and sociopolitical confounders overwhelm both disease and ergonomic measures in predicting the illness of work incapacity.[39, 40] It is very clear, however, that concerted mutual efforts must be made by health care practitioners, employers, politicians, and lawmakers to significantly impact the low back pain problem. Most importantly, the patient must begin to act as an informed consumer and participate in the development of reasonable treatment goals.

NATURAL HISTORY OF BACK PAIN

Low back pain remains a very common human condition that affects an estimated 80 percent of adults during some period in their life.[37] It has been widely suggested that the natural course for most low back pain is of a self-limiting nature, with the vast majority of individuals improving within 6 weeks or less. However, a less optimistic natural history suggests that only one-third of a population reporting back pain had symptoms less than a month, whereas another third reported pain lasting 1 to 5 months, and the remaining third reported pain lasting more than 6 months.[21] The natural history makes the study of intervention efficacy extremely difficult. However, this natural course of the low back pain problem suggests that one of the primary interventions that the clinician treating the patient with low back pain can offer is education for self-management strategies and encouragement of activity to give patients as much responsibility as possible for managing their back problem. This is especially important since recurrence rates for low back pain range from 60 to 85 percent.[76, 77, 78]

There are several factors that influence the natural history of acute low back pain. Early studies suggested that back pain onset is typically in the third decade, and the peak prevalence (prevalence referring to a specific point in time when the question, "Are you currently having back pain?" is asked) is during the fifth decade.[9] The prevalence of low back pain tends to decrease in males after the age of 55 years but females continue to show a slight increase, most likely due to the osteoporotic changes of the vertebrae.

Risk factors also influence the prevalence of back pain. Basic science studies that have demonstrated the beneficial effects of resistance and aerobic exercise on articular cartilage, ligaments, and tendons and the adverse effect that inactivity has on these musculoskeletal structures have been used to support the hypothesis that one's level of physical fitness is an important risk factor to be considered.[57] Cigarette smoking has been recognized as an important risk factor as smokers tend to report symptoms as more severe than nonsmokers.[44] Smoking is viewed as a risk factor because it is thought to interfere with intervertebral disc nutrition, results in poor oxygen transport, is associated with poor physical fitness, and is accompanied by continued bouts of coughing, which raises intra-abdominal pressure. Vibration is also known to be a risk factor for low back pain, as it appears to hasten fatigue failure of collagenous structures.[67]

The work environment also influences the natural course of low back disorders. Workers who view their jobs as boring, tedious, or dissatisfying have much less satisfactory recovery rates. Work relationships and interactions that the employee has with the employer and co-workers also significantly affect recovery.[7, 10] Likewise, the fewer personal-, job-, or family-related problems an individual has the greater chance that the injured worker with low back pain will return to work following acute low back injury.[46]

As suggested in the previous sections, low back pain is essentially a universal and self-limiting phenomenon and is so common that it can be considered a normal human occurrence.[83] By contrast, low back disability is a relatively recent phenomenon.[81] That is to say, although low back pain has been recognized and accepted as a fairly common occurrence, low back disability, as a distinct entity, has surfaced only in modern times. However, it is recognized that treating the patient with mechanical low back pain with activity decreases the disability, whereas treating the patient with prolonged rest, analgesics, and minimal activity increases the disability.[27] Furthermore, pain behaviors are inversely proportional to the amount of exercise done.[29] As a result, the most practical and cost-effective approach to the treatment of low back disorders is an active one that encourages an early return to activity.

This is an important change from previous methods emphasizing bed rest, medications, and passive modalities. One of the reasons for this important change in the focus of treatment is that an active approach minimizes the potential for the low back pain problem to develop into a chronic disability, which is resistant to successful management. Chronic disability becomes increasingly dissociated from its original physical basis.[28, 49, 81, 83]

An early return to activity as a result of restoration and improvement of function should be combined with biomechanical counseling to educate the patient in self-management strategies and ways to remain active and minimize the potential for reinjury. The quality of the educational process for self-management strategies, and the understanding the patient ultimately derives from such an education minimizes the potential for disability, because disability is the patient's subjective interpretation of the problem and his perception of its impact on his quality of life. One of the primary reasons for the escalation of the low back dilemma has been the difficulty in separating the predicament of low back pain from low back disability and predicting those patients with a propensity to disability. This treatment direction emphasizing patient education and promotion of activity helps to lessen the possibility for the conversion of low back pain into low back disability and is the current and future direction of successful management. Optimal treatment is now recognized as early and safe return to work and to the activities of daily living.[59]

As a result of this further understanding, the low back dilemma has been re-examined. We must acknowledge that currently there are few methods of localizing the exact source of low back pain. There is also a paucity of controlled trials that allow for a determination of the most effective forms of management. Furthermore, the response a patient has to treatment is rarely due only to the result of treatment intervention but is also influenced by social and psychological factors. Despite these shortcomings, the advances made in the natural and social sciences can and should be applied to managing the patient with low back pain.

BASIC PRINCIPLES OF MANAGING MECHANICAL DISORDERS

The previously stated activity-oriented approach utilized in the treatment of low back disorders parallels the approach used in the management of mechanical disorders for other areas of the musculoskeletal system. Clinical practice for mechanical disorders can be described briefly as (a) learning as much about the patient as possible through interview, history, and responses during the physical exam, (b) identifying the mechanics of injury, (c) recognizing the status of the injury, (d) recognizing the patient's psychological state, especially with regard to stressors in the person's life, (e) maximizing the potential for repair processes of the musculoskeletal tissues, (f) restoring function as rapidly as possible without reinjury in order to allow for functional healing, and (g) strengthening the musculofascial tissues surrounding the region.

These basic tenets of assessment and treatment have been the standard of care for injuries to the joints of the extremities, but have not been accepted as readily for the low back. In no other area of the body has there been such a plethora of traditional and nontraditional evaluation and treatment techniques. As a result, many patients develop a dependency on therapeutic interventions for symptomatic relief of low back pain at a much greater frequency than for any of the peripheral joints.

For example, the patient with an extremity joint injury is usually expected to alter his activities to avoid exacerbation of the problem. Many times he must accept the fact that this alteration of activities must be maintained for the rest of his life. He is made aware of his limitations occurring as a result of injury, and attempts to manage his own musculoskeletal problem with attention to activity modification and maintenance of strength necessary to support the injured area and help minimize the chance for further injury.

Many patients with mechanical low back pain behave differently and have a different set of expectations in part because of how the "system" treats them. They expect the therapeutic interventions to "cure" their back pain. They are given pathoanatomic diagnoses that are largely based on examiner bias rather than known clusters of signs and symptoms. These patients develop the thought process that the injured state of their low back is not really their problem, but rather the clinician's or system's problem. As a result of this type of thinking, "quick cures" are continually sought after by the clinician and patient alike: modalities to "heal" tissue, manipulation to free "locked" joints or "trapped" structures, mobilization to "release" soft tissues, surgery to "reconstruct" the low back anatomy according to a perceived normal structure, and specialty exercise devices—designed to "eliminate" pain.

These examples of treatment, and others with similar intent, are successful in only a small number of select patients; they are primarily methods to provide temporary relief of pain and have little impact on the long-range outcome. Such techniques alter the patient's perception of pain, rather than restore function. It is thought that if the pain is "taken away," function will automatically return. In most cases, these approaches are temporary solutions at best because the patient is not taught how to manage his own problem. What was once pain now becomes disability.

Contrast this with current methods of management for knee injury. Evaluation of the knee problem and therapeutic interventions to treat it are designed to restore function and teach the person the limits of activity. No matter what the therapeutic intervention, the desired outcome is increased function. A patient with a ligament injury, for example, accepts that he may have to modify his activity because his function will probably not be at the same level that it was before the injury.

Dilemma of Diagnosis for Activity-related Low Back Pain

Why is the approach to managing a peripheral joint injury different from the approach to managing low back pain? Certainly many answers and opinions have been offered. A case can be made, however, for the inability of the clinician to determine the exact source of pain in most low back pain syndromes. In the ideal clinical scenario, a set of symptoms and signs are related to a pathologic process involving a particular anatomical structure that is considered the pain source. A diagnosis is then made on the basis of the pathological process involving the anatomical structure—a pathoanatomic diagnosis. This ideal clinical scenario is not the norm in most cases of low back pain. Spratt et al. estimated that a precise diagnosis is unknown in 80 to 90 percent of disabling low back disorders.[72] Imaging techniques such as computerized tomography and magnetic resonance imaging are often used in an attempt to identify the anatomical structure at fault, but a true pathoanatomic diagnosis has been found in fewer than 15 percent of patients with low back pain.[60]

As a result of the dilemma of attempting to arrive at a pathoanatomic diagnosis, the Quebec Task Force Classification for Activity Related Spinal Disorders was developed.[71] *Activity-related spinal pain* is a term that refers to spinal disorders involving the connective tissues and muscular or neural elements as a result of injury, the aging process, or adaptive changes to the tissues. This classification focuses attention on the biomechanics of injury and the healing process and distinguishes these spinal disorders from those that occur as a result of lesions to the abdominal or pelvic viscera, or from medical conditions such as infection, systemic disease, or neoplasm. The primary emphasis of this textbook is on activity-related spine pain.

Although criticized in some circles because several of the diagnostic classifications are symptom- rather than pathoanatomically-based, the Task Force was a bold attempt to standardize the language used for diagnosis of low back disorders. The classification system accounts for the fact that structural abnormalities are often not identified in low back disorders and when structural abnormalities are found, there is questionable correlation to the signs and symptoms. The Quebec Task Force diagnostic classification scheme is based largely on symptom reports by the patient and the time frame for the problem (Table 1–2).

The standardization of the diagnosis is important. A standardized diagnostic scheme allows for an algorithm of care to be generated. It also allows for meaningful data relative to cost (e.g., cost/diagnosis, total cost of treatment) to be generated in a more accurate manner. At the present time, diagnoses for low back

Table 1–2. Quebec Task Force: Diagnostic Classifications

Localized Spinal Pain
Pain Radiating to Extremity—Proximally
Pain Radiating to Extremity—Distally
Pain Radiating to Extremity + Neurological Signs
Radicular Compression Presumed
Radicular Compression Confirmed
Spinal Stenosis Confirmed
Post Surgery < 6 Months
Post Surgery > 6 Months
Chronic Pain Syndrome
Other
Time Frames
7 days or less
> 7 days and < 7 weeks
> 7 weeks

(From Spitzer WO, Nachemson A et al: Scientific approach to the assessment and management of activity-related spinal disorders. A monograph for clinicians. Report of the Quebec Task Force on Spinal Disorders. Spine 12:S1–S59, 1987.)

pain are largely dependent on examiner bias. If a patient with low back pain sees three different health care professionals, there is a very good chance that three different diagnoses will be given. For example, a patient with activity-related low back pain seeking help may be given the idea that his pain is from an intervertebral disc or the sacroiliac joint, or is myofascial in nature. The problem with having several diagnoses attached to what appears to the patient to be one and the same problem is that it can elevate the patient's fear and distress because of the uncertainty of the pathoanatomic diagnosis. This has the potential of heightening patients' perceptions of the problems and consequently increasing their propensity toward disability. As pointed out previously, most low back disorders run a favorable course, but when given several diagnoses for what appears to be the same problem, the patient's concern becomes magnified.

Another reason that the approach in the treatment of low back disorders differs from that for the extremities is the inability to adequately rest an injured lumbopelvic region while remaining active. Many patients are unable to maximize their healing potential by using methods that have traditionally been successful in the management of extremity injuries. These include strategies such as remaining non–weight-bearing or using splints to render an area much less vulnerable to reinjury. In other words, the principles and techniques

used to optimize tissue repair capabilities and gradually restore function to allow injured tissue to heal along appropriate stress lines are more difficult to apply with low back disorders.

Treatment of the low back problem is changing, however, in response to the advances made in anatomy, biomechanics, and exercise physiology, and the increased understanding of soft tissue healing. New knowledge currently available allows us to understand the spine in ways not formerly appreciated. As we elucidate the structure and function in greater detail, new methods evolve of optimizing the potential for the healing process and restoring function. Treatment of the low back region can begin to approach the same practicality as treatment of the extremity.

The intent of this text is to integrate the sciences relevant to the lumbopelvic region, in a manner that invites a logical progression of assessment and treatment. It is readily apparent that passive therapeutic modalities and multiple surgical interventions are not effective in the long-term management of the problem. Prolonged rest and passive physical therapy modalities no longer have a place in the treatment of the chronic problem.[55] The successful clinician of the future will be one who can guide the patient through a rehabilitation process that most quickly and safely restores function in the most cost-effective manner, and measures success with outcomes that assess how treatment has affected quality of life measures.

INJURY AND REPAIR

In order to have a basis that provides direction for assessment and treatment, it is important to understand the processes of tissue injury and repair, and the biomechanics of the musculoskeletal tissues relative to these processes. A basic premise of this text is that, like the peripheral joints, the soft tissues as well as the cartilaginous and bony tissues of the spine all have the potential to be injured or adversely affected by age-related changes and the degenerative process. Although certainly not a novel thought, the concept of the soft tissues of the spine as a source of pain caused by injury is not as readily accepted as in the case of soft tissue injuries in the peripheral joints. Lesions of the intervertebral disc and the degenerative bony changes seen with the aging process are more typically considered the primary sources of mechanical low back pain than are the musculoskeletal tissues. Indeed, herniated nucleus pulposus and degenerative joint disease are two of the most common diagnoses given for injuries to the low back.

For the purposes of this text, it is helpful to refer collectively to the nonmuscular tissues of the spine as *specialized connective tissues.* Specialized connective tissues would include the articular cartilage associated with the joints, the components of the intervertebral discs, the bones, the ligamentous and fascial structures associated with the appendicular and axial skeleton, and the connective tissue elements of the muscle–tendon unit. Structural changes of the specialized connective tissues occurring as a result of injury- and age-related degenerative changes potentially alter function and are important aspects to consider when establishing realistic treatment goals for patients with low back pain.

Injury can be defined as the acute damage to or loss of cells and intracellular matrix; repair is defined as the replacement of damaged or lost cells and extracellular matrix with new cells and matrices.[85] Regeneration is a repair process in which new tissue that is structurally and functionally identical to the normal tissue is produced. Other repair processes, however, result in the formation of tissue not identical to the injured tissue.[79] The spine is comprised of many different types of tissues and, based on these operational definitions, any can sustain injury. Each tissue in turn has the potential to be repaired by mechanisms unique to its cellular composition and individual biochemistry.

Many factors come into play to determine whether the repair process will be of the regeneration type, or whether the injured tissue will be replaced by a dissimilar tissue. Two of the major factors that influence the result of this repair process are the availability of vascular supply and the extent of the injury. Tissues that are not typically thought of as having repair potential can undergo successful regeneration if the injury is sufficiently small. For example, muscle defects less than 3 g or articular cartilage defects less than 1 mm can successfully regenerate.[85]

However, injuries may occur in which the capacity for tissue regeneration is exceeded. In these instances the repair process for injured tissue results in the formation of a connective tissue scar. Replacement at the injury site with this type of tissue might be adequate in *approximating* the function of the tendon or ligament, but it will not be adequate for restoring the function of injured muscle, cartilage, or nerve tissue.

The healing process for tissues of the body typically begins with an inflammatory stage, followed by a second stage that entails cell and matrix proliferation, which forms a type of vascularized granulation tissue. During the second stage, collagen is synthesized and is initially distributed in a random pattern. Subsequent stages result in remodeling and maturation of the collagen to form a connective tissue scar, which completes the repair process.[79]

Connective tissue is thus vitally important in the repair processes of the musculoskeletal soft tissues as well as being the tissue comprising the specialized connective tissue. Connective tissue is also an integral part of the noninjured musculoskeletal tissues. The mechanical properties of connective tissue are such that the conflicting demands of mobility and stability are dependent on its health and integrity. This is especially evident with the spine, where the unique structure and functions of the intervertebral disc, joints, ligaments, and bones contribute to function. For these reasons a closer analysis of connective tissue is warranted.

CONNECTIVE TISSUE

There are many types of basic tissues in the human body. Tissues are formed by cooperating cells that are assembled in coherent associations and are bound together by fibrous and amorphous intercellular substances. The basic tissues of the body include epithelium, connective tissue, blood, muscle tissue, adipose tissue, and nervous tissue. Of particular interest for understanding mechanical disorders are the structure and function of connective tissue and muscle tissue, and the interrelations between the two.

Structure

Connective tissue can be divided into connective tissue proper and the highly specialized connective tissue subclasses. Connective tissue proper can be further subdivided into loose or dense connective tissue. Examples of dense connective tissue include tendon and ligament, and the specialized subclasses include cartilage and bone (Fig. 1–1). Despite the uniqueness of each type of connective tissue, they can be grouped under one family because of the similarity of the building blocks.

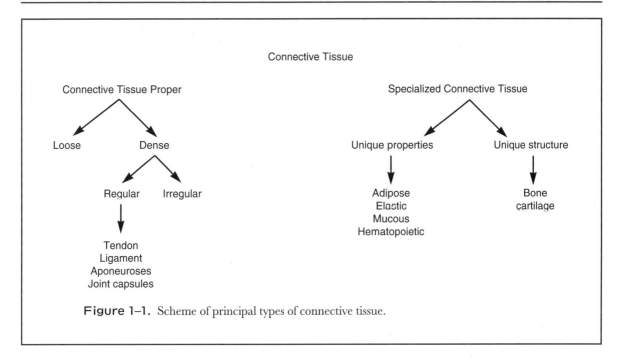

Figure 1–1. Scheme of principal types of connective tissue.

Connective tissues contain various concentrations of cells imbedded in an extracellular matrix. The matrix is composed of fibers and a ground substance. It is the distinct type of cell and the biochemical properties of the matrix that distinguish the type of connective tissue. Different types of proteins are synthesized by the cells and exist in various forms within the matrix. This determines the properties of the connective tissue. For example, the rigid structure of bone, the resiliency of cartilage, and the ability of connective tissue proper to yield are dependent on the aggregation of glycosaminoglycans and proteins to form the ground substance within the extracellular matrix.

Three types of fibers are seen in the various connective tissues: collagen, elastin, and reticulin. Collagen is the most abundant fiber type and has been further classified into subclasses.[24] The type of collagen synthesized is related to the specialized function of the connective tissue.

The orientation of the collagen also plays an important role in determining the function of the connective tissue. For example, the parallel arrangement of the collagen fibers, densely packed together, allows for the force of muscle contraction to be transmitted into and through the skeletal system with minimal elongation of the tendon. Because the tendon resists this deformation, it can be said that it has a certain stiffness. If the tendon lacked this stiffness, the force of muscle contraction would be diminished as it reached the bone. By comparison, the collagen of ligament is less highly ordered than tendon, yet its structural framework provides stiffness—resistance to deformation—to minimize movements in some directions while still allowing for movements in others.

The building block of collagen is tropocollagen, which consists of three polypeptide chains arranged in a triple helix (Fig. 1–2). The crosslinking of tropocollagen units enables collagen to have its great mechanical strength. Of particular importance in understanding the mechanics of the connective tissues is the wavelike undulations of the collagen fiber. This undulating phenomenon is known as "crimp."

Biomechanics: Stress–Strain and Hysteresis

The crimp of the collagen is one of the major factors behind the viscoelastic response of connective tissue and the characteristics of the stress–strain curve

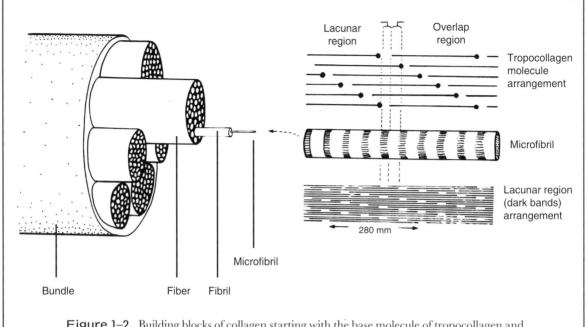

Figure 1-2. Building blocks of collagen starting with the base molecule of tropocollagen and its relationship to the collagen fiber.

(Fig. 1–3). It is thought to give the connective tissue a type of elasticity so that a structure such as a ligament behaves as a stiff spring as the crimp is straightened out by application of load.[30] The crimp is different for each kind of connective tissue, and consequently each tissue has a unique viscoelastic property.

The stress–strain curve graphically depicts the behavior of connective tissue as a stress is applied to the tissue. The curve starts with the toe region. In this range the connective tissue deforms easily, without the need for excessive force. The next region is the linear region, which represents the elastic stiffness of the connective tissue. If the applied forces are kept within this range, the tissue returns to its original shape. In this region crimp plays an important role. However, if the application of force increases beyond a certain point in the linear region, microtears of the tissue result. Finally, the stress–strain curve shows a rapid drop to zero if the force is further increased, and this represents failure of the connective tissue.

The biomechanics of connective tissue are important to consider because of the implications for injury. If the stress applied to the tissue is such that it exceeds

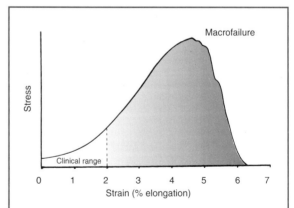

Figure 1–3. Stress–strain curve showing the amount of change and force imparted to collagenous structures. As a tensile force is imparted to the collagenous structure, the fibers straighten out or decrease the "crimp" (toe phase). As the force continues, the fibers arrange themselves in the line of the force. Microtearing occurs as the force continues until failure at approximately 6 to 8 percent of elongation.

the viscoelastic properties of the tissue, tissue failure results. This failure can be in the form of microscopic tears to the tissue or complete rupture of the tissue.

However, it is not only the strength of the collagen fiber but the condition of the intercellular matrix that is important. The collagen interacts with the ground substance to form a concentration proportional to the viscoelastic needs required by the specific tissue. The ground substance contains mucopolysaccharides in the form of glycosaminoglycan that aggregate with proteins to determine the viscosity of the ground substance. The protein–glycosaminoglycan structure, known as a proteoglycan, is one of the most important factors in maintaining the normal function of the tissues. Therefore, it is not only a change in the nature of the collagen but any change in the matrix that ultimately determine the viscoelastic properties of the tissue.

Because each type of connective tissue and specialized connective tissue has a unique allocation and arrangement of collagen, proteoglycans, and water,

the stress–strain curve is different for each tissue. Likewise, the same type of connective tissue (i.e., two ligaments from different areas) will show a difference in the stress–strain curve. The difference is due to the uniquely ordered structural matrix of each ligament, which depends on the area in which it is located and the stresses it must withstand.

The stress–strain curve is of special value in understanding the response of tissues to tensile stresses. However, the unloading of tissues is not a simple reversal of the stress–strain curve. Restoration of the tissue to its original length upon removal of the stress occurs at a lesser rate, and often to a lesser extent than the original elongation. There is an energy loss between the lengthening force and the recovery activity that is referred to as hysteresis (Fig. 1–4). As more chemical bonds are broken with applied stress, the greater the hysteresis. Instead of the tissue "rebounding" to its original length, it returns to a new length. Fig. 1–4 shows the tissue returning to a new level of strain. The

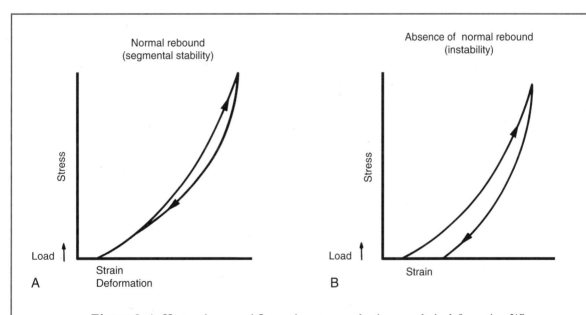

Figure 1–4. Hysteresis curve. *A,* Increasing stress on the tissue results in deformation. When the stress is removed, tissue rebounds to its resting length, although the rates of change between lengthening and return to resting length are different. *B,* With a change in tissue viscoelasticity, the strain change with increasing stress does not allow the tissue to return to its resting length. (From Porterfield JA, DeRosa C: Mechanical Neck Pain: Perspectives in Functional Anatomy. Philadelphia, WB Saunders, 1995.)

clinical significance of hysteresis is its relationship to instability. With a new, increased "set point" for the specialized connective tissues, stability between adjacent vertebral segments is now lessened and aberrational translational movements occur as a result of applied stresses. Connective tissue structures can only offer stability when the collagen framework is subject to tension. Note how the absence of normal rebound (change in the hysteresis curve) results in increased motion due to the increased tissue excursion necessary for tension to be generated within the collagen framework.

All connective tissues, therefore, have unique structural properties that help determine the functional capabilities and limitations of the tissue. Scar tissue, which is a form of specialized connective tissue, also displays properties that are different from the original tissue being replaced. These properties in turn result in altered function of the injured tissue.

In order to have a reference point from which to speculate on the potential impact of tissue injury, it is appropriate to select some of the specialized tissues and briefly discuss their function. With an understanding of normal structure and function, the result of injury to the tissues can be better appreciated. Although a detailed account of the structure and function of individualized tissues is beyond the scope of this book, some salient points are addressed to allow for the formulation of hypotheses concerning the assessment and management of mechanical disorders of the musculoskeletal system. These concepts can then be applied toward an understanding of lumbopelvic disorders.

LIGAMENTS AND JOINT CAPSULES

Ligaments and joint capsules typically consist of an array of closely packed collagen fibers that allow for their classification as dense connective tissue. Their fibrous composition allows for stabilization of the joints. They are also flexible and allow for joint movement. Because of the location of the ligaments and capsules and the directions of their fibers, motion can be restricted in one direction while ample movement is possible in another. Thus, the varied directions of joint motion are due in part to the orientation of the capsules and ligaments.

Ligaments and joint capsules function not only as support tissue but as a source of afferent input to the central nervous system. They have an important neurosensory function in providing afferent feedback to the central nervous system, allowing for conscious and unconscious proprioceptive and kinesthetic sense and the initiation of reflex activity of the musculature. The importance of afferent feedback from these structures has been recognized, especially with regard to initiating reflex activity of the musculature.[5, 32, 45, 66, 69, 87] Although caution must be taken to extrapolate research on the ligaments of the extremity to the low back, the evidence is strong that ligaments can play a major role in providing afferent stimulus to the central nervous system, and loss of this neural input owing to ligament injury significantly diminishes a person's proprioceptive capabilities.[5]

Therefore, ligaments are not simply passive structures but serve as important components of the reflex systems. Further research is necessary to quantify the influence that the receptors of the lumbar and sacroiliac joint capsules, as well as the receptors within the numerous support ligaments, have on motor control of the lumbopelvic region. It can only be speculated that significant damage to these connective tissue structures caused by low back injury results in altered proprioceptive input, which in turn leads to a modification of movement patterns.

Although repair processes are discussed below, it is important to note that because the ligament and capsule are a fairly thick connective tissue structure of specific length, the outcome from repair processes depends on the strength of tissue as well as the length of the newly repaired tissue. If the repaired ligament or capsule does not return to its appropriate length, then this laxity impedes the ability to stabilize joint motion. Additionally, if the ligament or capsule is immobilized too long, excessive shortening and stiffness ensues. In both cases the outcome is either a lack of shortening or excessive shortening of the ligament. Both processes alter joint mechanics and neural input. Combined, these have a potential effect on motor output.

ARTICULAR CARTILAGE

Articular cartilage is a highly specialized class of connective tissue with distinctive properties. It has a very high tensile strength and is resistant to compressive and shearing forces. At the same time it possesses some resilience and elasticity. The surface of articular cartilage is extremely smooth and relatively wear-resistant, and when combined with synovial fluid it provides an exceptionally low coefficient of friction between articulating surfaces. As with the other classes of connective tissue, it is the arrangement and types of specific proteoglycans, collagens, and cells, in association with water, that determine the properties of cartilage. A change in one of the structural components will alter articular cartilage function, and thus its capacity to accept the various stresses placed on it.

Proteoglycans contribute between 30 and 35 percent of the dry weight of cartilage.[56] They form the major macromolecule of the cartilage ground substance. The type of proteoglycans and the manner in which they are aggregated are important to the structural rigidity of the extracellular matrix. In addition, the viscoelastic properties of cartilage depend on the concentration of proteoglycans in solution.[85]

There is now good evidence that the structure and composition of the proteoglycans in articular cartilage change with age.[15] Because proteoglycans are important for maintaining cartilage stiffness, especially with regard to compression, and also contribute to the resilience of cartilage, an alteration in proteoglycan composition reduces these qualities.[41] This in turn alters the biomechanics of articular cartilage.

Articular cartilage contains different types of collagen (Fig. 1–5).[53] The properties of collagen provide the tissue with its tensile stiffness and strength. Type II collagen predominates, just as it does in normal nucleus pulposus. It is the combination of type II collagen in relation to proteoglycans that allows for and maintains an extremely high hydrated state, and thus makes this type of tissue well suited for compression stresses. The cyclic loading and unloading of the synovial joints squeeze water out of and back into the cartilage, and the removal of pressure rehydrates it.[38]

This rehydration phenomenon contributes to the cartilage nutrition due to fluid changeover. Although cartilage is described as an avascular structure, this is not entirely correct. What is actually meant is that the chondrocytes are located at a greater distance from the circulation as compared with other tissues.[84] Because of this vascular limitation, the contribution by rehydration is important in maintaining the health of the chondrocyte.

Chondrocyte health is important to consider because this cell is responsible for the existence and maintenance of the cartilage matrix. It is not known what signals the chondrocyte uses to alter the matrix. Understanding how the chondrocyte is signaled holds great promise in providing some of the answers related to cartilage repair.

MUSCLE TISSUE

The structure and function of muscle is detailed in Chapter 3. However, it is also important to briefly discuss muscle at this time with regard to injury. Muscle is a highly specialized tissue that has an elaborately organized vascular and nerve supply. Because of this high degree of specialization, extensive injuries of muscle cannot be adequately regenerated to original muscle tissue. If regeneration cannot occur, muscle atrophy, rather than fibrous tissue replacement or scarring, results.[85]

If the muscle lesion is small enough, then the satellite cells, which are normally present between the basal lamina and the muscle fiber, differentiate into myoblasts to begin the process of muscle regeneration.[11] The myoblasts are myogenic cells that fuse to form myotubules. Through a gradual process, differentiation into muscle fibers ultimately occurs.[80]

A complete functional repair of muscle would necessarily include restoration of the previous innervation pattern, including motor nerve supply and sensory innervation from the muscle proprioceptors. This is especially important to understand when considering the effects of abdominal or back surgery on spine function. Because normal muscle function also includes the development of appropriate vascular supply, this also becomes an important factor in determining whether the repair is complete. The restoration of muscle function after injury is critical because muscles are the motors that work with the fascial layers to direct the forces of weight-bearing and movement to bone and articular cartilage.

THE ATTENUATION OF TRUNK AND GROUND FORCES

With this brief overview of the structure and function of selected musculoskeletal and specialized con-

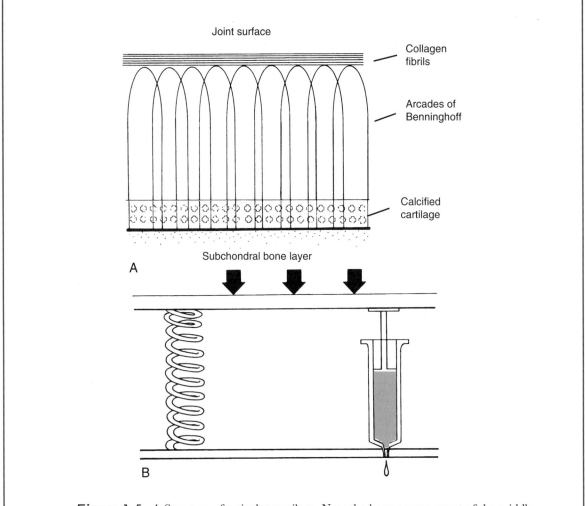

Figure 1–5. *A,* Structure of articular cartilage. Note the hoop arrangement of the middle layers of collagen. This structure permits function as shown in B. *B,* The mechanics of articular cartilage as shown in this sketch of a spring and syringe. As the cartilage is compressed, the descent is controlled by the hydraulics of the syringe and the rebound to normal height is dependent on the spring. This permits shock absorption and also fluid movement needed to maintain health of the tissue.

nective tissues, we can review how they work collectively to counteract the forces of weight-bearing and movement. The center of gravity in the human body lies just anterior to the second sacral vertebrae in the erect, standing posture. By analyzing the anatomical adaptations that have occurred in response to the development of the upright posture, the lumbopelvic region can rightfully be viewed as a hub of weight-bearing. Hub refers to a region into which trunk and ground forces converge and are attenuated by the musculoskeletal tissues. In later chapters the anatomy is described in detail and functional implications are discussed, but suffice it to say at this point that the lumbopelvic tissues appear to be extremely well designed for the maintenance of the upright posture.

What is meant by trunk and ground forces (Fig. 1–6)? The weight line of the head and trunk represents the trunk force component as it travels inferiorly into the lumbopelvic region. This weight line traverses the lumbar spine and sacrum as it courses downward through the body. The ground reaction forces are those forces generated as a result of the establishment of a closed kinetic chain when the lower extremity comes in contact with the ground. These forces are directed superiorly into the lumbopelvic region. The lumbopelvic tissues must safely attenuate the ground and trunk forces as they converge through the region. Musculoskeletal tissues, including those of the lumbopelvic region, function by transferring these forces to the surrounding tissues or directly absorbing the forces. Each musculoskeletal tissue functions differently, but it is the combined interactions of these tissues that permit the desired outcome.

How ground and trunk forces are attenuated is dependent on many factors, but one that should be considered when evaluating patients is body type. Each person is a combination of three basic body types: ectomorph, endomorph, and mesomorph (Fig. 1–7).[14]

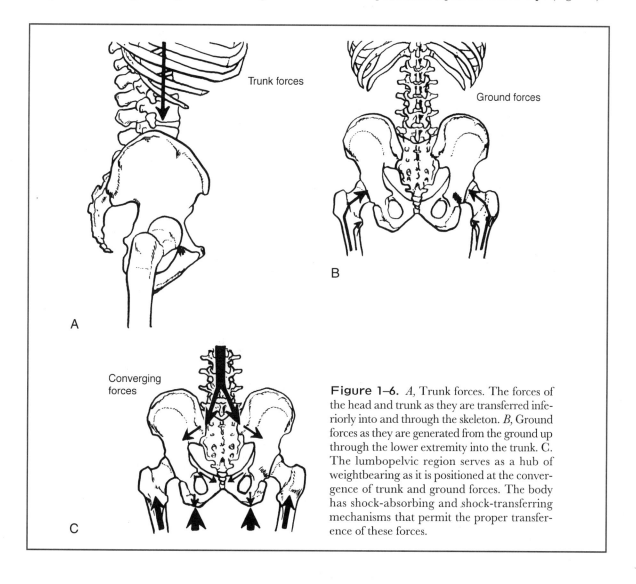

Figure 1–6. *A*, Trunk forces. The forces of the head and trunk as they are transferred inferiorly into and through the skeleton. *B*, Ground forces as they are generated from the ground up through the lower extremity into the trunk. C. The lumbopelvic region serves as a hub of weightbearing as it is positioned at the convergence of trunk and ground forces. The body has shock-absorbing and shock-transferring mechanisms that permit the proper transference of these forces.

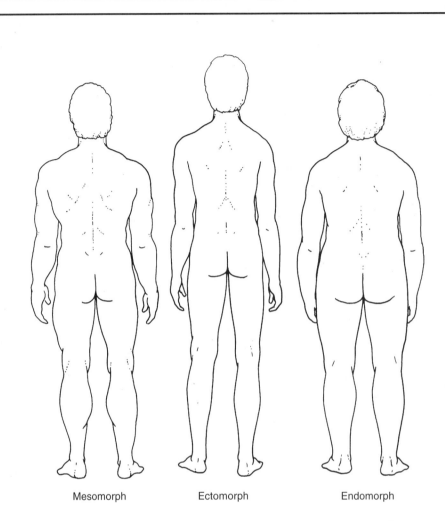

Mesomorph   Ectomorph   Endomorph

Figure 1–7. Examples of body types: ectomorph, endomorph, mesomorph. The ectomorph is a long, lean individual. The endomorph has difficulty in managing body fat and has an abundance of fatty tissue. The mesomorph is generally muscular. We are all combinations of these three body types and it is essential to assess tissue resilience and laxity as part of the evaluation process in patients.

The predominant ectomorph is the person who is long and lean and whose body weight seldom varies. His anthropometric features show a predominance of linearity and a relative fragility of body build; for example, the body type of the typical long-distance runner.

The predominant endomorph has a larger percentage of body fat and a difficult time maintaining a consistent body weight. His anthropometric features are more of corpulence and roundness. This body type typically possesses a great deal of joint mobility and is not as effective at sustaining the trunk and ground forces. We speculate that this lack of proper force transmission renders the supporting structures, especially the ligamentous tissue, vulnerable to injury.

As a result, this population is usually not as active in those activities that require the dispersement of large superincumbent and ground forces. When injured, this population can potentially present with instability problems in the weight-bearing structures.

The person whose body type is predominantly mesomorphic has a relative predominance of muscularity and less flexibility than the ectomorph. He does not readily attenuate the forces of gravity and movement but quickly transfers these forces through tissues. We speculate that this body type has the potential to overload the bony matrix and strain the stiffer connective tissues with excessive activity. The ground force is poorly dampened as it moves through the foot, ankle, knee, hip, and spinal regions. The mesomorph presents a clinical picture that is different from that of the predominant endomorph, for example, in that bony injury and frequent strains are more prominent. The mesomorph is more active, but generates forces that reach the physiologic limits of the optimal loading curve more quickly, with potential tissue breakdown as a result.

The analysis of body type is subjective. Most people have a body type that is represented along the continuum of all three body types. However, anthropometric features are an important clinical consideration in analyzing mechanical disorders of the musculoskeletal system. The relative body type of the patient must be identified because this information permits the clinician to make a judgment as to the manner in which the forces are passed through the region during the stresses of injury. As a "crossroads" of trunk and ground forces, the musculoskeletal tissues of the lumbopelvic region are vulnerable to sprain and strain injuries because they control the hub of weight-bearing. The tissues must respond appropriately to the demands of the activity without being damaged.

Often it is valuable to quickly examine the peripheral joints of the patient with low back pain to gain a sense of the connective tissue resilience and elasticity. For example, if a great deal of range of shoulder motion is present, the elbow joint easily reaches hyperextension and the metacarpal–phalangeal joints can be pushed to extreme hyperextension. It is then reasonable to assume that the connective matrix of that individual is very lax and allows for a great deal of joint play. Furthermore, it would be a logical assumption that the stability of the lumbopelvic articulations such as the bone—intervertebral disc interface, the capsular tissues related to the apophyseal joints, and the ligaments and capsule of the sacroiliac joint have the same degree of laxity, and hence the same potential for excessive joint play. One might assume that the same consequences of instability that are seen with the shoulder or knee as a result of connective tissue laxity occur in the low back, especially because the convergence of ground and trunk forces potentially results in aberrational motion between spinal segments.

TISSUE RESPONSES TO STRESS

Tissues of the musculoskeletal system have a common denominator: they all require the stimulus of nondestructive stresses to maintain their health. Nondestructive stresses refer to those forces of movement, weight-bearing, and muscle contraction that load the musculoskeletal tissues within their physiologic limits.

For example, cartilage nutrition,[59] muscle strength,[26] the strength of ligaments and their bony attachments, and tensile strength of tendon[74, 86] are all promoted with increased activity. Changes that improve the resilience of connective tissue structures include an increase in the diameter of collagen fiber bundles, higher collagen content,[73, 74] and an increase in the ultimate load capabilities of tendons secondary to changes at the bone insertion sites.[86] This underscores the importance of the interaction between muscle tissue and its connective tissue counterparts.

It is safe to assume that one of the contributing factors to maintaining musculoskeletal health is activity that places controlled stresses on these tissues. Exactly *how* these stresses provide the signal for cellular activity that results in such effects as increased fibril size, connective tissue stiffness, and tissue strength is not known.

By comparison, immobilization has deleterious effects on the musculoskeletal tissues. Changes include loss of water content, altered proteoglycan concentrations, and a decreased overall strength of the tissue. As a result, deterioration of cartilage, tendons, ligaments, and muscle occurs.[2, 13, 17, 23, 51]

Figure 1–8 illustrates the concept of optimal versus destructive loading patterns of musculoskeletal tissues. As implied with the graph, there is an optimal loading range of tissues that helps maintain optimal health of the tissue. This is represented by the middle portion of the graph. When the various forces of weight-bearing and movement, coupled with the forces exerted by

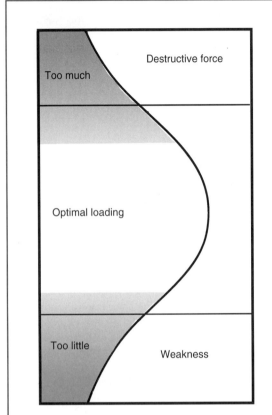

Figure 1–8. Optimal loading zone of tissues illustrating the concepts of physiological loading capacity and potentially destructive load zones. Tissue breakdown occurs as a result of either insufficient or excessive loading.

lative microtrauma. Muscle fiber necrosis has been demonstrated after conditions of intense training and prolonged activity.[34,42] Potential tissue destruction occurs in both instances because the physiological capacity of the tissue tolerance to loading has been exceeded.

Another example of overloading occurs with prolonged, asymmetrical stresses. In these instances the magnitude of the force is not as important as the length of time that the force is applied. The repetitive stresses result in an accumulation of microscopic insults to the tissue. A well-known example is the long-term articular cartilage changes in one compartment of the knee after unilateral meniscectomy of that same compartment. After the meniscectomy the loading patterns of the knee joint articular cartilage are altered, and degeneration patterns such as articular cartilage damage and subchondral bone changes result.[18,68] Frontal plane asymmetry leading to asymmetrical loading patterns of the hips results in degenerative changes of the articular cartilage of the hip joint.[33] Such stresses to the specialized connective tissues of the spine with asymmetrical loading patterns are described later in this text.

ALTERING THE OPTIMAL LOADING ZONE

The physiological capacity of tissues to accept load is altered by three main factors (Fig. 1–9). The first is *age*. With the aging process there is change in both the type and the aggregation patterns of proteoglycans. The tissues change both structurally and functionally as we age. For example, in articular cartilage, chondroitin sulfate content decreases and the aggregations of proteoglycans become smaller.[15] These changes alter the water-binding capacity of the molecule and thus its shock-attenuating capacity.

Changes in the proteoglycan and collagen makeup also affect the properties of the specialized connective tissues. Factors known to influence structural and mechanical properties of ligaments and their insertions are age and mechanical stress.[85] Because of *age-related changes*, the matrix becomes more fibrous and the viscosity is increased. This in turn alters the mobility and failure rate of the tissues. These do not represent the only changes of the aging process, however; aging ultimately decreases the ability of the tissue to withstand the magnitude and duration of forces that were formerly tolerated.

way of muscle contraction, remain within the optimal loading range, the health of the tissue is assured.

Conversely, musculoskeletal tissues weaken from overuse or disuse. If the forces to the tissues exceed the upper limit of the optimal loading zone, tissue breakdown results. The destructive stimulus dosage can be in the form of a single high-impact loading such as that experienced with a fall or a motor vehicle accident. Rapid impact loading can result not only in fracture of the cartilage but can also cause cartilage swelling and a change in the proteoglycan and collagen association in the cartilage matrix. Tissue breakdown may also occur with prolonged, excessive overloading, such as seen with overtraining or cumu-

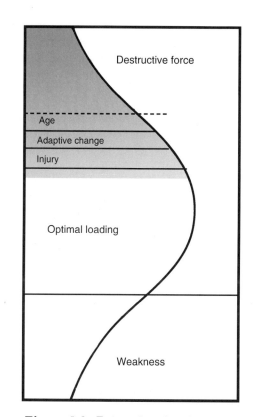

Figure 1-9. Factors that alter the optimal loading zone: injury, age, and adaptive changes.

The second factor that alters the upper limit of the optimal loading zone is *adaptive change*. A clinical example might best demonstrate this phenomenon. The person who leads a sedentary lifestyle exhibits structural adaptive changes over the course of many years. He may develop shortened hamstring and anterior hip muscles and tight hip joint capsules from prolonged sitting, and a weakened or stretched abdominal wall. These structural changes are compounded by body composition changes that also occur as we age. The average person gains 1 pound of total body weight per year and loses 1 percent of muscle strength per year after age 25. This further accentuates the adaptation of the musculoskeletal tissues.

When this person presents to the clinician with the first episode of low back pain, he does not often relate the physical changes over the past years as the precursor to the mechanical disorder giving rise to pain. Rather, the focus is on the single episode that initiated the painful syndrome. Adaptive changes in the form of connective tissue shortening and muscle weakness reduce the musculoskeletal system's tolerance to stresses. Recognition of these changes is important because they influence the treatment approach. This point is discussed more fully in Chapters 5 and 6.

The third factor that alters the loading capacity of the tissues is *injury*. After the musculoskeletal tissue is damaged, healing begins. As this process continues, the end result is repair with a tissue related in structure but different from the original tissue that was damaged. The repair process, however, does not typically restore the tissue to its former loading capacity. As an example, after injury to the medial collateral ligament of the knee, the tensile strength returns to only 50 to 70 percent of the original, preinjured tensile strength.[31, 86] There is no reason to suspect that ligamentous healing in the lumbopelvic region is markedly different. Indeed, it may be even harder to develop a strong, functional repair, since it is difficult to immobilize this region with the same efficacy as the shoulder or knee joint. Because of the convergence of trunk and ground forces in the lumbopelvic region, this area is vulnerable to multiple stresses. It can be speculated that the stages of repair will proceed, provided that destructive stimuli are kept from the area. One of the keys to management is minimizing the chances for these destructive stimuli to reach the region. Significant injuries can ultimately result in permanent impairment, which can lead to adaptive changes, recurring pain, and loss of function.

Age and injury also influence the proprioceptive activity in the musculoskeletal tissues. Because some of the receptors are highly specialized connective tissue structures themselves, injury to the ligament, tendon, or joint capsule might also damage the receptor. Additionally, as a person ages, the number of proprioceptors related to the tissues decreases. The combination of these changes probably alters the afferent input to the central nervous system.

These three factors (age, adaptive changes, and injury) alter musculoskeletal tissue tolerance to stresses. As a result, a stimulus that was formerly nondestructive to the area may now be destructive or injurious. There is, in effect, a new and now lowered maximal limit of tissue tolerance.

The lower end of the graph depicted in Figure 1–8 remains relatively consistent in its position. As mentioned above, it is recognized that if the tissues of the musculoskeletal system do not have physiologic stresses applied to them, they undergo degenerative changes. This results in weaker tissue that is unable to properly attenuate forces, and predisposes the region to injury and the potential for the cyclic pattern of injury–pain–reinjury.

So the critical issue is determining how much stress is too much, and how much exceeds the physiologic capacity for the musculoskeletal tissues. It is a well-accepted axiom that the tissues of the musculoskeletal system not only develop, but heal, in accordance with the stresses placed on them. Perhaps the most well-known example of this phenomenon is Wolff's law.[65] This law states that bone is laid down according to the stresses placed on it. Bone thickens at those points where the stresses are greatest and thins at the areas where the load is diminished. The trabecular pattern forms as a result of the various compression and tensile forces imparted to the bone. Specialized cells—the osteoblast and the osteoclast—are available to carry out this task. Specialized connective tissues of the musculoskeletal system and muscle also respond to the same basic principle. For example, the connective tissues of the ligament, tendon, and matrix of muscle respond to the stresses of activity by making the necessary adaptations to the increased demands.

Muscle tissue is also capable of making adaptations as a result of the stresses incurred. For example, muscle tissue changes both anatomically and biochemically in response to demands placed on it. Endurance training increases the capacity of the mitochondria to generate adenosine triphosphate aerobically by oxidative phosphorylation, and also increases the number and size of the mitochondria.[54] This is a response to the type of training demands placed on the muscle. Even the skin follows this basic principle of adaptation as it adapts to the frictional stresses of weight-bearing by forming a callus at that point where the overload occurred. Essentially all of the musculoskeletal tissues respond to the various long-term stresses placed on them by adaptation. This response has been described as a specific adaptation to imposed demand (SAID).[4] The SAID principle is an acronym used to relate the effects of sports conditioning and training. It indicates that conditioning and training are directed toward the specific demands of a given sport. It is an important concept because it provides a basis for the rehabilitation of most musculoskeletal disorders, and does not necessarily have to be limited to sports. The goal with

rehabilitation programs for mechanical disorders is to prepare the body for the various stresses it may face. It is not exercise per se that results in a "cure." Instead, rehabilitation programs that emphasize activity (a form of musculoskeletal training) stimulate the adaptations necessary to meet imposed demands. Later in the text the concept of training is discussed in its rehabilitation context. Suffice it to say, at this point that connective tissue and muscle adaptations in response to training occur, a more active lifestyle becomes a reachable goal.

Therefore, the clinician's goal in the management of mechanical disorders is to identify the injury status of the tissues and provide a treatment plan designed to do the following:

1. Optimize the environment to heal the wound
2. Maintain the relations of the injured tissues to the noninjured tissues
3. Maintain the health of the noninjured tissues
4. Introduce nondestructive forces to help assure functional healing to the injured tissues
5. Prevent the application of excessive forces to the injured tissues

Although these objectives are more fully explored in Chapter 6, they should be mentioned in the context of the SAID principle. Understanding the SAID principle is especially important and is one of the major reasons that a more active approach to managing mechanical low back disorders is preferred. The inability to effectively carry out this plan of care for a musculoskeletal tissue injury leads to various forms of tissue dysfunction, such as contracture, adhesion, laxity, and diminished function, and we speculate that it subsequently alters neurophysiologic feedback.

Mismanagement also results in frequent reinjury, mainly because of the dysfunction of the region, and chronic symptoms. Prevention of the syndrome, and, more important, prevention of disability from a mechanical low back disorder, is facilitated by prompt, accurate identification of the injury and the beginning of a goal-oriented, supervised rehabilitation program. These types of programs are best designed by a professional who is skilled in the analysis of human movement, recognizes the three-dimensional relations of anatomical structures, understands the processes of tissue healing, and begins to direct the responsibility of managing the syndrome of activity-related low back pain to the patient.

PATHOMECHANICS OF ACTIVITY-RELATED LOW BACK PAIN

As mentioned previously, it is often not possible to precisely name the anatomic structure that is at fault in low back disorders. A diagnosis is essential, but the terminology that is used should take into account that it may be counterproductive to leave the patient with the impression that there is certainty with such a diagnostic "guess." In this textbook, we will emphasize a pathomechanical approach to assessment, rather than a pathoanatomical one. A diagnostic classification scheme is presented in Chapter 5.

It may be of greater clinical utility to think in terms of injury mechanisms leading to structural failure or the new optimal loading zones of tissue that occur as a result of injury and degeneration. The consequences of injury—those factors leading to diminished function—are primarily mechanical in nature. For example, a force applied to the outer annular ring of the intervertebral disc that exceeds the viscoelasticity of that tissue causes a permanent elongation of that structure. A sprain of an annular ring has occurred and it no longer functions normally. This is much like the example of the knee joint injury in which the viscoelasticity of the anterior cruciate ligament is exceeded and permanent elongation of the ligament results. The ligament has been sprained, and the manner in which forces are accepted by other tissues in the knee is now altered. The degenerative processes of the surrounding tissues are hastened. We can safely assume that the sprained annulus fibrosus will also alter the normal force acceptance in the lumbopelvic region.

The alteration of mechanics owing to injury is the case with any tissue in the lumbopelvic region. The biomechanics of this region require an interplay of multiple joints, especially the lumbar zygapophyseal, sacroiliac, and hip joints, their connective tissue restraining elements, and muscular effort at both a conscious and a reflex level. If the mechanical forces applied to the lumbopelvic region are not attenuated by these multiple tissues, then the mechanical threshold of the tissue may be exceeded. The rich nociceptive system in this region is then stimulated by mechanical deformation or chemical irritation of the nociceptors (see Chapter 2).

Therefore, the concept that is presented in this text is that it does not matter what tissue is involved in the cause of mechanical low back pain—of greatest importance is the abnormal or excessive force(s) that converge on a region and chemically and/or mechanically stimulate the nociceptive system and result in pain. We suggest that altering the magnitude and mechanism of force convergence into the region of injury, and affecting the chemical environment and fluid stasis surrounding injured tissue, might be the unifying elements between the various treatment techniques being used for low back pain. Reflex responses caused by modality or manual techniques may influence the central nervous system in such a way that the resultant response by the muscular system influences joint mechanics. Manual or surgical techniques attempt to remove an offending force or alter the way forces reach the area. Active and passive range of motion alter fluid stasis and modify the biochemical milieu.

When viewed in this manner, the "technique" becomes less important than the science. For this reason a major portion of this text is devoted to the three-dimensional aspects of the normal anatomy and the relations that tissues have with one another, both structurally and functionally. If the clinician has this understanding, then the assessment of the biomechanics of human movement can be more directly related to evaluation and treatment of mechanical low back pain.

Knowledge of mechanical low back disorders has matured beyond past notions that all back pain is from the intervertebral disc, or the zygapophyseal joints, or is all myofascial in nature, or that we often have only an isolated injury. If we can identify the nociceptive stresses, especially during a patient's activities of daily living, and minimize these stresses while allowing the person to stay active, then the healing process will more readily occur. In effect, one of the goals of treatment for any mechanical injury is to provide an optimal healing environment.

The clinician and the patient are thus challenged to identify the forces that are stimulating the nociceptive system and reproducing symptoms, and to control and alter the way that they reach the lumbopelvic region. It is extremely important that the patient have an active role in this management. Less than 2 percent of his waking time is spent in treatment. The clinician must convince the patient of the importance of the other 98 percent of his waking time with respect to managing his own syndrome. Anything less invites failure and patient-dependency on the health care professional. The clinician's responsibility is to understand the details of the functional anatomy of the region to allow for a purposeful evaluation and the development of a valid treatment protocol, and to educate patients in self-management strategies for their activity-related low back disorder.

SUMMARY

In this chapter we briefly reviewed selected epidemiological aspects of low back pain and the important differences between low back pain and low back disability. As a hub of weight-bearing, the low back is susceptible to compressive, tensile, and shear stresses, due to ground and trunk forces. Age, injury, and adaptive change alter the capacity of the specialized connective tissues to tolerate these stresses. Once the integrity of the specialized connective tissues is compromised, they do not regenerate but instead go through a repair process that leaves them less able to tolerate stresses. In the subsequent chapters, the various aspects of the functional anatomy will be detailed to provide the reader with an understanding of how the lumbopelvic tissues respond to this convergence of trunk and ground forces. With a working knowledge of the functional anatomy of the region and the expected responses of tissue to injury, a logical progression of evaluation and treatment can be formulated.

REFERENCES

1. Aaron H, Schwartz WB: Rationing health care: The choice before us. Science 247:418, 1990.
2. Akeson WH, Woo SL-Y, Amiel D, et al: The connective tissue response to immobility: Biochemical changes in periarticular connective tissue of the immobilized rabbit knee. Clin Orthop 93:356, 1973.
3. Andersson GBJ: Epidemiologic aspects of low back pain in industry. Spine 10:482, 1985.
4. Arnheim DD: Modern Principles of Athletic Training. St. Louis, C.V. Mosby, 1985.
5. Barrack RL, Skinner HB, Buckley SL: Proprioception in the anterior cruciate deficient knee. Am J Sports Med 17:1, 1989.
6. Benn RT, Kelsey J, White AA: Epidemiology and impact of low back pain. Spine 6:133, 1980.
7. Bergenudd E, Nilsson B: Back pain in middle age: Occupational workload and psychologic factors. Spine 13:58, 1988.
8. Berkowitz M, Greene C: Disability expenditures. American Rehab 15(1):7, 1989.
9. Biering-Sorenson F: Low back trouble in a general population of 30, 40, 50, and 60 year old men and women: Study design, representatives and basic results. Dan Med Bull 29:289, 1982.
10. Bigos SJ, Battie MC, Spengler DM, Fisher LD, Fordyce WE, et al: A longitudinal prospective study of industrial back injury reporting. Clin Orthop and Rel Research 279:21, 1992.
11. Bischoff R: A satellite cell mitogen from crushed adult muscle. Dev Biol 115:140, 1986.
12. Boden SC, Davis DO, Dina TS, Patronas NJ, Wiesel SW: Abnormal magnetic scans of the lumbar spine in asymptomatic subjects. A prospective investigation. J Bone Joint Surg (Am) 72:403, 1990.
13. Bortz WM: The disuse syndrome. West J Med 141:691, 1984.
14. Brooks GA, Fahey TD: Exercise Physiology: Human Bioenergetics and Its Applications. New York, John Wiley & Sons, 1984.
15. Buckwalter JA, Kuettner KE, Thonar EJM: Age-related changes in articular cartilage proteoglycans: Electron microscopic studies. J Orthop Res 3:251, 1985.
16. Cats-Baril WL, Frymoyer JW: the Economics of Spinal Disorders, in Frymoyer J ed. The Adult Spine. Raven Press, New York, 1991, p.101.
17. Cooper RR: Alterations during immobilization and regeneration of skeletal muscle in cats. J Bone Joint Surg 54A:919, 1972.
18. Cox JS, Cordell LD: The degenerative effects of medial meniscus tears in dogs' knees. Clin Orthop 125:236, 1977.
19. Cypress BK: Characteristics of physician visits for back symptoms: a national perspective. Am J Public Health 73:389, 1983.
20. Deyo RA, Andersson G, Bombardier C, Cherkin DC, et al: Outcome measures for studying patients with low back pain. Spine 19:2032S, 1994.
21. Deyo RA, Tsui-Wu Y-J: Descriptive epidemiology of low back pain and its related medical care in the United States. Spine 12:264,1987.
22. Ellwood PM: Shattuck Lecture. Outcomes management: A technology of patient experience. N Eng J Med 318:1549, 1988.
23. Enneking WF, Horowitz M: The intra-articular effects of immobilization on the human knee. J Bone Joint Surg 54A:973, 1972.
24. Eyre DR: Collagen: Molecular diversity in the body's protein scaffold. Science 207:1315, 1980.
25. Fairbank JCT, Couper J, Davies JB, O'Brien JP: The Oswestry Low Back Pain Disability Questionnaire. Physiotherapy 66:271, 1980.
26. Faulkner JA: New perspectives in training for maximum performance. JAMA 205:741,1986.
27. Fordyce WE, Brockway JA, Bergman JA, Spengler D: Acute back pain: A control group comparison of behaviourial vs. traditional management methods. J Behav Med 9:127, 1986.
28. Fordyce WE, Fowler RS, Lehmann JF, DeLateur BJ: Some implications of learning in problems of chronic pain. J Chron Dis 21:179, 1968.
29. Fordyce WE, McMahan R, Rainwater G, et al: Pain complaint–exercise performance relationship in chronic pain. Pain 10:311, 1981.
30. Frank C, Amiel D, Woo SL-Y, et al: Normal ligament properties and ligament healing. Clin Orthop 196:15, 1985.

31. Frank C, Woo SL-Y, Amiel D, et al: Medial collateral ligament healing: A multidisciplinary assessment in rabbits. Am J Sports Med 11:379, 1983.

32. Freeman MAR, Wyke B: Articular reflexes at the ankle joint: An electromyographic study of normal and abnormal influences of ankle–joint mechanoreceptors upon reflex activity in the leg muscles. Br J Surg 54:990, 1967.

33. Friberg O: Clinical symptoms and biomechanics of lumbar spine and hip joint in leg length inequality. Spine 8:643, 1983.

34. Friden J, Sjostrom M, Ekblom B: Myofibrillar damage following intense eccentric exercise in man. Int J Sports Med 4:170, 1983.

35. Frymoyer J, Cats-Baril WL: An overview of the incidence and costs of low back pain. Orthop Clin North Am 22:263, 1991.

36. Frymoyer JW, Cats-Baril W:Predictors of low back pain disability. Clin Orthop 221:89, 1987.

37. Frymoyer JW: Back Pain and Sciatica. N Engl J Med, 318:291, 1988.

38. Gradisar IA, Porterfeld JA: Articular cartilage. Top Geriatr Rehabil 4:1, 1989.

39. Hadler NM: Regional musculoskeletal diseases of the low back. Cumulative trauma vs. a single incident. Clin Orthop Rel Res 221:33, 1987.

40. Hadler NM: The predicament of backache (editorial). J Occup Med 30:449, 1988.

41. Harris ED Jr, Parker HG, Radin EL, et al: Effects of proteolytic enzymes on structural and mechanical properties of cartilage. Arthritis Rheum 15:497,1972.

42. Hikida RS, Staron RS, Hagerman FC, et al: Muscle fiber necrosis associated with human marathon runners. J Neurol Sci 59:185,1983.

43. Hodgson TA, Meiners MR: Cost of illness methodology: A guide to current practice and procedures. Milbank Mem Fund Q 60(3):429, 1982.

44. Kelsey JL, Githens PB, O'Connor T, et al: Acute prolapsed intervertebral disc: An epidemiologic study with special reference to driving automobiles and smoking. Spine 9:608, 1984.

45. Kennedy JC, Alexander IJ, Hayes KC: Nerve supply of the human knee and its functional importance. Am J Sports Med 10:329, 1982.

46. Lancourt J, Kettelhut M: Predicting return to work for lower back pain patients receiving worker's compensation. Spine 17:629, 1992.

47. Leavitt SS, Johnston TL, Beyer RD: The process of recovery. Industr Med Sur g 40(No. 1, p.7; No.2, p.5), 1972.

48. Lehman TR, Spratt KF, Lehmann KK: Predicting long term disability in low back injured workers presenting to a spine consultant. Spine 18:1103, 1993.

49. Loeser JD, Fordyce WE: Chronic pain. In Carr JE, Dengerink HA (eds): Behaviourial Science in the Practice of Medicine. New York, Elsevier, 1983.

50. Main CJ, Waddell G: The assessment of pain. Clin Rehab 3:267, 1989.

51. Mayer TG, Gatchel RJ, Kitchino N, et al: Objective assessment of lumbar function following industrial injury. Spine 10:482, 1985.

52. Mayer TG, Gatchel RJ: Functional Restoration of Spinal Disorders: The Sports Medicine Approach. Philadelphia, Lea & Febiger, 1988.

53. Mayne R, Irwin MH: Collagen types in cartilage. In Kuettncr KE, Schleyerbach R, Hascall VC (eds): Articular Cartilage Biochemistry, p. 38. New York, Raven Press, 1986.

54. McArdle WD, Katch FI, Katch VL: Exercise Physiology: Energy, Nutrition, and Human Performance. Philadelphia, Lea & Febiger, 1986.

55. Mooney V: Where is the pain coming from? Presidential address for International Society for the Study of the Lumbar Spine. Spine 12:754, 1987.

56. Muir IHM: The chemistry of the ground substance of joint cartilage. In Sokoloff L (ed): The Joints and Synovial Fluid, Vol. 2, p. 27. New York, Academic Press, 1980.

57. Nachemson A: Advances in low-back pain. Clin Orthop 200:266, 1985.

58. Nachemson A: Chronic pain: The end of the welfare state? Qual Life Res 3(suppl.l):S11, 1994.

59. Nachemson A: Work for all, for those with low back pain as well. Clin Orthop 179:77, 1983.

60. Nachemson AL: Advances in low back pain. Clin Orthop 200:266, 1985.

61. Nordby E: Epidemiology and diagnosis in low back injury. Occup Health Safety 50:38, 1981.

62. Patrick DL, Erickson P: Health Status and Health Policy: Quality of Life in Health Care Evaluation and Resource Allocation. New York: Oxford University Press, 1993.

63. Praemer A, Furner S, Rice DP: Musculoskeletal Conditions in the United States. Park Ridge IL, American Academy of Orthopaedic Surgeons, 1992.

64. Roland M, Morris R: A study of the natural history of back pain, Part I: Development of a reliable and sensitive measure of disability in low back pain. Spine 8:141, 1983.

65. Salter R: Textbook of Disorders and Injuries of the Musculoskeletal System, 2nd ed. Baltimore, Williams & Wilkins, 1983.

66. Schultz RA, Miller DC, Kerr CS, et al: Mechanoreceptors in human cruciate ligaments: A histological study. J Bone Joint Surg 66A:1072, 1984.

67. Seidel H, Heide R: Long term effects of whole body vibration: A critical survey of the literature. Int Arch Occup Environ Health. 58:1, 1986.

68. Shapiro F, Glimcher MJ: Induction of osteoarthrosis in the rabbit knee joint: Histologic changes following meniscectomy and meniscal lesions. Clin Orthop 147:287, 1980.

69. Skinner HB, Barrack RL, Cook SD: Age-related decline in proprioception. Clin Orthop 184:208, 1984.

70. Spengler D, Bigos S, Martin N, et al: Back injuries in industry: A retrospective study. Overview and cost analysis. Spine 11:241,1986.

71. Spitzer WO, Nachemson A: Scientific approach to the assessment and management of activity-related spinal disorders. A monograph for clinicians. Report of the Quebec Task Force on Spinal Disorders. Spine 12:S1, 1987.

72. Spratt KF, Lehman TR, Weinstein JW et al: A new approach to low back examination: behavioral assessment of mechanical signs. Spine 15:96, 1990.

73. Stone MH: Implications for connective tissue and bone alterations resulting from resistance exercise training. Med Sci Sports Exerc 20 (suppl):S162, 1988.

74. Tipton CM, James SL, Mergner W, et al: Influence of exercise on strength of medial collateral knee ligaments in dogs. Am J Physiol 218:894, 1970.

75. Tipton CM, Matthes RD, Maynard JA, et al: The influence of physical activity on ligaments and tendons. Med Sci Sports 7:165, 1975.

76. Troup JDG, Foreman TK, Baxter CE, Brown D: The perception of back pain and the role of psychophysical tests of lifting capacity. Spine 12:645, 1987.

77. Troup JDG, Marting JW, Lloyd DCE: Back pain in industry: A prospective survey. Spine 6:61, 1981.

78. Valkenburg HA, Haanen HCK: The epidemiology of low back pain. In: White AA III, Gordon SL, eds. American Academy of Orthopaedic Surgeons symposium on idiopathic low back pain. St. Louis, Mosby p.9, 1982.

79. van der Muelen JCH: Present state of knowledge on processes of healing in collagen structures. Int J Sports Med 3:4, 1982.

80. Vracko R, Benditt EP: Basal lamina: The scaffold for orderly cell replacement: Observations on regeneration of injured skeletal muscle fibers and capillaries. J Cell Biol 55:406, 1972.

81. Waddell G, Main CJ, Morris EW, et al: Chronic low back pain, psychological distress and illness behavior. Spine 9:209, 1984.

82. Waddell G, Main CJ: Assessment of severity in low back disorders. Spine 9:204, 1984.

83. Waddell G: A new clinical model for the treatment of low-back pain. Spine 12:632, 1987.

84. Williams PL, Warwick R: Gray's Anatomy, 36th Br. ed. Philadelphia, W.B. Saunders, 1986.

85. Woo SL-Y, Buckwalter JA: Injury and Repair of the Musculoskeletal Soft Tissues. American Academy of Orthopedic Surgeons, Park Ridge, Illinois, 1988.

86. Woo SL-Y, Ritter MA, Amiel D, et al: The effects of exercise on the biomechanical and biochemical properties of swine digital flexor tendons. J Biomech Eng 103:51, 1981.

87. Wyke B: Neurological aspects of low back pain. In Jayson M, ed: Lumbar Spine and Back Pain, p.189. New York, Grune & Stratton, 1976.

CHAPTER 2

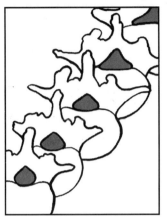

NEUROMECHANICAL AND NEUROCHEMICAL BASES OF LUMBOPELVIC PAIN AND DYSFUNCTION

INTRODUCTION

Understanding low back pain requires a basic understanding of the vast influences of the nervous system on lumbopelvic function and pain mechanisms. The complete scope of such neural influences remains relatively unknown, and what was understood previously is reinterpreted as new knowledge emerges. The neuromechanical and neurochemical bases of low back pain are perhaps the most dynamic of the many fields of study related to lumbopelvic disorders.

The extent of nervous system influences is too large to be presented in a text of this nature, but certain aspects of the neurosciences, especially as they relate to disorders of the spine and the perpetuation of low back pain, need to be addressed. In everyday clinical practice, many aspects of neuroanatomy and neurophysiology are applied in the evaluation process and in interpretation of assessment findings. In addition, treatment strategies attempt to alter pain perception and impact neuromotor function, both clearly having broad neural implications for patients suffering from low back disorders. This chapter focuses primarily on those aspects of the neurosciences relevant to the phenomena of low back pain and lumbopelvic function. In particular, the innervation of lumbopelvic tissues, the details of the nerve root complex, and the inter-

action between the sensory and motor aspects of motor behavior are discussed.

The innervation of the lumbopelvic tissues and the contributions of the various elements of the nervous system to motor control illustrate the synergistic behavior of the trunk and extremity musculature and the importance of the sensory system in movement patterns. Muscle is an effector organ because it converts neural commands into a desired force. This force contributes to movement or stability. To generate smooth, purposeful motor activity, information from the various sensory receptors must be channeled into the central nervous system to allow appropriate interactions between motor control centers and the activities of different muscles.

Mechanical low back pain alters this afferent–efferent balance and, in the broadest sense, many patients who suffer from low back pain can be viewed as having movement disorders. Various treatment regimens emphasize pain modulation, sensory stimulation, or motor enhancement, singly or in combination. These regimens seek to increase neuromuscular efficiency to improve psychophysical outcome. The object of the short discourse on the lumbopelvic neural sciences presented in this chapter is to promote recognition of the common threads among the various regimens used for treating low back pain.

LOW BACK PAIN: PATHOANATOMICAL AND BIOCHEMICAL INFLUENCES

Despite the vast toll that low back pain has taken on society, the question of what actually makes a patient's spine painful is far from fully answered. Advances in the knowledge of spinal anatomy and mechanics, innervation of spinal tissues, and the effects of aging, degeneration, and injury of the spine have certainly contributed to an understanding of the low back pain phenomenon. However, investigation has largely focused on the contributions of structural or mechanical abnormalities to the onset and propagation of low back pain. For example, mechanical or structural explanations for low back pain include intervertebral disc fragments distorting the nerve root complex or posterior longitudinal ligament, facet osteophytes compressing the nerve root at the region of the intervertebral foramen, excessive strain at the apophyseal joint capsule, and compromise of the spinal canal contents from lumbar spinal canal stenosis.

Largely because structural abnormalities are often poorly correlated with painful spine syndromes (see Chapter 4), nonstructural causes of low back pain have been sought. There is increasing evidence that inflammatory, vascular, and immunological factors play major roles in the initiation and propagation of low back pain. A more complete picture of low back pain thus includes structural, mechanical, inflammatory, immunologic, and vascular mechanisms. Low back pain is most likely the result of both pathoanatomical and biochemical influences, and it clearly involves a complex pathophysiological process with symptoms and signs emanating from biochemical changes in the tissues. It has been suggested that in the future, analyzing blood plasma to determine such biochemical changes may become an important diagnostic procedure for chronic low back pain.[16]

LOW BACK PAIN: TISSUE SOURCES

Tissues supplied by free nerve endings, the *nociceptors*, are considered to be potential sources of pain. The activation of nociceptors occurs by mechanical, chemical, or thermal stimuli. Mechanical and chemical stimuli are the primary means of nociceptor activation in activity-related low back pain syndromes.

Nociceptors play key roles in the cascade of reactions contributing to the overall inflammatory processes accompanying tissue injury (Fig. 2-1). Chemicals such

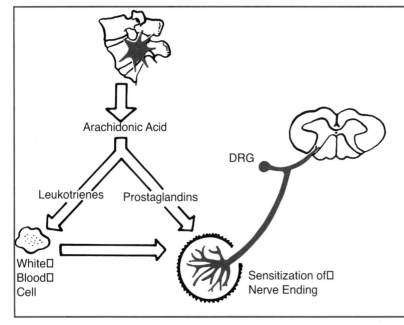

Figure 2–1. Nociceptors serve as chemical mediators of pain and contribute to the inflammatory process. Nociceptive endings are stimulated and sensitized by chemicals released as a result of tissue injury. Neuropeptides synthesized by nociceptive neurons are released both at the tissue site of injury, where they facilitate the inflammatory process, and at the dorsal horn of the spinal cord, where they make synaptic connections with local neurons.

as bradykinins, prostaglandins, serotonin, histamine, and leukotrienes released at the site of injury from mast cells, injured cells of the tissue, and blood vessels act to increase the excitability of the nociceptive sensory nerve endings. Such chemicals arising from these non-neural tissues and cells have the ability to propagate pain via stimulation of the nociceptive nerve endings.[81] Upon exposure to these chemical mediators, some nociceptive nerve endings become sensitized, that is, their threshold response to stimuli is lowered, resulting in hyperalgesic states.[81]

A further role of the nociceptors is to respond effectively to the chemical stimuli released from non-neural cell and tissue mediators of inflammation by releasing neuropeptides and other neuromodulators from their nerve endings. These neuropeptides function to increase the excitability of adjacent nociceptors, facilitate tissue repair, and further modulate the inflammatory process.[64] Thus, the nociceptors not only serve the function of providing sensory information to the central nervous system regarding tissue injury but also contribute to the inflammatory and healing processes.

How do the nociceptors contribute to inflammatory and healing processes? Various neuropeptides (Table 2-1), such as substance P and calcitonin gene-related peptide, are synthesized in the dorsal root ganglion of the nociceptive neuron and travel to the terminal endings via axoplasmic transport along the axon cylinder.[43] The neuropeptides are then released from the nociceptive nerve endings into the tissue site, facilitating chemical reactions that result in increased vascular permeability and increased attraction of polymorphonuclear leukocytes and monocytes to the region of injury and inflammation. The neuropep-

tides further act to stimulate the function of leukocytes and monocytes. Additionally, neuropeptides contribute to repair processes in injured tissues.

Pain, inflammation, and various nervous system elements are thus tightly interwoven, and the nervous system plays a key role in the inflammatory response to injury. Tissue injury activates both the neurogenic and non-neurogenic systems by activating the pain system, resulting in a cascade of events contributing to tissue repair.

Many different tissues of the lumbar spine are supplied with nociceptors. These include muscle and fascia with associated connective tissue and blood vessel frameworks; the lumbar apophyseal and sacroiliac joint capsules; support ligaments such as the supraspinous, interspinous, and anterior and posterior longitudinal; the ligamentum flavum; the periosteum of the vertebrae; the intervertebral disc; the dorsal root ganglion; the nerve root complex; the dura mater; and the vasculature associated with the spinal canal.

Muscle

Despite the prevalence of diagnoses of myofascitis, fibrositis, and fibromyalgia, the role of muscle as a source of pain remains controversial. Muscles contain a large population of small myelinated and unmyelinated nerve fibers responsible for pain and mechanoreceptor feedback to the central nervous system. A wide range of etiological factors related to muscles as a source of pain can arise from muscle mechanics. Such factors include ruptures of muscle from excessive strain, muscle contusions, syndromes of overuse of spinal muscles, delayed muscle soreness, and muscle spasm occurring as sequelae to intervertebral disc or joint injury.

Fibromyalgia has been linked to depression, illustrating the association between psychological factors, psychosocial stresses, and muscle response.[32] This association is especially relevant when considering the frequency of muscle spasm and trigger point findings in patients who are unable to adequately manage the various psychological stresses they may experience.

Pain occurring as a result of muscle involvement may arise from release of neuropeptides into the muscle, ultrastructural damage to the muscle from excessive loads,[74] delayed inflammatory changes following prolonged use,[61] accumulation of noxious agents when there is decreased blood flow to the muscle, and irri-

Table 2–1. Neuropeptides Occurring in Primary Afferent Neurons

Substance P
Somatostatin
Calcitonin gene-related peptide
Cholecystokinin-like substance
Vasoactive intestinal peptide
Gastrin-releasing peptide
Dynorphin
Enkephalin
Neurotensin
Angiotensin II
Galanin

tation of pain receptors within the walls of the blood vessels of muscles.[84] Local biochemical events within the muscle tissue rather than tissue disruption are more likely the cause of pain from muscle, although the precise neurophysiological pathways are unknown.

Apophyseal Joint

The capsule of the apophyseal joint contains free and encapsulated nerve endings, and the free nerve endings are thought to subserve a nociceptive function.[6] Several investigators have demonstrated that back pain can be experimentally induced in subjects by direct stimulation of the lumbar apophyseal joints.[51, 55, 58] In addition to joint capsule and capsular ligament involvement due to injury, increased mechanical stress, or disease, the pain from lumbar apophyseal joints has also been ascribed to articular cartilage breakdown, resulting in osteoarthrosis and its consequent pain.[11, 21, 44] Various patterns of mechanical loading have also been noted to increase mechanical stress on the lumbar apophyseal joint. Increased loading between the articulating facets and the laminae of subjacent vertebrae with lumbar hyperextension may exceed joint loading capacity and result in early degenerative changes in the joint.[87] Despite this understanding of lumbar joint mechanics, carefully controlled clinical trials suggest that there are very few clinical features that reliably discriminate among patients with pain of apophyseal joint origin and pain from other causes.[73]

Sacroiliac Joint

The sacroiliac joint is supplied with nociceptors from spinal segments L2 to S4 and thus may serve as a source of low back and buttock pain.[2] Diagnostic injections have been noted to relieve low back pain in selected patients, further suggesting that the sacroiliac joint may serve as a source of pain.[24] In addition to implications that mechanical perturbations of the sacroiliac joint may result in pain, pathological processes such as spondyloarthropathies, infections, and crystal-induced arthropathies may cause sacroiliac joint pain.[14]

Spinal Dura

Despite implications that intervertebral disc protrusion mechanically compressing the dural tissue sur-

rounding the nerve roots is a source of low back pain, the exact nature and function of spinal dura innervation remain relatively unknown. Nerve fibers are sparsely placed throughout the spinal dura. The sinuvertebral nerve, which carries autonomic nerve fibers as well as somatic fibers, supplies several structures within the spinal canal, including the ventral aspect of the dura mater (see below).[20, 31] The paucity of nerve fibers in the dura, however, suggests it has only a limited role in pain propagation.[41] The question remains as to which sensory modality the nerve fibers ramifying through the spinal dura subserve.

Dural ligaments are also present within the spinal canal; they serve to fix the dura and nerve roots to the posterior longitudinal ligament and the periosteum of the vertebral body. The nerve root is also fixed at the region of the intervertebral foramen. Such attachments can result in distortion of the nerve root complex when it is subjected to the mechanical pressure of intervertebral disc herniation.[76]

Intervertebral Disc

The outer aspect of the intervertebral disc (primarily the outer one-third to one-half of the annulus fibrosus), and the posterior longitudinal ligament, which reinforces the posterior aspect of the disc, contain free nerve endings.[8, 88] These free nerve endings contain substance P and calcitonin gene-related peptide, which are synthesized in the sensory nerve fibers and are responsible for transmitting pain.[3, 82]

Mechanical stimulation of the posterior aspect of the intervertebral disc has been noted to produce low back pain in clinical trials.[42] The afferent pathways of discogenic pain are primarily from branches of the sinuvertebral nerve (described below), which also carry sympathetic nerve fibers. This suggests that the pain from intervertebral disc disease may be mediated in part by the sympathetic nervous system, much like the pain seen with diseases of the abdominal and pelvic viscera.[60]

Additional nerve supply to the disc is from the ventral and grey rami (which supply the posterolateral aspect of the disc), the ascending and descending branches of the grey rami (which supply the lateral aspect of the disc), and the branches from the sympathetic plexus adjacent to the vertebral body supplying the anterior aspect of the disc, including the anterior longitudinal ligament.[6] As noted above, the remaining posterior aspect of the annulus fibrosus and the posterior longitudinal ligament are innervated by the sinuvertebral nerve.

Because nerve fibers with their free nerve endings and receptors have been found within the annulus, it is tempting to speculate on their function. Certainly pain from mechanical or chemical irritation of the free nerve endings appears reasonable, and thus annular injury may result in primary discogenic pain. Primary discogenic pain typically has broad, ill-defined boundaries[34]: the patient usually describes a broad, nonspecific band across the back or gluteal region. The pain may spread into the upper posterior or posterolateral thigh and across the abdomen. Maitland[50] described the quality of pain as "distressing, wearing, sickening and depressing." This is a different quality of pain from the aching and discomfort of injured ligamentous structures.

The innervation of the disc and the possibility of a receptor system associated with nerve endings ramifying within the disc also suggest a proprioceptive function for the intervertebral disc. The various compressive, torsion, and tensile stresses on the annulus as a result of movement and muscle contraction have the potential to stimulate these nerve endings when applied in a variety of spatial and temporal patterns. Although conclusive evidence for the neural functions of the disc is still lacking, Farfan[22] suggested that it is tempting to conceive of the disc as serving as one of the largest sense organs in the body that influence postural mechanisms. This idea is based on the premise that afferent neurologic information produced by forces on the disc results in reflex connections with neurons involved in the motor pathways controlling the skeletal muscle of the trunk and extremities. Motor activity is modified, resulting in postural changes and adaptations to the various forces placed on the spine.

Ligaments

Mechanical stimulation of a ligament in the form of excessive stretching or deformation results in accumulation of strain energy within the neural endings. This ligament distortion activates the nociceptive endings embedded within the ligament. Chemical stimuli, such as substances released from injured cells within the ligament or chemicals that diffuse into the ligament from surrounding injured tissues, may also result in activation of the nociceptive nerve endings.

In addition to the capsular ligaments, the ligamentum flavum and the anterior and posterior longitudinal, supraspinous, and interspinous ligaments are supplied with free nerve endings. Of these, the posterior longitudinal ligament appears to have the greatest density of nerve endings.[85]

Dorsal Root Ganglion

The dorsal root ganglion is situated just beneath the vertebral pedicles and is adjacent to the superior facet of the lumbar vertebrae. Nervi nervorum ("nerves supplying nerves") on the dorsal root ganglion serve as mechanically sensitive nociceptors. Posterolateral disc herniations or osteophytes in the region of the intervertebral foramen can mechanically compromise the dorsal root ganglion, resulting in pain because of the mechanosensitivity of the ganglion. The dorsal root ganglion as a source of pain is markedly different from the nerve root complex. Nerve roots are not normally sensitive to mechanical stimulation unless they are the site of inflammation. The dorsal root ganglion, on the other hand, appears to be a key potential source of pain because it is sensitive to mechanical stimulation even in the absence of inflammation.

Nerve Root

Although the formation and function of the nerve root are discussed below in some detail, the nerve root is included in this section on painful tissues to emphasize its role in pain syndromes. Diseases of the spine such as intervertebral disc disease, facet osteoarthrosis, segmental instability resulting in perturbations to the nerve root complex, and spinal canal stenosis are just several of the clinical entities thought to be associated with nerve root pain and dysfunction.

Compression or tension of the nerve root by itself, however, does not typically result in nerve root pain.[25, 35, 83] There must also be concurrent inflammation of the nerve root for symptoms to arise.[68] It has been suggested that protruded or extruded discal material contains substances that could biochemically irritate and alter nerve root function, such as glycoproteins,[52] immunoglobulins,[65] phospholipase A2 (which is known to promote inflammation and is present in high concentrations in the intervertebral disc),[70] and hydrogen ions.[59] In addition to the symptoms of pain, clinical signs of nerve root involvement must be correlated with the pain pattern (Tables 2-2 and 2-3). In the absence of nerve root irritation, pain ceases when mechanical stresses are placed on the nerve root. Conversely, when an inflamed nerve root is subjected to compression or tension, pain occurs. This is more fully described below.

Referred Pain

A discussion of the tissue origins of pain would not be complete without a review of the concept of referred pain. It is well recognized that low back pain with concurrent lower extremity pain is not necessarily due to nerve root involvement. Experimental studies have demonstrated that nearly all lumbopelvic tissues are capable of causing localized back pain, as well as pain that is felt in the lower extremities. Irritation of the zygapophyseal joint capsule, sacroiliac joint, dura mater, low back musculature, annulus fibrosus, and interspinous ligaments has been shown to give rise to symptoms in the lower extremities as well as in the low back.[23, 39, 46, 55, 58] Likewise, disorders of the pelvic or abdominal viscera may give rise to a perception of pain in the back or lower extremities.

In relation to low back disorders, pain perceived in the lower extremities owing to involvement of the lumbopelvic tissues or viscera is typically known as *referred pain*, whereas pain from involvement of the nerve root complex itself is referred to as *radicular pain*. One of the distinguishing features between referred pain and radicular pain is that in referred pain patterns, the spine pain is typically more aggravating than the lower extremity pain, whereas in radicular pain patterns, the pain in the lower extremity is more disconcerting and aggravating than the spine discomfort (Table 2-2). Additionally, the dull, poorly localized discomfort of referred pain contrasts with the sharper, localized pattern of radicular pain.

Because pain interpretation is highly subjective, a neuroanatomical pathway for referred pain would be

Table 2–3. Nerve Root Compression
Reflex changes
Muscle weakness
Muscle atrophy
Sensory loss over defined dermatome

difficult to define precisely. Cyriax has given referred pain the simplest definition by calling it "pain felt elsewhere than at its true site".[19] Although this definition is adequate as a working clinical description, it only describes the phenomenon as perceived by the patient and observed by the clinician. Little is known about the definitive pathways and multitude of central nervous system synapses that are probably involved in referred pain patterns.

The central nervous system, rather than the peripheral nervous system, is largely responsible for referred pain. As stated by Grieve,[30] "pain happens within the central nervous system, and does not reside in the damaged locality, though it may be perceived so." That is, the subjective experience of pain is the result of processing of the afferent impulse at the levels of the spinal cord, brain stem, and cerebral cortex. The painful stimulus activates many pools of neurons at all levels of the central nervous system, all of which contribute to the perception of referred pain.

Referred pain is well recognized and has given rise to the various dermatome, myotome, and sclerotome charts. These charts are occasionally referred to because embryologic segmentation is thought to be a predictor for patterns of referred pain. Although such charts may be helpful in some instances, segmental overlap is common, and it is still not possible to definitively determine the tissue of injury solely based on a distinct referred pain pattern.

In the strictest sense, pain from irritation of the nerve root or nerve root complex can also be considered referred pain because symptoms are felt at a distance from the source of irritation. The dura mater of the spinal canal, the nerve root sleeve, and the nerve root itself are pain—sensitive structures that are innervated by the sinuvertebral nerve (see below) and have the potential to refer pain to distal regions. However, the clinician usually classifies pain in the lower extremities that results from involvement of the nerve root as radicular pain, and involvement of any other lumbopelvic tissue or viscera that results in pain felt at a distance from its source as referred pain. This distinc-

Table 2–2. Nerve Root Irritation
Pain below the knee
Straight-leg raise reproduces leg pain
Excessive pain irradiation with gentle spinal motions
Leg pain greater than back pain
Leg pain in clearly demarcated region

tion, although not anatomically precise, will be kept for its clinical utility.

INNERVATION OF THE LUMBOPELVIC TISSUES

General Concepts: Nerve Roots, Spinal Nerve, and Rami

The previous section focused on several important tissues supplied with nociceptive nerve endings that are felt to be potential sources of pain and potential pain referral patterns when irritated, injured, or damaged. This section focuses primarily on the pathways by which nociceptive and mechanoreceptive endings deliver afferent information to the central nervous system, as well as the pathways used by the efferent nerve fibers to supply spinal musculature.

In the spinal canal, motor and sensory information for human behavior is carried by individual nerve roots.

Nerve rootlets attached to the spinal cord converge to form the dorsal and ventral roots, and these nerve roots then merge to form the spinal nerve. The spinal nerve is an extremely short segment of nerve and is the first point at which the sensory fibers (from the dorsal root) and motor fibers (from the ventral root) intermingle. From the spinal nerve outward, the motor and sensory components intertwine and travel together by way of the ventral and dorsal rami (Fig. 2-2). Therefore, although the dorsal and ventral roots are largely involved with sensory and motor information, respectively, the dorsal and ventral rami carry both motor and sensory information. It is these rami that ultimately give rise to peripheral nerves, which directly innervate the lumbopelvic tissues.

The branching of the spinal nerve into dorsal and ventral rami occurs immediately upon exit of the spinal nerve from the intervertebral foramen. The ventral rami pierce the psoas major muscle and merge with ventral rami from other lumbosacral levels to form the lumbosacral plexus (Fig. 2-3). Some of the branches of

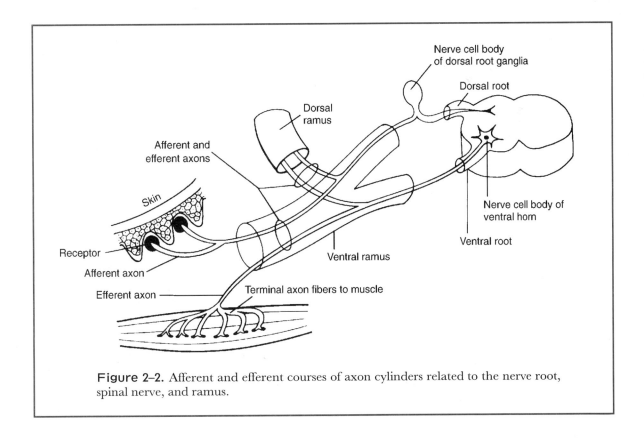

Figure 2–2. Afferent and efferent courses of axon cylinders related to the nerve root, spinal nerve, and ramus.

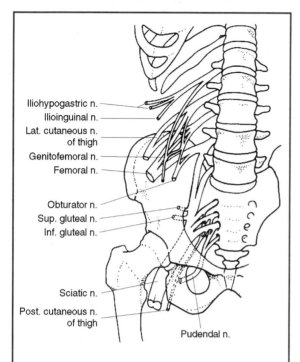

Figure 2–3. The lumbosacral plexus with its motor and sensory branches. Direct branches of the plexus innervate the psoas muscle as the plexus courses through the muscle. Portions of the lumbosacral plexus lie directly anterior to the sacroiliac joint.

The Dorsal Ramus

The dorsal ramus branches from the spinal nerve, turns posteriorly, and then courses through the tissues of the back. The L5 dorsal ramus is longer and has a more tortuous course than the other dorsal rami, because it follows the alar and dorsal surfaces of the sacrum.[9] Both the afferent information originating in the lumbopelvic tissues and being transmitted to the central nervous system and the efferent information originating in the central nervous system and being transmitted to the muscles of the lumbopelvic region must traverse rami.

Figure 2-4 illustrates the path of the dorsal ramus and its associated branches. The two largest divisions are the medial and lateral branches. Bogduk and associates[9] noted that careful dissection of the medial and lateral branches of the dorsal rami can reveal a third branch, the intermediate branch. This branch appears to be an intermediate branch of the lateral ramus, but

the ventral rami directly innervate the psoas major, psoas minor, and quadratus lumborum muscles, whereas others give rise to the numerous peripheral nerves that ultimately innervate the lower extremity. Cutaneous nerves to the lower extremity are also derived directly from the lumbosacral plexus or branch from the peripheral nerves of the lumbosacral plexus.

The ventral rami are primarily concerned with the motor and sensory innervation of the lower extremity. However, the dorsal rami and their branches assume great importance with regard to the innervation of the various low back tissues. They are responsible for nearly all of the motor and sensory innervation of the posterior elements of the lumbopelvic region, including the spinal extensor muscles, ligaments of the spine, joint capsules, and intervertebral disc, which warrants a closer inspection of their anatomical makeup and function.

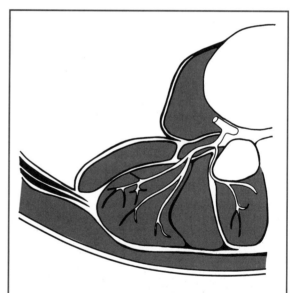

Figure 2–4. The path of the dorsal ramus. The medial branch of the dorsal ramus courses inferior to the apophyseal joint, and the lateral branch courses through the erector spinae muscle. (Adapted from Korr IM [ed]: The Neurobiologic Mechanisms of Manipulative Therapy. New York: Plenum Press, 1978.)

for the purposes of this discussion, only the lateral and medial branches are considered.

The medial branch of the dorsal ramus innervates the lumbopelvic tissues that are medial and adjacent to a parasagittal plane through the zygapophyseal joints (Fig. 2-4). Tissues that occupy the area between the spinous processes and the longitudinal plane of the zygapophyseal joints include the multifidus, interspinalis, and intertransversarii musculature and the apophyseal joint structures. All are therefore innervated by the medial branch of the dorsal ramus. Small-caliber axons from branches of the medial branch of the dorsal ramus have also been identified in the supraspinous and interspinous ligament, ligamentum flavum, and the thoracolumbar fascia.[66, 86]

The medial branch of the dorsal ramus provides an abundant neural supply to the apophyseal joint capsule. Nerve endings include high-threshold slow-conducting nerve fibers and low-threshold fast-conducting fibers, suggesting both nociceptive and proprioceptive functions of these nerve endings. Small-caliber primary afferent axons containing neuropeptides such as substance P and calcitonin gene-related peptide have also been noted to ramify within the joint capsule.[1, 5] The

presence of such fibers supports the contention that the apophyseal joints can be a source of low back pain.

Tissues that are lateral to the apophyseal joint plane are innervated by the lateral branches of the dorsal ramus. They include the iliocostalis and longissimus divisions of the superficial and deep erector spinae and the thoracolumbar fascia (Fig. 2-5).[6] The lateral branches of the dorsal rami of L1, L2, and L3 eventually become cutaneous in their course through the iliocostalis and longissimus muscles to supply the skin and are referred to as the superior cluneal nerves.[36] These nerves pierce the superficial fascia above the iliac crest and descend to supply the skin over the buttock. The middle cluneal nerves are the lateral branches of the dorsal rami of the first three sacral nerves. They extend more laterally to innervate skin toward the region of the greater trochanter (Fig. 2-6).

This description of tissues innervated by the medial and lateral branches of the various dorsal rami indicates that both sensory and motor innervation are provided by these nerves. The motor innervation to many of the skeletal muscles of the low back, such as the superficial and deep erector spinae and multifidus, and the nociceptive, proprioceptive, and kinesthetic sensory

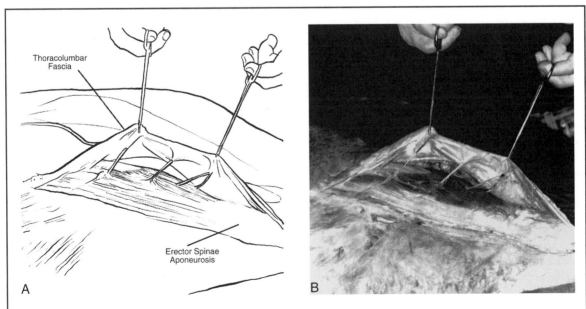

Figure 2–5. *A* and *B,* The lateral branch of the dorsal ramus is seen piercing the erector spinae muscle and entering the reflected thoracolumbar fascia.

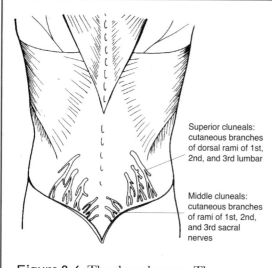

Figure 2–6. The cluneal nerves. These nerves contribute to the cutaneous innervation of the posterior pelvis and hip regions.

Superior cluneals: cutaneous branches of dorsal rami of 1st, 2nd, and 3rd lumbar

Middle cluneals: cutaneous branches of rami of 1st, 2nd, and 3rd sacral nerves

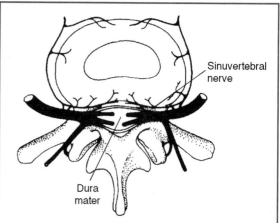

Sinuvertebral nerve

Dura mater

Figure 2–7. The sinuvertebral nerve originates from the distal pole of the dorsal root ganglion or the proximal portion of the spinal nerve, then courses back through the intervertebral foramen to supply structures within the spinal canal.

qualities from the joint structures, osseous elements, and soft tissues of the low back are carried by branches of the dorsal rami. An understanding of this innervation is important to an appreciation of the anatomic pathways that are used for sensory feedback and muscle activity and that contribute to motor control.

Sinuvertebral Nerves

Because of the increasing recognition of the role the degenerative disc plays in many low back pain syndromes, the sinuvertebral nerve has been subject to detailed investigation.[38] This important nerve branches from the distal pole of the dorsal root ganglion or the initial portion of the spinal nerve and then traverses a path back through the intervertebral foramen (Fig. 2-7). The sinuvertebral nerve is primarily responsible for innervating structures within the spinal canal. Also known as the recurrent nerve or the nerve of Luschka, it is often joined by branches from the grey ramus communicans of the sympathetic chain ganglion. Small autonomic branches of sympathetic nerves also enter the intervertebral canal independent of the sinuvertebral nerve. Using highly refined staining techniques, Groen et al. have suggested that the sinuvertebral nerve is almost exclusively derived from the

ramus communicans, which underscores the sympathetic nervous system contribution to the sinuvertebral nerve.[31]

Structures within the spinal canal, such as the ventral aspect of the dura mater, epidural vasculature, posterior longitudinal ligament, posterior aspect of the annulus fibrosus, and venous plexus, as they enter the vertebral body are innervated by the sinuvertebral nerve.[6] As the nerve enters the intervertebral foramen, it typically divides into ascending and descending branches, and from these branches the ventral aspect of the dura mater is innervated. The sinuvertebral nerve gives off a plexiform mass of nerve fibers supplying the posterior longitudinal ligament (Fig. 2-8). This innervation is especially dense over the region of the posterior longitudinal ligament, which forms an expansion over the intervertebral disc.

The complexity of the sinuvertebral nerve is revealed on examination of the nerve fibers that form its substance. Cross-sectional studies of the nerve show small and moderately large myelinated fibers. The smaller fibers, which are most likely postganglionic nerve fibers from the sympathetic chain ganglion that lie adjacent to the vertebral bodies, are autonomic fibers mediating the smooth muscle of the vascular elements of the spinal canal. The larger fibers most likely involve proprioceptive function, especially

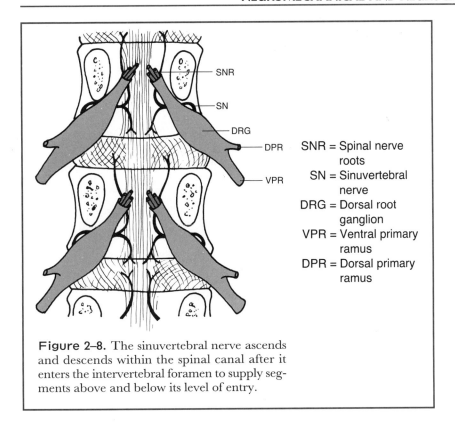

SNR = Spinal nerve
roots
SN = Sinuvertebral
nerve
DRG = Dorsal root
ganglion
VPR = Ventral primary
ramus
DPR = Dorsal primary
ramus

Figure 2–8. The sinuvertebral nerve ascends and descends within the spinal canal after it enters the intervertebral foramen to supply segments above and below its level of entry.

because the posterior longitudinal ligament contains numerous encapsulated nerve endings. The bulk of the nerve endings related to the sinuvertebral nerve are unencapsulated free nerve endings that are considered to subserve nociception.[34, 62] Because these nerves do not innervate skeletal muscle structures, their fibers are primarily afferent, carrying sensory qualities such as nociception and proprioceptive feedback to the central nervous system, with secondary functions of efferent motor supply to the smooth muscle of the vasculature.

Nerve Roots

After Mixter and Barr's[57] report in 1934, the nerve root and its relation to the intervertebral disc received great attention. The results of that study were interpreted as demonstrating that the major mechanism behind the clinical syndromes of low back and leg pain was compression of the nerve roots by the protruded intervertebral disc.

In subsequent years, research into the structure and function of the nerve root has led to a clearer understanding of its unique nature. In addition, the osseous and nonosseous tissues that surround it have also been more completely described. Recognition is now given to the fact that structures other than the disc can adversely influence the nerve roots in their path from the spinal canal to the intervertebral foramen. Detailed descriptions of the meningeal coverings, pedicle of the vertebrae, lateral recess, zygapophyseal joint, transforamenal ligaments, and the contents within the intervertebral foramen are now available, and these structures have been investigated as to their potential influence on nerve root function. The purpose of this section is to detail the anatomy of the nerve root and the structures it interacts with along its course and then consider its role in low back pain.

As pointed out above, the ventral and dorsal nerve roots serve as the motor and sensory pathways, respectively, that link the central nervous system with the tissues and organs of the body. Because the spinal cord ends opposite the intervertebral disc between the second and third lumbar vertebrae, the nerve roots must be progressively longer to make their exit at the spinal level below their respective vertebrae.[4] In the lumbosacral region, these elongated roots form the cauda equina, which traverses the lower lumbar vertebral spinal canal (Fig. 2-9). The obliquity of the course of the nerve roots gradually increases as it proceeds inferiorly. The first and second lumbar nerve roots have an angle of inclination of 70 to 80 degrees; the third and fourth, 60 degrees; the fifth, 45 degrees; and the first sacral nerve root, 30 degrees.[10]

The nerve roots are formed by a series of rootlets that are attached to the spinal cord and converge to form the fibers of the nerve root cylinder (Fig. 2-10). The ventral nerve root and the typically larger dorsal nerve root then stream toward the intervertebral foramen, where they merge to form the spinal nerve.[77] Just medial to this merging, the dorsal root ganglion presents as a distinct swelling of the dorsal root. A nerve root sheath (discussed below) invests the nerve roots and the dorsal root ganglion (Fig. 2-11).

In their simplest description, all nerve roots, spinal nerves, rami, and peripheral nerves are organized bundles of cellular processes that extend from nerve cell bodies. These cellular processes are axon cylinders, also referred to as nerve fibers. The nerve cell bodies that give rise to these axon cylinders are located in the ventral horn of the spinal cord and in the dorsal root ganglion.[68] The name given to an axon cylinder (nerve root, spinal nerve, ramus, or peripheral nerve) is determined by the anatomic region in which that axon cylinder is located (Fig. 2-12).

The lumbar and sacral nerve roots travel within the subarachnoid cistern and ultimately pierce the dura as they exit the intervertebral foramen (Fig. 2-13). The nerve roots serve as the link between the central nervous system (spinal cord) and the peripheral nervous system (spinal nerves and their associated rami).

The nerve root's response to mechanical stresses is different from the dorsal root ganglion's response and is explored in the next section. In the lumbosacral region, the space around the nerve root is widest in

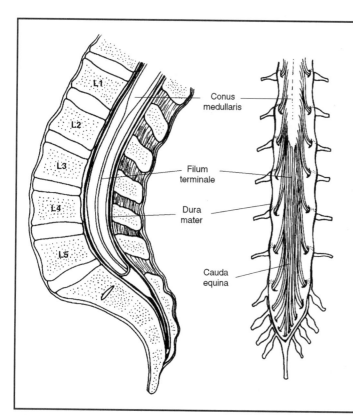

Figure 2–9. Cauda equina. *A,* Sagittal view showing the relation between the dural sac and the vertebral canal. *B,* Nerve roots within the dural sac.

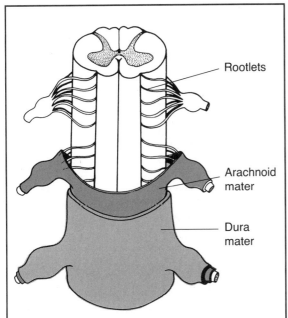

Figure 2–10. Formation of nerve roots by a series of rootlets. The meningeal layers have been cut away to show the rootlets attaching to the spinal cord.

the spinal canal and narrowest in the intervertebral foramen.[33] As the nerve roots course through the spinal canal, the space is typically wide and unobstructed. As the roots approach the intervertebral foramen, the exit narrows considerably. At the intervertebral foramen, the nerve roots are supported and cushioned by fat—containing connective tissue.[79] Transforamenal ligaments also bridge the opening of the intervertebral foramen.[7] Nevertheless, there is still ample room for the nerve root and its associated vasculature in the intervertebral foramen.

DORSAL ROOT GANGLION

With the pathway the nerve roots traverse more clearly defined, some detail of the dorsal root ganglion can now be added. As previously mentioned, the dorsal and ventral roots approach the intervertebral foramen within the dural sheath. The dorsal root ganglion is usually located in the approximate center of the foramen.[68]

The dorsal root ganglion is composed of nerve cell bodies of various sizes.[45] Various neuropeptides are manufactured and reside in these cell bodies, but their physiological roles have not been fully elucidated. The processes that extend from the nerve cell bodies travel in opposite directions: one process travels toward the spinal cord through the dorsal roots, and the other travels toward the periphery through the spinal nerves.

At the terminal end of the peripheral processes (those processes destined for the peripheral tissues) are the various receptors of the joints and tissues, such as the articular mechanoreceptors, muscle spindles, Golgi tendon organs, and nociceptors (Fig. 2-14). Quite simply, the cell bodies for all sensory receptors are locat-

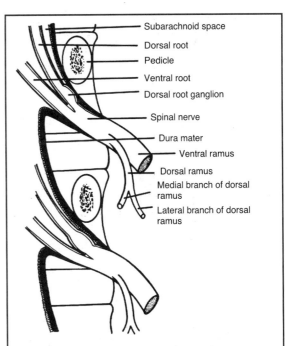

Figure 2–11. The dorsal and ventral nerve roots merge to form the spinal nerve. Just medial to the point at which the two roots come together is the dorsal root ganglion. This ganglion is the distinct swelling on the dorsal root that is the location of cell bodies giving rise to the axons of the dorsal root and axons of the spinal nerve and both rami. The dural sheath (thecal sac) can be seen ending as a blind sac just distal to the dorsal root ganglion (Adapted from Bogduk N, Twomey LT: Clinical Anatomy of the Lumbar Spine. New York: Churchill Livingstone, 1987.)

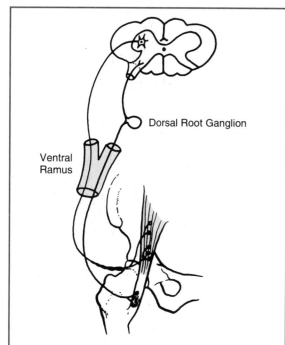

Figure 2–12. Afferent and efferent courses of the axon cylinders related to the nerve root, dorsal root ganglion, spinal nerve, and rami.

ed together in the dorsal root ganglion, and they use the central process, which is the dorsal root, to convey their information to the central nervous system. Normal function is such that stimulation of the receptor initiates an action potential that travels along the peripheral process toward the cell body in the dorsal root ganglion. From the cell body, the action potential then travels along the dorsal nerve root and into the dorsal horn of the spinal cord.

The action potential traveling through the dorsal nerve root initiates the release of neurotransmitters at the dorsal horn of the spinal cord that interact with synaptic endings of various neurons in the spinal cord. These neurotransmitters are peptides that are synthesized in the nerve cell bodies of the dorsal root ganglion. Axoplasmic transport is one of the primary methods of moving the transmitter from the cell body to the synaptic ending of the axon.

The dorsal root ganglion is a mechanically sensitive structure in comparison with the nerve root. Thus, there is a major difference between compression of

the normal nerve root and compression of the normal dorsal root ganglion. Compression of the normal dorsal root ganglion results in repetitive depolarization of the nerve cell bodies that constitute it.[37] This increased nerve cell activity results in generation of action potentials. The increase in afferent activity to the spinal cord may initiate the neural pathways responsible for eliciting pain and may also alter the sensorimotor reflex activity that contributes to the contractile state or resting tension of muscle. In the broadest sense, such increased dorsal root activity "sensitizes" the central nervous system.

AXOPLASMIC TRANSPORT AND NERVE ROOT FUNCTION: IMPLICATIONS FOR LOW BACK DYSFUNCTION

The cell bodies of the dorsal root ganglion are anatomically unique structures in the nervous system and deserve special mention. Although they appear to give rise to only one axon that bifurcates into two branches, they actually derive from bipolar cells whose two processes fused during embryonic development. One branch is the peripheral axon, which is attached to the receptors in the periphery, and the other is the central axon, which contributes to the formation of the dorsal root.[72] Recognizing that the axon cylinder is a cellular extension of the nerve cell body is important in understanding how the nerve cell provides the necessary neuronal proteins to the axon terminals. In addition, used materials can be returned to the cell body for either degradation or restoration and reuse.

Axoplasmic transport is an important physiological function of the nerve cell. Amino acids taken up by the nerve cell bodies can be incorporated into proteins that can then be transported distally through the axon cylinders to reach the presynaptic terminals. This movement of proteins and substrates from the cytoplasm of the cell body through the cytoplasm of the axon is known as axoplasmic transport. The communication to and from the cell body is therefore vitally important for the integrity of the nerve fiber.

The relation of the physiological process of axoplasmic transport to mechanical low back pain is not immediately apparent, until the site of the cell bodies of the dorsal root ganglion is recognized. Their location in the lumbosacral region in particular leaves them vul-

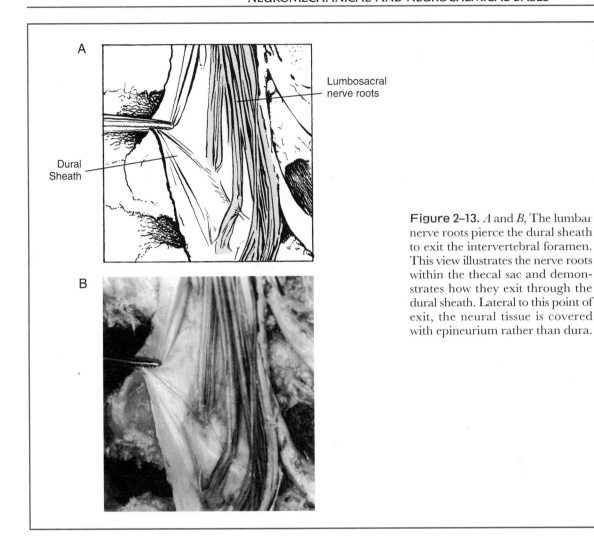

A

Lumbosacral
nerve roots

Dural
Sheath

Figure 2–13. *A* and *B*, The lumbar nerve roots pierce the dural sheath to exit the intervertebral foramen. This view illustrates the nerve roots within the thecal sac and demonstrates how they exit through the dural sheath. Lateral to this point of exit, the neural tissue is covered with epineurium rather than dura.

B

nerable to injury, which potentially compromises this important function. The vulnerability of the dorsal root ganglion is such that dorsal root ganglion injury potentially alters axoplasmic transport physiology and thus interferes with dorsal nerve root function. Injured dorsal nerve roots in turn alter the type and quality of information that reaches the dorsal horn of the spinal cord.

What are these relations between cell body location, axoplasmic transport, and nerve root function that can be integrated into a discussion of mechanical low back pain? The axon cylinder, an extension of the cell body, depends on axoplasmic transport to ensure its proper function, because it uses the various proteins synthesized in the cell body for its synaptic activity. The nucle-

us of the nerve cell body is essential for the synthesis of proteins, which can then be carried by this axoplasmic flow to replace proteins that have been degraded owing to nerve cell activity.

Because the cell body is so important for proper nerve cell function, the location of the dorsal root ganglion is of special significance in the lumbosacral region (see Fig. 2-11). Located in the intervertebral foramen or immediately subjacent to the pedicle of the vertebrae, the cell bodies of the dorsal root ganglion are easily subjected to mechanical stresses. As mentioned earlier, the unique nature of the dorsal root ganglion is such that each nerve cell body has two axon cylinders. One extends centrally to the spinal cord and the

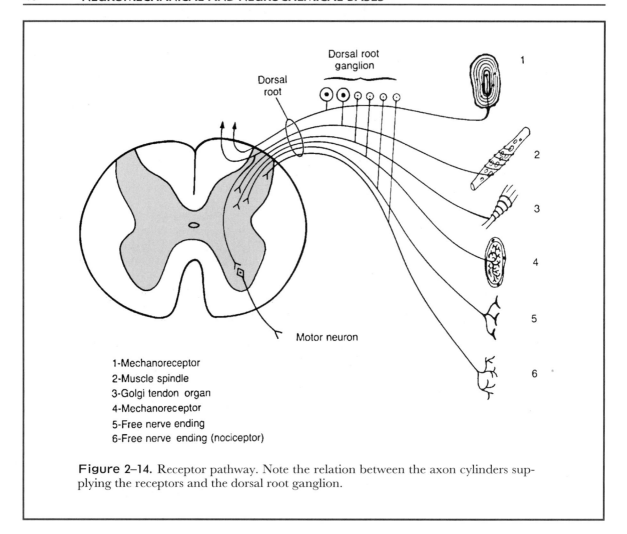

Figure 2–14. Receptor pathway. Note the relation between the axon cylinders supplying the receptors and the dorsal root ganglion.

other extends peripherally to the receptors located in the tissues. Altered axon (nerve fiber) function can occur as a result of injury to these nerve cell bodies because of interference with the axoplasmic transport process. The cell bodies that reside in the ventral horn of the spinal cord are equally as important, from the perspective of axoplasmic transport, as the cell bodies of the dorsal root ganglion; however, they are not located in as vulnerable a position.

The discussion above centered on injury to the cell body. If the nerve root itself is injured, then interference with its normal function, owing to interruption of axoplasmic transport, also results. Therefore, two mechanical causes can interfere with axoplasmic trans-

port: damage to the axon cylinder (the nerve root itself) and injury to the cell bodies (dorsal root ganglion or ventral horn cell). Injury of either nerve root potentially alters the sensory or motor system.[40]

THE NERVE ROOT SLEEVE

The nerve root is closely invested with a very thin covering of pia mater. Outside of this closely investing sheath are the cerebrospinal fluid and the meninges. For each nerve root, the subarachnoid space ends at approximately the region of the dorsal root ganglion

(Fig. 2-11). The nerve root invaginates the arachnoid and dura mater close to the intervertebral foramen, at which point the dural covering becomes the epineurium of the peripheral nerve. The meningeal covering (dura and arachnoid) that invests the nerve root in its course toward the intervertebral foramen is referred to as the dural sleeve.

The nerve root, with its pial covering, must pierce the arachnoid and dura mater in the path from the spinal canal through the intervertebral foramen. The very thin arachnoid layer closely adheres to the inner surface of the dura. By adhering to the inner aspect of the dura in this way, a subarachnoid space is created around the nerve roots. The cerebrospinal fluid that bathes the nerve roots is contained in this space. The vasculature and cerebrospinal fluid are responsible for nourishing these nerve root structures.

The anatomic pathway the nerve root takes from the lateral aspect of the dural (thecal) sac to the intervertebral foramen is the nerve root canal.[10] In this path from spinal canal to intervertebral foramen, the roots are anterior to the lamina, ligamentum flavum, and zygapophyseal joint and posterior to the intervertebral disc and vertebral body. The roots also lie immediately subjacent to the vertebral pedicle.

Narrowing of this nerve root canal is termed *lateral canal stenosis* or *lateral recess stenosis*, and constrictive alteration in the dimensions of the spinal canal is *spinal canal stenosis*. Such constrictions can occur as a result of a wide range of space-occupying conditions, such as hypertrophy of the ligamentous tissues in the spinal canal, inflammatory conditions, tumors, osteophytes, and segmental instability. Any structure along the border of the nerve root canal or within the spinal canal can be involved.[33]

The lumbar spinal canal in cross section is typically triangular in shape, with the base of the triangle anteriorly placed (Fig. 2-15). It is the anterolateral corners of this triangle that serve as the lateral recess of the spinal canal. The lateral recess is a markedly restricted area accommodating the nerve roots. Most intervertebral disc pathologies occur at the posterolateral margin of the disc, which is in the same immediate environment as the anterolateral corner of the spinal canal—the lateral recess. The pressure from a herniated disc occurs anteriorly on the nerve root, compressing the root posteriorly against the lumbar facet or the pedicle. The resulting lateral canal stenosis may produce varying degrees of radiculopathy.

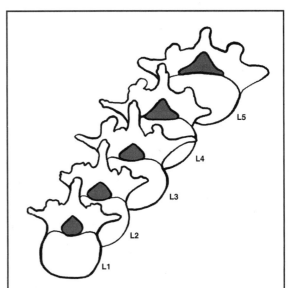

Figure 2–15. The triangular shape of the lumbar spinal canal is such that the base of the triangle is anteriorly placed. This renders the nerve roots occupying the anterolateral corners of the canal vulnerable to potential stresses from posterolateral protrusions of the intervertebral disc.

The vulnerability of the nerve root is quite different at the region of the intervertebral foramen, where the nerve root complex with its nerve root sleeve cover and blood vessels exit and enter the spinal canal. In the lumbar region, the transverse height of the intervertebral foramen ranges from 12 to 19 mm. By comparison, the transverse diameter may be as little as 7 mm. The anterior–posterior dimensions of the intervertebral foramen has a greater potential to compromise the nerve root complex than the superior–inferior dimension. Segmental instability may be associated with nerve root inflammation, pain, and neurologic deficit because of the limited anterior–posterior diameter of the intervertebral foramen. This is most apparent in spondylolisthesis.[26]

In the lumbar spinal canal, the nerve roots float freely within the subarachnoid space of the thecal sac. Because of their mobility within this space, they can escape mechanical stresses. The symptoms of spinal stenosis that are associated with compressive phenomena are most likely due to arterial compromise within the canal rather than direct compression of the cauda equina.[71] Therefore, compression of the lumbosacral nerve roots in the spinal canal is not as common as compromise within the lateral canal. The nerve roots are also vulnerable at these lateral recesses because they pick up a close investment of dura as they exit laterally through the thecal tube. This dural sleeve becomes attached to the nerve root close to the region of the intervertebral foramen. This fixation to the dura reduces the mobility of the roots and their ability to escape mechanical stresses.

At the region of the intervertebral foramen, the mobility of the dural sleeve itself is limited because the root sleeves may be anchored to the adjacent pedicle. Motion of the lumbar nerve root complex is therefore also limited.[58, 76] Additionally, the anatomy of the intervertebral foramen and the tentlike shape of the dural sleeve preclude any excessive motion of the dura. A small excursion of the dural sleeve in an inferior and lateral direction, as might occur with a traction force to the root, effectively "plugs" the intervertebral foramen (Fig. 2-16).[79] This plugging of the intervertebral foramen by the dura mater is comparable to attempting to pull an A-frame tent through a doorway. The top of the tent can move a short distance through the doorway, but eventually the body of the tent plugs the doorway and prevents any further movement.

The nerve root is dynamic, and elongation and changes in the direction of the roots of the cauda equina occur during movement.[48] Movement results in traction forces on the nerve root and its dural sleeve, and the unique method of dural investment and fixation helps to minimize the chance of nerve root avulsion from the spinal cord. However, this also leaves the nerve root with its dural sleeve vulnerable to mechanical forces, because the limited mobility in the region of the intervertebral foramen does not allow easy escape from these forces.

Even though the dura mater is a tough, fibrous tissue, the nerve roots are still considered more vulnerable than the peripheral nerves to potentially damaging insults such as tensile and compression forces and chemical irritation. The nerve roots lack the protective epineural and perineural coverings found in the peripheral nerves.[78, 79] The connective tissue matrix of the epineurium and perineurium, with their fat cushions, offers the peripheral nerve a mechanism for protection against various mechanical stresses. The nerve root lacks this protection.

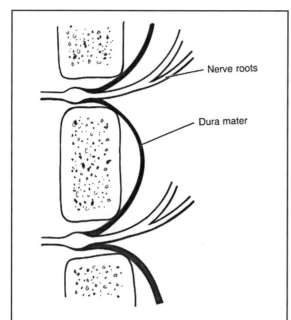

Figure 2–16. Protective function of the dura mater as it plugs the intervertebral foramen to minimize the potential for nerve root avulsion when a tensile force is imparted to the spinal nerve.

NERVE ROOT AND DORSAL ROOT GANGLION NUTRITION

The nerve root is subjected to many mechanical stresses throughout daily activities. For example, lumbar hyperextension should theoretically place a compressive force on the nerve roots. Kicking the leg out straight places a tensile stress on the sciatic nerve and lumbosacral nerve roots. Observation of a person performing the activities of daily living, however, reveals that a painful response does not occur every time the spine is extended or the leg is placed forward.

Yet, in some people with radicular signs or symptoms, even the slightest extension movement of the lumbar spine appears to increase compression on the nerve root, or a straight-leg raise of only 30 degrees appears to increase nerve root tension. The resulting painful response appears disproportionate to the apparent force on the nerve root. Why are these nerve roots more responsive to mechanical stress, and what is the difference between normal and injured nerve roots?

The lumbosacral roots have some unique and clinically important characteristics that give insight into this question. Parke and Watanabe[63] noted that the lumbosacral nerve roots are structurally, vascularly, and metabolically unique regions of the nervous system. They are distinct structures when compared with the peripheral nerves. The neural fibers of the nerve roots are freestanding tracts, and they do not become incorporated into nerve bundles until they pierce the dural sheath.[63] Recall how the rootlets attach to the spinal cord and eventually form nerve fiber bundles. A tight, compact nerve bundle structure does not begin to form until the root gets closer to the intervertebral foramen. The rootlets and freestanding fibers more closely resemble spinal cord tissue than peripheral nerve tissue. The nerve roots are not only functionally distinct but also anatomically different from the peripheral nerves.

The difference between the nerve roots and peripheral nerves is also illustrated when comparing how nutritional elements reach them. The vascular supply to the nerve roots more closely resembles the vascular supply to the spinal cord than that to the peripheral nerve tissue. Vasculature to the lumbosacral roots relies on circulation stemming from the vascular plexus of the spinal cord. This vasculature follows the rootlets outward to partially nourish the nerve root. In addition, the peripheral and central portions of the nerve roots, including the rootlets, also receive nourishment from branches of the lumbar segmental arteries. These lumbar arteries are located outside the intervertebral foramen and send small branches back through the foramen. These small vessels give rise to a microvascular system that combines with vessels from the spinal cord to provide a vascular supply to the nerve root complex.

This circulation, however, accounts for only a portion of the nutritional source for the nerve root. The other nutritional source is via percolation of the cerebrospinal fluid into the nerve root complex. This is a major physiologic difference between the nerve root and the peripheral nerve, which by comparison obtains nearly all of its nutrition from the vasculature.[63, 69]

The contribution of the cerebrospinal fluid, which bathes the nerve roots, is quite extensive. Nutrients diffuse from the cerebrospinal fluid through the thin covering of pia mater and into the nerve root. Because diffusion of metabolites into the nerve root serves as a mechanism allowing nutrients into the nerve roots, inflammatory conditions associated with the nerve root

or other spinal canal elements potentially impede this mechanism and therefore adversely affect the nerve root. Nerve root compression affects the ability of the cerebrospinal fluid to percolate along the nerve roots. If both the circulation and cerebrospinal fluid percolation are compromised, nutritional mechanisms become markedly reduced.[18] These factors are of fundamental importance in understanding the concepts of lumbosacral nerve root ischemia, nerve root irritation caused by an inflammatory process, and the biomechanics of the nerve root and associated vasculature.

NERVE ROOT AND DORSAL ROOT GANGLION PAIN MECHANISMS

With this basic understanding of anatomy, nerve root pain mechanisms can be further developed. In experimental studies in which compressive forces were applied to noninjured nerve roots, MacNab[49] noted that the subjects experienced numbness and paresthesia but did not complain of pain. The healthy nerve root appears to be protected from eliciting a painful response when subjected to mechanical stresses. Even though the nerve root has close relations with many tissues in the path from the spinal canal to the intervertebral foramen, there appears to be a safeguard against continuous pain that may result from forces on the nerve root.

Smyth and Wright,[75] however, studied nerve roots that had been previously injured as a result of intervertebral disc lesions. In their experiments, pain did result from forces placed on the injured roots. The difference between these two experiments is that stress was placed on noninjured nerve roots in one instance and on injured nerve roots in another, with different experimental outcomes.

McCarron and coworkers[56] shed further light on this aspect of injured nerve roots and, in particular, inflammation of the nerve roots. In their experiments with a homogenate of nucleus pulposus material, they were able to demonstrate that the nucleus pulposus acts as a chemical or an immunogenic irritant to the nerve root. The nerve roots and dural sac showed various degrees of inflammatory response, ranging from edema and fibrin formation to increased vascularity and regional fibrosis, when exposed to this nucleus pulposus material. Inflammation or fibrosis of the root presents a physical impediment to the diffusion of nutrients from the cerebrospinal fluid through the membrane of the nerve root. This in turn leads to neuroischemic conditions that prevent or delay the delivery of essential nutrients normally supplied by the microvasculature. An alteration in the nutritional status of the nerve root can result in minor damage to the axons. There is good evidence that axonal damage can cause mechanical sensitivity at the traumatized region and alter the spontaneous and evoked activity of the damaged axon segment and its dorsal root ganglion.[15, 37, 47]

Therefore, there is a strong suggestion that it is not the mechanical pressure alone that causes the phenomena of nerve root pain, but rather an abnormal chemical environment of the nerve root that alters electrical activity. The mechanical stresses lower the depolarization threshold, with resultant action potentials, which in turn initiate the nociceptive response (Fig. 2-17). In the majority of patients, pain will resolve with nonoperative treatment despite evidence of continued compression.[26, 80]

In recalling the osseous and nonosseous elements the nerve root must traverse, it should be apparent that an inflammatory response caused by injury of any of the tissues along the pathway has the potential to alter the function of the nerve root by changing its nutritional status. Injury to any of these other tissues yields the same effect on the nerve root: altered nutritional status, an inflammatory response, and an irritated nerve root. The potential for inflammation in the spinal canal is great owing to the rich vascular plexus surrounding the posterior longitudinal ligament (Fig. 2-18).

In summary, the major clinical considerations for involvement of the nerve root complex based on its structure and function include the following:

1. Inflammatory conditions of the nerve root complex;
2. Fibrotic, scarred nerve roots with a resultant potential for decreased percolation of nutrients from the cerebrospinal fluid of the subarachnoid space and into the nerve root;
3. Neuroischemia of the root complex;
4. Injury or mechanical irritation of the dorsal root ganglion;
5. Relative immobility of the nerve root and sheath at the region of the nerve root canal that leaves it potentially vulnerable to abnormal forces.

The mechanisms of pain associated with the nerve root include *nerve root compression* and *nerve root irritation*. The clinical phenomenon of nerve root compression is most easily explained based on the current understanding of axon function. Compression of the axon cylinder alters its conduction capabilities. Consequently, signs of nerve root dysfunction are expected when the nerve roots themselves are compressed. This compressive phenomenon can occur at any point along the pathway from the spinal canal to the intervertebral foramen.

In addition to noting pain location and pain pattern to determine radicular involvement, a neurological screen that examines sensory and motor root function should be included in all low back examinations. Table 2-4 lists sample tests for a nerve root screening examination that provide information about the integrity of the lumbosacral nerve roots and alert the clinician to possible neurological involvement. These tests are further described and incorporated into the complete low back examination described in Chapter 5. These neurological tests are designed to evaluate

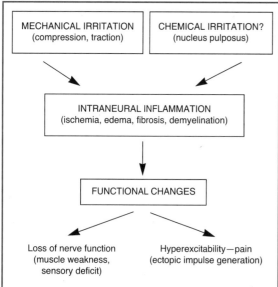

Figure 2–17. Mechanical and biochemical factors that result in nerve root pathology. (From Rydevik B, Garfin S: Spinal nerve root compression. In Szabo RM [ed]: Nerve Compression Syndromes—Diagnosis and Treatment. Thorofare, NJ: Charles B. Slack, 1989.)

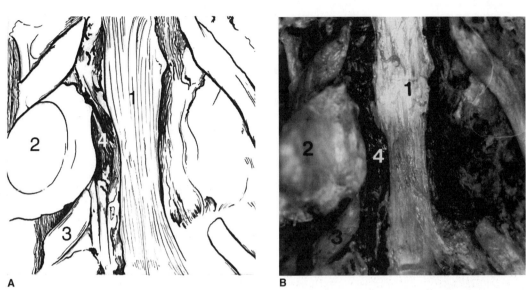

Figure 2–18. *A* and *B*, The posterior longitudinal ligament and posterior aspect of the disc have a rich venous plexus associated with them. Note the intimate relationship between the posterior longitudinal ligament (1), disc facet of the apophyseal joint (2), and nerve root (3). The rich vascular network (4) suggests an environment capable of inflammation and increase in the fluid environment as a result of inflammatory conditions. (From DeRosa C: Integration of the Objectives of Treatment for Low Back Pain with Lumbar Spine Anatomy. Ph. D. Thesis, Union Institute, Cincinnati, OH, 1993.)

altered reflex activity, muscle weakness or wasting, and paresthesia and numbness in a clearly demarcated area. Because the tests are not used to evaluate pain, they tend to provide objective data, although a certain amount of subjectivity is inherent in any sensory test or request for motor activity.

Whereas nerve root compression results in changes in axon function that are, in many cases, measurable, nerve root irritation is not as clearly understood. Recall the discussion above pointing out that compression of the normal nerve root does not typically result in pain. However, the injured or irritated nerve root does give rise to pain when it is subjected to mechanical distortion. This increased sensitivity is the direct result of an inflammatory process of the nerve root.

Different mechanical stresses can be placed on the irritated nerve root and its accompanying investments. One of the most common tests used in the evaluation of the sensitivity of the nerve root complex is the straight-leg raise test. With nerve root irritation, leg pain may be exacerbated as the lower extremity is raised. By incorporating internal rotation and adduction of the hip during the straight-leg raise test, an even greater tensile force is placed on the nerve roots by way of the sciatic nerve.[12] This increased tensile force placed on the nerve root is due to the course the sciatic nerve takes as it travels lateral to the ischial tuberosity (Fig. 2-19). This bony protuberance acts as a fulcrum during the maneuver. Other methods to increase the tensile force on the nerve root include ankle dorsiflexion and manual compression by the examiner in the popliteal fossa.

Maitland[50] described the "slump test," which maximally stresses the dural sheath and the nerve roots (Fig. 2-20). This test exerts a cephalad and caudally directed force on the dura mater and additionally places a tensile stress on the nerve roots of the lower extremity.[50] From the sitting position, the patient slumps

Table 2–4. Screening Examination for Nerve Root Compression

Test	Roots Evaluated
REFLEXES	
Quadriceps	L3–L4
Tibialis posterior	L4–L5
Gastroc-soleus	S1–S2
MUSCLE	
Hip flexors	L2–L3
Quadriceps	L3–L4
Anterior tibialis	L4
Extensor hallucis longus	L5
Peroneals	S1–S2
Gastroc-soleus	S1–S2
Hamstrings	L4–L5
Gluteus maximus	L5-S1
SENSORY	
Medial side of leg/foot	L4
Lateral side of leg/foot	L5
Posterior/posterolateral leg or thigh	S1–S2

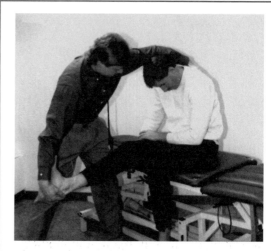

Figure 2–20. Slump test as described by Maitland.[50]

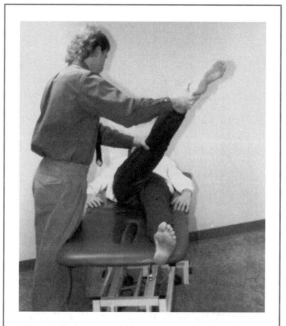

Figure 2–19. Adding hip adduction and internal rotation to the straight-leg raise test increases the tensile stress on the lumbosacral nerve roots.

forward, which flexes the thoracic and lumbar spine. Overpressure is applied through the shoulders to increase the flexion force. Head and neck flexion are then added to the position. While the patient maintains this position, the knee is extended and the ankle dorsiflexed (Chapter 5). The test is instructive in the mechanics of the nerve roots and their coverings within the spinal canal and intervertebral foramen. The examiner has the ability to decrease or increase the tension on the dura or nerve roots by varying the degree of neck flexion or knee extension, or any other component of the final position. The relation between the pain response of the patient and the varying amounts of tension can be used to assess the degree and severity of nerve root irritation.[50]

THE MECHANORECEPTOR SYSTEM AND ITS ROLE IN MOTOR CONTROL

From a practical standpoint, it is helpful to divide neural function into two components: the sensory, or afferent, information that reaches the central nervous system from the tissues themselves and the motor, or efferent, information that leaves the central nervous system to innervate the effectors. Connections between these two systems are universally accepted; however, the detailed nature of the synapses and pathways through the spinal cord, brain stem, and cerebral cortex is not fully known. This section focuses primarily on the receptor system and its influence on motor behavior.

The components of the afferent system can be subdivided into the receptors located within the tissues and the peripheral sensory nerves that carry information toward the spinal cord. For the purpose of discussing the receptor system in relation to lumbopelvic function and dysfunction, the receptors can be further subdivided into (a) nociceptive receptors, (b) skin and articular (joint) mechanoreceptors, and (c) receptors in the muscle and muscle–tendon units (muscle spindles and Golgi tendon organs).

Using the lumbopelvic tissues as an example, a centripetal pathway from the tissue receptor to the spinal cord can be detailed. The receptors, when activated by an appropriate stimulus of adequate magnitude, initiate an action potential that progresses through the nerve fibers of the medial or lateral division of the dorsal rami, the dorsal ramus itself, the spinal nerve, the dorsal root, and finally into the dorsal horn of the spinal cord. Three examples of this centripetal flow of information from the tissues to the spinal cord are shown in Figure 2-21. These three pathways describe the common route used by the nociceptors, the articular mechanoreceptors, and the muscle spindles. Even though the sensory modality is different in each case, the afferent pathway to the dorsal horn of the spinal cord is similar. In the spinal cord, the individual sensory modality is sorted into different tracts that influence other spinal cord levels as well as the brain stem, cerebellum, basal nuclei, and cerebral cortex.

Mechanical low back pain can develop as a result of an abnormal movement pattern that loads the tissue

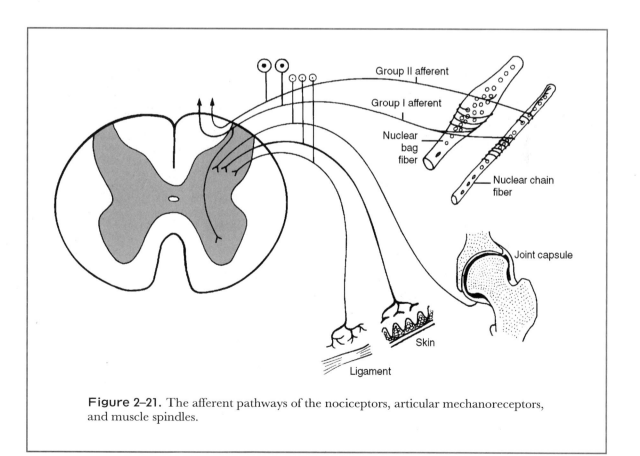

Figure 2–21. The afferent pathways of the nociceptors, articular mechanoreceptors, and muscle spindles.

at levels that exceed tissue tolerance. Following injury, a movement pattern may continually stress the lumbopelvic tissues above their tolerance. Changes in movement patterns become critical when tissue is injured because these changes have the potential to increase or decrease the destructive forces on injured tissue. In this regard, focusing on mechanical low back pain as a movement disorder redirects the emphasis of evaluation and treatment.

Both reflex and conscious control of movement patterns occurs because the articular mechanoreceptors, muscle spindles, and Golgi tendon organs convey sensory information to the central nervous system. These receptors play a unique role in influencing motor output because they provide proprioceptive and kinesthetic information. This information becomes the basis for motor control when it is processed at the various levels of the central nervous system. It is important for the clinician managing mechanical low back pain to be aware of the relation between these receptors and motor output because it is the scientific foundation for the various exercise, training, ergonomic, and back education programs used in the management of this problem.

Mechanoreceptors are biological transducers that take a mechanical stimulus and convert it into electrical energy. This electrical energy initiates central nervous system responses. The multiple types of skin and joint receptors work together in both temporal and spatial summation patterns and inform the central nervous system of joint activity.[67]

The muscle spindles and Golgi tendon organs are also mechanoreceptors that provide important sensory information to the central nervous system. Because of their anatomical location, these receptors can convey information regarding the changing status of muscle activity. They play a major role in the conscious appreciation of proprioception and kinesthesia. For example, joint angle is estimated from information about muscle length provided by the muscle spindle receptors.[53]

It is important to note the distinction between sensory information delivered to the central nervous system that does not reach consciousness and sensory information that reaches conscious awareness, because they are entirely different phenomena. Not all sensory information reaches conscious appreciation levels. Even though the articular receptors described previously deliver their information to the central nervous system, they are not the only contributors to the conscious aspects of proprioception and kinesthesia. Conscious awareness is also in part a result of muscle spindle activity with contribution by the articular receptors.[27, 28, 54] However, because many of our motor programs occur and are influenced by central nervous system activity at the subcortical level, afferent activity from all receptor sources is important because of their influence on the various motor centers of the spinal cord and brain.

The muscle spindles do not contribute directly to overall muscle tension; however, indirectly they play a major role. Because the spindle has contractile properties, it can shorten when stimulated by the gamma motor neuron. This contraction distorts the spindle, which subsequently results in afferent discharge to the central nervous system. The sophistication of the muscle spindle system is such that the two types of spindle fibers (bag and chain) differ in the types of contraction they can exhibit: slow contractions of the spindle are produced by the bag fibers, and fast contractions are produced by the chain fibers.[17] By having a variation of spindle contractions, distortion of the receptor portion of the spindle occurs at different rates and provides a variety of unique afferent information regarding the status of the muscle to the central nervous system.

Because the muscle spindle is arranged in parallel with the muscle fiber, it increases its rate of discharge whenever the muscle is stretched. The different types of spindle receptor allow it to be responsive to changes in the length of muscle as well as to the rate at which the changes in length occur. When the alpha motor neuron causes the extrafusal muscle fibers to contract, the tension on the muscle spindle activity tends to decrease because it is being unloaded. However, because there is coactivation of the alpha and gamma motor neurons, the spindle, which is also contracting owing to gamma motor neuron firing, maintains some degree of tension rather than becoming completely unloaded.

The Golgi tendon organs are connective tissue capsules located at the musculotendinous junction. Approximately 15 to 20 skeletal muscle fibers enter the capsule. The Golgi tendon organ is thus oriented in series with the muscle. Because of this anatomical arrangement, the Golgi tendon organ is activated by stretching the muscle, contracting the muscle, or both. The afferent nerve of the Golgi tendon organ enters the capsule and branches many times. As the muscle contracts or stretches, the collagen framework of the Golgi tendon organ becomes distorted. This distortion causes the axons to fire, and a flow of afferent information toward the central nervous system begins.

The Golgi tendon organ has a high threshold when activated by passive stretch. It was originally believed that the role of the Golgi tendon organ was protective in that it prevented the muscle from producing excessive tension by inhibiting the motor neurons innervating the homonymous and synergistic muscles. It is now recognized that these receptors are extremely sensitive to muscle contraction and provide important feedback to the central nervous system, differentiating the degree of muscle tension during contraction. Because they are located at the musculotendinous junction and are related to 15 to 20 extrafusal muscle fibers, it is conceivable that the force produced by just one motor unit can be recorded by these receptors.[13] Therefore, the Golgi tendon organ responds not only to the degree of stretch placed on the tendon but also to any contraction by the muscle. As the muscle contracts, various gradations of force are used, depending on the desired results. These various gradations are sensed by the Golgi tendon organ, which in turn informs the central nervous system. A feedback loop evolves in which motor control is adjusted at the spinal cord, brain stem, and cerebral cortex levels.

The Golgi tendon organ, like the muscle spindle, also delivers afferent information to the cerebellum and assists in the regulation of motor output. The cerebellum is known to exert influence over the spinal cord, various nuclei of the brain stem that give rise to motor tracts, and the cerebral cortex, from which the corticospinal tracts originate.

The receptor system has been briefly described to provide the basis for a more comprehensive understanding of its influence on motor behavior. Consideration must be given to how the receptor system and muscles work as a unit. It is interesting to note, for example, that the pools of alpha motor neurons that innervate the skeletal muscle are in the same immediate location in the spinal cord as the gamma motor neurons that innervate the muscle spindle. Both pools are thus under the direct influence of central motor tracts and the multiplicity of sensory stimuli that arise from the tissues. Smooth movement requires an integration of and balance between the afferent and the efferent aspects of motor behavior.

Afferent information is especially important in the timing and shaping of motor patterns. In the treatment of low back disorders there is a need to include proprioceptive and kinesthetic awareness training of spinal positions and movements, especially those postures that have the potential to stimulate the nociceptive receptors in injured tissues.

To allow the patient to successfully manage his low back problem, it is necessary that he recognize the vulnerable positions of his lumbopelvic region that allow destructive forces to occur. The first step in restoring function in the rehabilitation process is teaching the patient what a vulnerable position for his particular spinal problem might be. These vulnerable and invulnerable positions are determined by the clinician during the evaluation process (see Chapter 5). The patient needs to develop proprioceptive awareness as to which positions are vulnerable and which invulnerable for his particular injury. Subsequent strengthening exercises are futile without development of this proprioceptive sense because the patient will continually invite reinjury. Training in this manner recognizes the importance of the afferent input reaching the central nervous system.

As a muscle is trained, changes in its resting tension can be seen. Although these changes are partly due to a remodeling of the muscle, a certain degree of central nervous system activation also occurs. Carew and Ghez[17] compared the tension of the muscle with that of a spring. With a thicker spring, the stiffness increases (see Chapter 3). The stiffness of the muscle can also be increased by increasing the neural outflow to it. Recall that this neural outflow affects the gamma as well as the alpha motor systems. The gamma system plays a large part in biasing the spindle toward an increased sensitivity to movement. This increased potential for awareness of movement by the sensory receptors is in part a training mechanism in itself.

The central nervous system also makes important changes with proper exercise programs. This training is the result of an enhanced balance between the afferent sensory and efferent motor systems. Sensitivity toward movement is an important component of proprioceptive and kinesthetic strength training. Diminished proprioceptive feedback is characteristic of sedentary living and results in a reduction of the sensitivity of the spindle secondary afferents in antigravity muscles.[29] Recognition of this is probably the unifying element behind the myriad back education programs now available. These programs teach the patient awareness of spine postures (proprioceptive awareness) and ultimately require a significant degree of muscle activity (muscle training).

Because all patients do not have similarly injured tissues, and the nociceptive response varies owing to the different degree of mechanical or chemical irritation of the nociceptors, standardized treatment programs have little to offer the patient in the way of self-management. Consideration must be given to the importance of the afferent neurology of the region rather than simply teaching every patient to maintain one particular spine position or exercise one muscle group. Management in this manner ignores basic neurophysiology; that is, the person moves in a motor pattern appropriate for his strength, coordination, and connective tissue makeup. In any case, the low back pain patient has a movement pattern that perpetuates the nociceptive response. Recognition of this balance between afferent and efferent neurobiology is essential to understanding the function of the lumbopelvic region.

SUMMARY

The purpose of this chapter was to familiarize the clinician with selected aspects of neuroanatomy and neurophysiology of the lumbopelvic region. In particular, functional considerations were presented in a manner intended to stimulate the clinician to fully consider the importance of afferent neurobiology in the evaluation and treatment of lumbopelvic disorders. The new paradigm to add to our past knowledge of anatomy and mechanics is a biochemical one.

Neuromechanical and biochemical elements of lumbopelvic problems especially underscore the scientific foundations of pain and function. The treatment approach to dealing with low back pain is rapidly changing to a focus on function to alter the disability. As in rehabilitation of the extremities, optimal function is not simply "efferent" in nature—that is, absolute strength or aerobic capacity—but includes such factors as coordination, balance, motor learning, and self-management strategies. This suggests the important influence of the nervous system for optimal function. An early and safe return to activity after injury is just as important in maintaining central nervous system health as it is in maintaining musculoskeletal health. We suggest that restoration of function include an integration of the neuromusculoskeletal systems.

REFERENCES

1. Ahmed M, Bjurholm A, Kreicbergs M: Neuropeptide Y, tyrosine hydroxylase and vasoactive intestinal polypeptide-immunoreactive nerve fibers in the vertebral bodies, disc, dura mater, and spinal ligaments in the rat lumbar spine. Spine 18:268,1993.
2. Alderink GJ: The sacroiliac joint: A review of anatomy, mechanics and function. J Orthop Sports Phys Ther 13:71,1991.
3. Ashton IK, Roberts S, Jaffray DC, Polak JM, Eisenstein SM: Neuropeptides in the human intervertebral disc. J Orthop Res 12:186, 1994.
4. Barr M: The Human Nervous System. Philadelphia: JB Lippincott, 1988.
5. Beaman DN, Graziano GP, Glover RA, Wojts EM, Chang V: Substance P innervation of lumbar spine facet joints. Spine 18:1044, 1993.
6. Bogduk N: The innervation of the lumbar spine. Spine 8:286, 1983.
7. Bogduk N: Clinical Anatomy of the Lumbar Spine. New York: Churchill Livingstone, 1987.
8. Bogduk N, Tynan W, Wilson AS: The innervation of the human lumbar intevertebral discs. J Anat 132:39, 1981.
9. Bogduk N, Wilson AS, Tynan W: The human lumbar dorsal rami. J Anat 134:383, 1982.
10. Bose K, Balasubramaniam P: Nerve root canals of the lumbar spine. Spine 9:16, 1984.
11. Bough B, Thakore J, Davies M, Dowling F: Degeneration of the lumbar facet joints. Arthrography and pathology. J Bone Joint Surg [Br] 72:275, 1990.
12. Breig A, Troup JDG: Biomechanical considerations in the straight leg raising test. Spine 4:243, 1974.
13. Brodal A: Neurological Anatomy Related to Clinical Medicine. New York: Oxford University Press, 1981.
14. Brower AC: Disorders of the sacroiliac joint. Surg Rounds Orthop 13:47, 1989.
15. Burchiel KJ: Effects of electrical and mechanical stimuli on two foci of spontaneous activity which develop in primary afferent neurons after peripheral axotomy. Pain 18:249, 1984.
16. Cameron BM, VanderPutten DM, Merril CR: Preliminary study of an increase of a plasma apolipoprotein E varioan associated with peripheral nerve damage. Spine 20:581, 1995.
17. Carew TJ, Ghez C: Muscles and muscle receptors. In Kandel ER, Schwartz JH (eds): Principles of Neural Science. New York: Elsevier, 1985, p. 443.
18. Cornefjord M, Takahashi K, Matsui H, et al: Impairment of nutritional transport at double level cauda equina compression. Neuro-Orthopaedics 13:107, 1992.
19. Cyriax J: Textbook of Orthopaedic Medicine, vol.1. London: Baillière Tindall, 1978.
20. Edgar MA, Nundy S: Innervation of the spinal dural mater. J Neurol Neurosurg Psychiatry 29:530, 1966.
21. Eisenstein SM, Parry CR: The lumbar facet arthrosis syndrome—Clinical presentation and articular cartilage changes. J Bone Joint Surg [Br] 69:3, 1987.
22. Farfan HF: Mechanical Disorders of the Low Back. Philadelphia: Lea & Febiger, 1973.
23. Feinstein B, Langton JNK, Jameson RM, Schiller F: Experiments on pain referred from deep structures. J Bone Joint Surg [Am] 36A:981, 1954.

24. Fortin JD, Dwyer AP, West S, Pier J: Sacroiliac joint: Pain referral maps upon applying a new injection/arthrography technique. Part II: Clinical evaluation. Spine 19:1483, 1994.

25. Garfin SR, Rydevik BL, Brown RA, Sartoris DJ: Compression neuropathy of spinal nerve roots—A mechanical or biological problem? Spine 16:162, 1991.

26. Garfin SR, Rydevik B, Lind B, Massie J: Spinal nerve root compression. Spine 20:1810, 1995.

27. Goodwin GM, McCloskey DL, Matthews PB: The contribution of muscle afferents to kinesthesia shown by vibration induced illusions of movement and by the effects of paralysing joint afferents. Brain 95:705, 1972.

28. Goodwin GM, McCloskey DL, Matthews PB: The persistence of appreciable kinesthesia after paralysing joint afferents by preserving muscle afferents. Brain Res 37:326, 1972.

29. Gowitzke BA, Milner M: Scientific Basis of Human Movement. Baltimore: Williams & Wilkins, 1988.

30. Grieve G: Referred pain. In Grieve G (ed): Modern Manual Therapy of the Vertebral Column. Edinburgh: Churchill Livingstone, 1986, p. 233.

31. Groen GJ, Baljet B, Drukker J: The innervation of the spinal dura mater: Anatomy and clinical implications. Acta Neurochir 92:39, 1988.

32. Hadler NM: A critical appraisal of the fibromyositis concept. Am J Med 81 (Suppl 3A):26, 1986.

33. Hasue M, Kikuchi S, Sakuyama Y, Ito T: Anatomic study of the interrelation between lumbosacral nerve roots and their surrounding tissues. Spine 8:50, 1983.

34. Hirsch C, Inglemark B, Miller M: The anatomical basis for low back pain. Acta Orthop Scand 33:1, 1963.

35. Hitselberger WE, Witten RM: Abnormal myelograms in asymptomatic patients. J Neurosurg 28:204, 1968.

36. Hollinshead WH, Rosse C: Textbook of Human Anatomy. Philadelphia: Harper & Row, 1985.

37. Howe JF, Loeser JD, Calvin WH: Mechanosensitivity of dorsal root ganglia and chronically injured axons: A physiological basis for the radicular pain of nerve root compression. Pain 3:25,1977.

38. Humzah MD, Soames RW: The inevertebral disc: Structure and function. Anat Rec 220: 337, 1988.

39. Kellgren JH: Observations on referred pain arising from muscle. Clin Sci 3:175, 1938.

40. Kelly JP: Reactions of neurons to injury. In Kandel E, Schwartz J (eds): Principles of Neural Science. New York: Elsevier, 1985, p. 187.

41. Kumar R, Berger RJ, Dunsker SB, Keller JT: Innervation of the spinal dura. Spine 21:18, 1996.

42. Kuslich SD, Ulstrom CL, Michael CJ: The tissue origin of low back pain and sciatica: A report of pain response to tissue stimulation during operations on the lumbar spine using local anesthesia. Orthop Clin North Am 22:181, 1991.

43. Lee Y, Takami K, Kawai Y, et al: Distribution of calcitonin gene-related peptide in the rat peripheral nervous system with reference to its co-existence with substance P. Neuroscience 15:1227, 1985.

44. Lewinnek GE, Warfield CA: Facet joint degeneration as a cause of low back pain. Clin Orthop 213:216, 1986.

45. Lieberman AR: Sensory ganglia. In Landon DN (ed): The Peripheral Nerve. London: Chapman & Hall, 1976, p. 182.

46. Lippit AB: The facet joint and its role in spine pain. Spine 9:746, 1984.

47. Loeser JD: Pain due to nerve injury. Spine 10:232, 1985.

48. Louis R: Vertebroradicular and vertebromedullar dynamics. Anat Clin 3:1, 1981.

49. MacNab I: The mechanism of spondylogenic pain. In Hirsch C, Zotterman Y (eds): Cervical Pain. Oxford: Pergamon, 1972, p. 89.

50. Maitland G: Vertebral Manipulation, 5th ed. London: Butterworth, 1986.

51. Marks RC, Houston T, Thulbourne T: Facet joint injection and facet nerve block: A randomized comparison in 86 patients with chronic low back pain. Pain 49:325, 1992.

52. Marshall LL, Trethewie ER: Chemical irritation of the nerve root in disc prolapse. Lancet 11:320, 1973.

53. Martin JH: Receptor physiology and submodality coding in the somatic sensory system. In Kandel ER, Schwartz JH (eds): Principles of Neural Science. New York: Elsevier, 1985, p. 301.

54. Matthews PB: Where does Sherrington's "muscular sense" originate? Muscles, joints, corollary discharges? Annu Rev Neurosci 5:189,1982.

55. McCall IW, Park WM, O'Brien JP: Induced pain referral from posterior lumbar elements in normal subjects. Spine 4:441, 1979.

56. McCarron RF, Wimpee MW, Hudkins PG, Laros GS: The inflammatory effect of the nucleus pulposus: A possible element in the pathogenesis of low back pain. Spine 12:760, 1987.

57. Mixter WJ, Barr JS: Rupture of the intevertebral disc with involvement of the spinal canal. N Engl J Med 211:210, 1934.

58. Mooney V, Robertson J: The facet syndrome. Clin Orthop 115:149, 1976.

59. Nachemson A: Intradiscal measurements of pH in patients with lumbar rhizopathies. Acta Orthop Scand 40:23, 1969.

60. Nakamura S, Takashi K, Takahashi Y, Morinaga T, et al: Origin of nerves supplying the posterior portion of the lumbar intevertebral discs in rats. Spine 21:917, 1996.

61. Newham DJ: The consequences of eccentric contractions and their relation to delayed onset muscle pain. Eur J Appl Physiol 57:353, 1988.

62. Parke WW: Applied anatomy of the spine. In Rothman RH, Simeone FA (eds): The Spine, 3rd ed. Philadelphia: WB Saunders, 1992, p. 35.

63. Parke WW, Watanabe R: The intrinsic vasculature of the lumbosacral nerve roots. Spine 10:508, 1985.

64. Payan DG, McGillis JP, Renold FK, et al: Neuropeptide modulation of leukocyte function. Ann NY Acad Sci 496:182, 1987.

65. Pennington JB, McCarron RF, Laros GS: Identification of IgG in the canine intervertebral disc. Spine 13:909, 1988.

66. Rhalmi S, Yahia L'H, Newman N, Isler M: Immunohistochemical study of nerves in lumbar spinae ligaments. Spine 18:264, 1993.

67. Rowinski M: Afferent neurobiology of the joint, In Gould JA (ed): Orthopaedic and Sports Physical Therapy, 2nd ed. St. Louis: CV Mosby, 1990, p. 49.

68. Rydevik B, Brown M, Lundborg G: Pathoanatomy and pathophysiology of nerve compression. Spine 9:7, 1984.

69. Rydevik B, Holm S, Brown MD, Lundborg H: Nutrition of the spinal nerve roots: The role of diffusion from the cerebral spinal fluid. Trans Orthop Res Soc 9:276, 1984.

70. Saal JS, Franson RC, Dobrou R, Saal JA, White AH, Goldthwaite N: High levels of inflammatory phospholipase A2 activity in lumbar disc herniations. Spine 15:674, 1990.

71. Schonstrom N, Hansson T: Pressure changes following constriction of the cauda equina. An experimental study in situ. Spine 13:385, 1988.

72. Schwartz JH: The cytology of neurons. In Kandel ER, Schwartz JH (eds): Principles of Neural Science, 2nd ed. New York: Elsevier, 1985, p. 27.

73. Schwartzer AC, Aprill AN, Derby R, et al: Clinical features of patients with pain stemming from the lumbar zygapophyseal joints. Spine 19:1132, 1994.

74. Sejerstedt OM, Westgaard RH: Occupational muscle pain and injury. Eur J Appl Physiol 57:271, 1988.

75. Smyth J, Wright V: Sciatica and the intevertebral disc, an experimental study. J Bone Joint Surg [Am] 40A:1401, 1959.

76. Spencer DL, Irwin GS, Miller JA: Anatomy and significance of fixation of the lumbosacral nerve roots in sciatica. Spine 8:672, 1983.

77. Sunderland S: Avulsion of nerve roots. In Vinken PJ, Bruyn GW (eds): Handbook of Clinical Neurology, vol. 25. Injuries of the Spine and Spinal Cord, New York: Elsevier, 1975, p. 393.

78. Sunderland S: Nerves and Nerve Injuries, 2nd ed. Edinburgh: Churchill Livingstone, 1978, ch. 4.

79. Sunderland S: Traumatized nerves, roots and ganglia: Musculoskeletal factors and neuropathological consequences. In Korr IM (ed): Neurobiologic Mechanisms of Manipulative Therapy. New York: Plenum Press, 1978, p. 137.

80. Weber H: Lumbar disc herniation. A controlled prospective study with ten years of observation. Spine 2:131, 1983.

81. Weinstein J: Anatomy and neurophysiologic mechanisms of spinal pain. In Frymoyer J (ed): The Adult Spine, Raven Press: New York, 1991, p. 602.

82. Weinstein J, Claverie W, Gibson S: The pain of discography. Spine 13:1344, 1988.

83. Weisel SW, Tsourmas N, Feffer HL, Citrin CM, Patronas N: A study of computer assisted tomography: 1. The incidence of positive CAT scans in an asymptomatic group of patients. Spine 9:549, 1984.

84. Wyke B: The neurology of low back pain. In Jayson MIV (ed): The Lumbar Spine and Back Pain. London: Pitman, 1980, p. 265.

85. Wyke B: The neurology of low back pain. In Jayson MIV (ed): The Lumbar Spine and Back Pain, 2nd ed. Kent, UK: Pitman Medical Publishing, 1980.

86. Yahia LH, Garzon S, Strykowski H, Rivard CH: Ultrastructure of the human interspinous ligament and ligamentum flavum: A preliminary study. Spine 15:262, 1990.

87. Yang KH, King AI: Mechanism of facet load transmission as a hypothesis for low back pain. Spine 9:557, 1984.

88. Yoshizawa H, O'Brien JP, Smith WT, Trumper M: The neuropathology of intervertebral discs removed for low back pain. J Pathol 132:95, 1980.

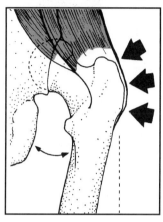

CHAPTER 3

LUMBOPELVIC MUSCULATURE: STRUCTURAL AND FUNCTIONAL CONSIDERATIONS

MUSCLE STRUCTURE

Skeletal muscle is one of the most complex of all musculoskeletal tissues. It consists of muscle cells, muscle-specific extracellular matrix, and an elaborate network of nerves and vessels. Normal muscle function depends not only on the integrity of the muscle cells but also on the nerve and vessel networks and mechanical loading capabilities.[60] To better understand the function of muscle, structure will be briefly reviewed. Once structure is described, generalizations regarding the diverse roles of muscle will be considered. From this general framework of reference, inferences regarding the specific functions of the lumbopelvic musculature can then be developed.

Muscle is constructed of various proteins of which actin and myosin represent approximately 84 percent of the total.[33] The proteins form a unit that has the ability to shorten, lengthen, and vary its state of stiffness (stiffness = resistance to deformation) on demand of the central nervous system.

Actin is a double helix protein with the troponin and tropomyosin proteins located within it. Actin surrounds the larger myosin protein in a hexagonal manner (Fig. 3–1). Myosin contains cross-bridges that are the linkage points between the actin and myosin proteins, and the interaction between these two proteins permits the actin to slide over the myosin.[33] This mechanism is described below.

When viewed under low magnification, the skeletal muscle appears as alternating dark and light bands owing to the configuration and overlap of the various proteins of the muscle. Attached to the sarcolemma of the cell is the Z line, which helps to physically stabilize the muscle cell. The functional unit of the muscle cell, the sarcomere, is the repeating unit between two Z lines (Fig. 3–2). Sarcomeres are placed end-to-end to form muscle filaments. The filaments are grouped together to form myofibrils, which in turn are further organized into groups to form muscle fibers and then organized into a specific muscle (Fig. 3–3). The magnitude of this structural complex is noted by Vander and associates who state that a "single muscle fiber 100 μm in diameter and 1 centimeter long contains about 8000 myofibrils, each myofibril consisting of 4500 sarcomeres. This results in a total of 16 billion thick and 64 billion thin filaments in a single fiber."[54]

The connective tissue covering of a muscle fiber is the endomysium. Groups of muscle fibers are further organized into bundles, or fasciculi, that are also encased in a connective tissue covering called the perimysium. Finally, the connective tissue that covers the complete muscle is known as the epimysium (Fig. 3–4). The connective tissues of the muscle become fused

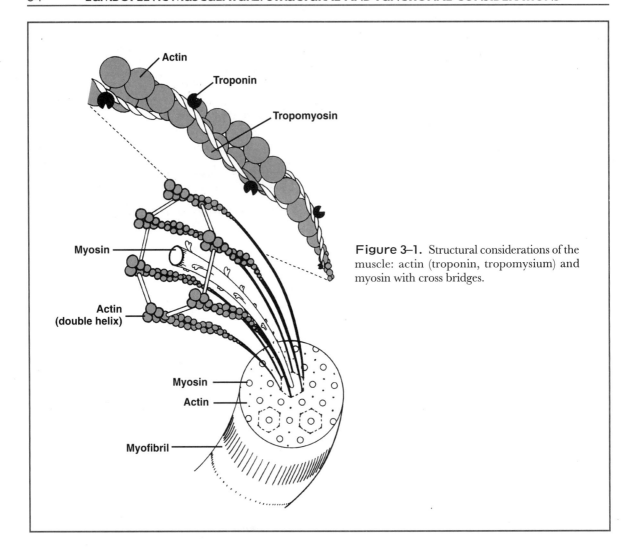

Figure 3–1. Structural considerations of the muscle: actin (troponin, tropomysium) and myosin with cross bridges.

together at the terminal ends of the muscle and form a parallel arrangement of specialized connective tissue termed the tendon. Intimately related to the structural arrangement of muscle and tendon are specialized receptors known as the muscle spindle and the Golgi tendon organ. These receptors communicate the status of the muscle and tendon to the central nervous system by way of afferent nerve fibers (see Chapter 2).

MUSCLE CONTRACTION

Muscle contraction is a complex activity that involves interplay between the nervous, muscular, and skeletal systems. Because muscle contraction depends on signals from the central nervous system, its physiology is detailed below, starting at the anterior horn cell.

The cell body of a motor neuron located in the anterior horn of the spinal cord gives rise to an axon, which exits the central nervous system and travels peripherally to innervate skeletal muscle fibers. This axon, or nerve fiber, has numerous terminal branches which then innervate different muscle fibers. Through this branching network, a single nerve innervates many individual muscle fibers. The motor nerve and the muscle fibers that it innervates are referred to as a motor unit. For some muscles the ratio of muscle fibers to nerve is large, whereas in others it is quite

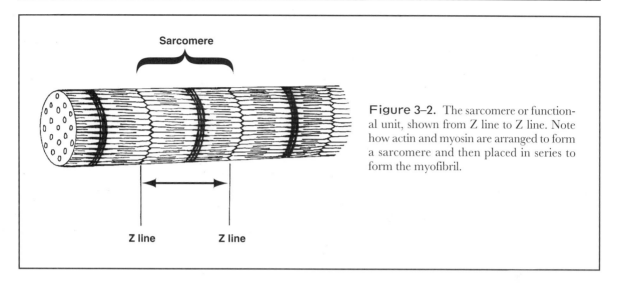

Figure 3–2. The sarcomere or functional unit, shown from Z line to Z line. Note how actin and myosin are arranged to form a sarcomere and then placed in series to form the myofibril.

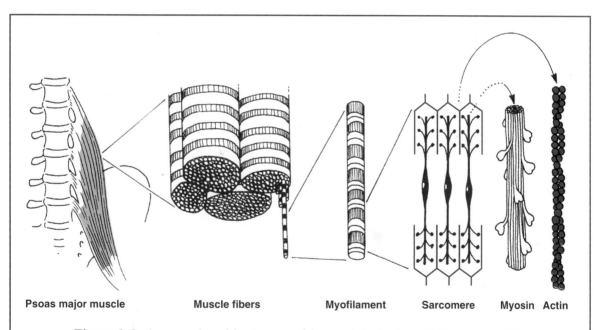

Psoas major muscle   Muscle fibers   Myofilament   Sarcomere   Myosin Actin

Figure 3–3. A progression of the structure of the muscle beginning with the actin (small filament) and myosin (large filament) molecule, grouped to form the muscle myofibril (grouped filaments), further grouped into four muscle fibers (grouped myofibrils) and then within the structure of the psoas major muscle.

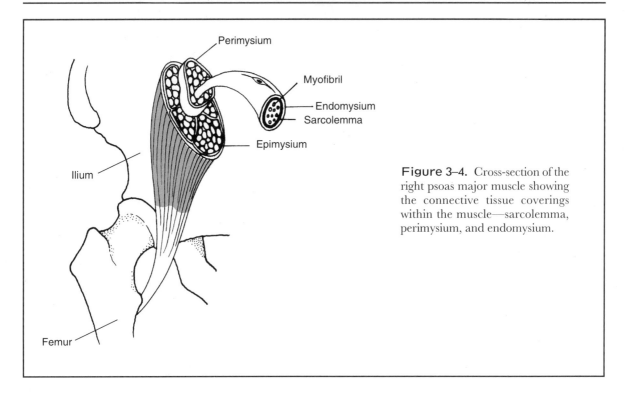

Figure 3–4. Cross-section of the right psoas major muscle showing the connective tissue coverings within the muscle—sarcolemma, perimysium, and endomysium.

small. For example, the precise control of the eye muscles requires that one neuron control only 10–15 muscle fibers; in larger muscles, such as the gluteus maximus, one neuron may control 2000–3000 muscle fibers. The difference in the various ratios allows for varying degrees of precision to be available to the muscle.

The action potential travels distally along the axon of the efferent motor neuron until it reaches the presynaptic membrane at the neuromuscular junction. The neuromuscular junction is the interface between the nerve and muscle that forms the motor end-plate. Here the electrical impulse is converted to a chemical stimulus by neurotransmitters that are stored in the presynaptic membrane. Acetylcholine is the principal neurotransmitter released into the cleft of the neuromuscular junction. When acetylcholine combines with receptors in the postsynaptic membrane of the muscle fiber, the permeability of the fiber to sodium and potassium is altered. The resultant changes in the intracellular and extracellular ion concentrations cause the muscle cell membrane to be depolarized.

The frequency of this synaptic transmission can be modulated by other neurotransmitters, such as epinephrine and enkephalin.[26] The modulation also depends on other factors, such as the temporal and spatial summation of the impulses traversing the efferent motor nerve. Once depolarization occurs at the postsynaptic membrane, it is rapidly conducted across the surface of the muscle cell and into the muscle fiber by way of the transverse tubule system (T tubules). The action potential travels past sleevelike structures known as the sarcoplasmic reticulum that surround the myofibril (Fig. 3–5). Calcium is stored in the lateral sacs of the sarcoplasmic reticulum.

Excitation of the sarcoplasmic reticulum membrane triggers the release of the calcium into the contractile proteins of the muscle. The initial effect of this activity influences two of the regulatory proteins bound to actin: troponin and tropomyosin. Calcium interacts with the troponin protein that resides on the actin molecule. As the troponin is activated by the release of calcium, it changes shape and essentially pulls tropomyosin, which is situated end-to-end along the

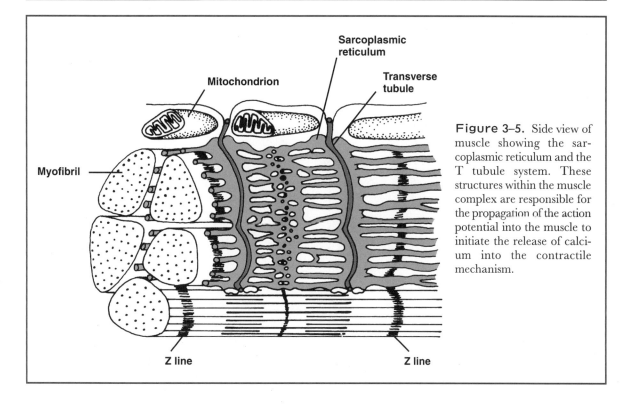

Figure 3–5. Side view of muscle showing the sarcoplasmic reticulum and the T tubule system. These structures within the muscle complex are responsible for the propagation of the action potential into the muscle to initiate the release of calcium into the contractile mechanism.

actin molecule, partially covering a binding site, away from the myosin binding site so that attachments between actin and myosin can develop.

At the attachment of myosin to actin a breakdown of adenosine triphosphate (ATP) to adenosine diphosphate (ADP) and inorganic phosphate takes place, releasing the energy stored in ATP. This energy release results in a force that causes a movement or swiveling of the myosin cross bridge, which effectively creates a sliding of the actin over the myosin.[25] The amount of calcium released determines the number of active sites that are available for the cross-bridges to develop.

As the actin slides over the myosin, the myofibril shortens. The force developed by the sliding mechanism is transmitted across the Z line to the connective tissue matrix of the muscle into the tendon and then into the bone. This connective matrix has an individually variant elasticity, a property that ultimately affects the efficiency of the contractile mechanism and the muscle's ability to meet tension requirements. This physical property of muscle is known as series elasticity (Fig. 3–6).

NEUROMUSCULOSKELETAL INTEGRATION

As mentioned earlier and in Chapter 2, the muscular system is under the direct control of the central nervous system. This has several functional implications. The muscular system is influenced by the afferent input received by the central nervous system from the various receptors. This receptor input comes from a variety of sources, including the muscle spindles, Golgi tendon organs, and skin, joint capsule, and ligament mechanoreceptors. This afferent receptor information helps regulate efferent motor output. Of clinical importance is the afferent input from nociceptors activated in injured tissues. Afferent input to the central nervous system as a result of tissue injury often results in increased reflex activity of musculature in order to protect the joint from further damage or nociceptive activity. Reflex muscle guarding and increased motor activity of the spinal musculature is often seen in patients with spine pain. Potential reasons for this increased activity are discussed below when individual

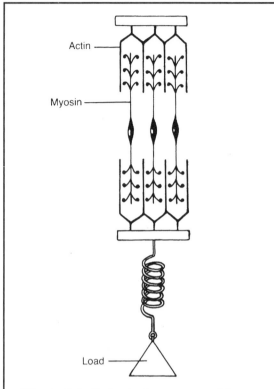

Figure 3–6. Series elastic component of the muscle. The muscle contraction (actin sliding on myosin) increases connective tissue tension of the muscle (spring) to impart a force to the tendon, fascia, ligament, and periosteum as it reaches the bone, resulting in movement. The elastic qualities of the connective tissue matrix play a role in the efficiency of the muscle contraction, i.e., the more elastic the connective tissue with the muscle and tendon, the more the muscle must contract in order to impart the force to the bone.

manner that depends on both afferent feedback to the central nervous system and efferent output to the muscles. All types of muscle contraction not only affect the movement of the bone, but also generate forces to the intramuscular fascia (perimysium and endomysium), the extramuscular fascia (muscular septa, thoracolumbar fascia, abdominal fascia, and fascia lata), the tendon, and the periosteum. Muscle activity also directs forces through tissues that are designed to absorb and transfer them such as the articular cartilage, bone, and the intervertebral disc. Finally, muscles themselves can act as shock absorbers and in fact may be one of the most important shock absorbing tissues in the human body. Eccentric muscle activity, such as muscle action occurring during running and walking gait, is largely shock absorption and force attenuation. Without neuromuscular control of these functions it would not be possible to perform coordinated movements—especially those associated with increased external loads—without tissue injury.

A healthy, optimal functioning muscular system helps assure that a nondestructive load-bearing pattern travels through the specialized connective tissues by continually adjusting to the variety of forces to which the connective tissues are subjected. As muscles fatigue, control or coordination of the load-bearing process is altered.[4, 38] The uncontrolled loading of spinal tissues, either by single impact or prolonged overloading, increases the potential for injury and degeneration. Muscle action, regulated by afferent and efferent neuromodulation results in dynamic stabilization which plays a role in the way in which the musculoskeletal system adapts to the asymmetrical loads of movement.[43]

The muscles of the trunk function as prime movers and stabilizers of the spine. Stabilizing or controlling the load-bearing pattern is impossible without a continuous barrage of afferent information from the environment. Successful stabilization is fixing one part of the skeleton while permitting movement of surrounding parts. This is largely a subconscious and involuntary process. The afferent neural input is channeled into the central nervous system and processed to influence motor output. It is only then that contraction in correct muscle sequence becomes possible.

The central nervous system in effect "sets" the muscle for the appropriate action as a result of the afferent input. This muscle activity is typically controlled by the spinal cord, brain stem, cerebellum, and cerebral cortex. Training and reconditioning programs not only

muscles related to the lumbopelvic region are detailed. The important point to consider at this time is muscle guarding when found during evaluation of the patient. It may be beneficial, and the use of modalities to decrease muscle activity may leave the injured tissues less protected from further injury.

Most descriptions of muscle activity concentrate on the analysis of movement during a concentric contraction that brings the insertion of the muscle toward the origin. In addition to this function, muscle also contracts eccentrically and isometrically in a controlled

initiate anatomic and biochemical changes in muscle but also affect change at the central nervous system level.

MECHANICS OF MUSCLE

To assist in understanding the role of the musculature in the lumbopelvic unit, the mechanical nature of muscle will be briefly considered. Muscle tension has been compared with the physical properties of springs (Fig. 3–7).[9] This is a useful analogy because it provides us with an understanding of how the various muscles, with their size, fiber direction, and contractile capabilities, might contribute to lumbopelvic stability.

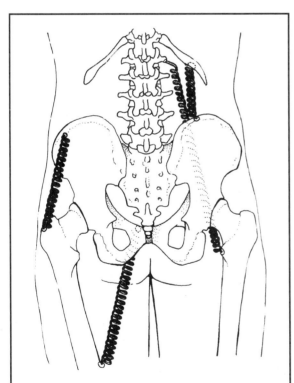

Figure 3–7. Posterior view of the lumbopelvic region showing the right quadratus lumborum muscle, right iliopsoas muscle, left gluteus medius muscle, and left femoral adductor muscles as springs replicating a mechanical model of lumbopelvic stability.

Springs are mechanical devices with stored energy. From an engineering perspective, they have a certain stiffness. Stiffness can be defined as a resistance to deformation; that is, the greater the degree of stiffness of the spring, the more difficult it is to change the spring's shape. Increasing the stiffness of a structure makes it more difficult for an outside force to deform the structure. The energy from this outside force would instead be stored as potential energy. Viewing muscles as springs allows us to better understand the role of muscles as shock absorbers.

A spring also has the ability to restore itself to its original length after it has been stretched. As the spring is stretched, the tension within the spring increases. Stiffness of the spring is a function of the difference in the length over the difference in the tension. In other words, as the spring is stretched, a resistance or stiffness develops by virtue of the increase in length.

Muscles behave in the same manner as they are passively or actively stretched, or as the efferent activity to the muscle is increased. The muscle has a resting tension, sometimes referred to as muscle tone, that is under direct influence of the central nervous system. This resting tension is equivalent to stiffness. The efferent output of the central nervous system increases or decreases the muscle's resting tension, depending on the summation of excitatory and inhibitory activity within the central nervous system. For example, when a person bends forward and toward their left side, the musculature on the right side of the lumbopelvic region is elongated, and an eccentric muscle contraction helps control the movement. At the same time, the muscle must maintain a functional length to allow it to effectively contract concentrically and assist in returning the spine to an upright position (Fig. 3–8). Excess stiffness can also lead to pathologic states of motor behavior, such as rigidity and spasticity; however, detailed discussion of these central nervous system disorders are beyond the scope of this text.

Excitatory and inhibitory balance is directly influenced by the receptor system. For example, a key function of the gamma motor system is to shorten the muscle spindle, thereby increasing the sensitivity to length changes that occur in the muscle. As another example, injury to any structure within the lumbopelvic region increases the nociceptive afferent input into the central nervous system, which may result in a new (enhanced) set point of muscle tension that can cause a resistance to movement.

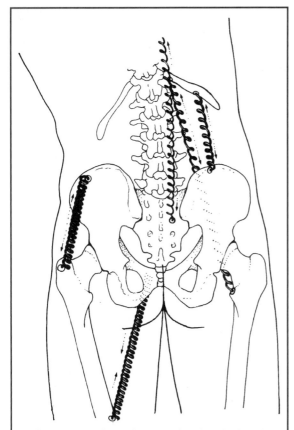

Figure 3–8. Posterior view showing the lengthening of the right posterior lumbopelvic muscles (illustrated as springs) as the trunk is forward bent and side bent to the left. Note the different states of muscle contraction (isometric, concentric, and eccentric) required for the trunk to move into this direction and hold that position.

greater muscle tension is required to move the load and a greater number of fibers must contract.[54]

Tension produced by the muscle contractions depends on four variables.[54] The first is the action potential frequency or the frequency–tension relation. This variable relates to time delay between the contraction stimulus and the muscle contraction. As the frequency of the action potential increases, the level of muscle tension increases to the point of maximal achievable tension.

The second variable that determines muscle tension is the length–tension relation of the muscle. Every muscle has an optimal length at which it can produce the maximal amount of tension. The further the muscle length is from this optimal point, the less tension it is able to produce with contraction.

The third variable is the duration of the activity and degree of fatigue. The longer the time required for the muscle to contract, the less its ability to maintain or produce muscle tension. The exact causes of fatigue are unknown, but there is good evidence that the excitation coupling reaction at the cross-bridge may be the site of certain types of fatigue.[4]

The last variable that determines muscle tension is related to the type of muscle fiber. Different fiber types produce different amounts of muscle tension. For example, type II fibers produce greater tension but have decreased endurance capabilities. Conversely, type I aerobic fibers produce lower amounts of tension but have greater endurance capabilities.

MUSCLE TENSION AND FORCE ATTENUATION

The neuromechanical properties of the muscles that surround the spine control the manner in which forces are transferred and absorbed by the axial skeleton. The ability of the muscle to dynamically produce tension to stabilize a specific body segment such as the lumbar spine and pelvis, so that another body part such as the lower extremity can move, has significant clinical relevance, especially when developing a treatment plan for the injured patient (see Chapter 6).

The resting state of muscle stiffness (resting tension) and the ability of the central nervous system to continually alter the set-point of muscle tension in response to changing loads (active tension) are the key aspects of dynamic stabilization. The muscle's attachments and the effect that resting tension and active tension have

The central nervous system can alter muscle tension or the force output by varying the number of fibers contracting and the tension produced by that muscle fiber. The number of contracting fibers is proportional to the number of motor units activated and the number of fibers within each motor unit. Recruitment of the motor neurons depends on the load that must be overcome. The size principle states that the smaller motor units are initially called on to contract and are followed by the contraction of the larger motor units that increase total muscle tension. As the load increases,

on intervening tissues because of these attachments are important to consider. The interaction of lumbopelvic muscles with the three fascial systems—thoracolumbar fascia, fascia lata, and abdominal fascia—are especially important when considering the roles that muscle plays in spine conditions. The lumbopelvic muscles not only attach directly to these important fascial structures and exert tension via their pull but are also encased within the fascial envelopes. Thus, tension-generating ability from muscles pulling on the fascia, and hypertrophy of the muscles within the fascial envelope, are important aspects to consider when developing an exercise program for musculature of the lumbopelvic region. Because of the muscle's ability to generate tissue tension in a very controlled manner, it can act as a true shock absorber in the attenuation of ground and trunk forces. The functional implication is that the muscle with an enhanced set-point is more reactive to a given stimulus, and the increased stiffness allows it to be more effective as a shock absorber. We suggest that one of the results of resistance exercises is to allow for this set-point to be more reactive to continually changing loads affecting the skeletal tissues.

Injury can occur when the contractile and noncontractile tissues are unable to control the forces of gravity and movement that results in exceeding the viscoelastic capacity of the specialized connective tissues. Forces applied to the specialized connective tissues with increased magnitude and speed, or a lesser force imparted over an excessive period of time, can render the connective tissue matrix vulnerable to disruption, which minimizes the ability of the connective tissues to stabilize the bony segments. Once deformation or structural alteration of the connective tissue takes place, excessive or abnormal movements can occur between spinal segments if the muscles are unable to stabilize the area. Altered mechanics can cause further deformation of the tissues, and if tissue damage results, the nociceptor system is activated. It is at this point that the stabilization of the bony elements increasingly relies on the actions of the muscles related to the spinal segments.

It is important for the clinician dealing with low back pain to understand the relations between contractile and noncontractile tissues in the lumbopelvic region as they work together to assure nondestructive loading. The lumbopelvic anatomy should be readily visualized in order to assess the tensile, compressive, torsional, and shear forces directed into and through the tissues during movement.

Without a three-dimensional appreciation of the functional anatomy of this region, effective evaluation and treatment of the low back are difficult. Once the clinician gains an understanding of the functional anatomy of the trunk, logical and effective treatment programs can be implemented, especially those utilizing exercise as the focus of treatment.

MUSCLE AND FASCIAL NETWORKS OF THE LUMBOPELVIC REGION

One of the best examples of the intricacies of neuromuscular regulation mechanisms is the lumbopelvic complex, which requires an integration of the musculature of the lumbar spine, abdomen, pelvis, and hips. In addition, muscles such as the latissimus dorsi and scapular retractors acting over the shoulder girdle influence lumbopelvic mechanics. Although the intervertebral discs are often considered to be shock absorbers for the spine, it is actually the musculature that is responsible for shock absorption.[24] This section of the chapter details the muscles of the lumbopelvic region, and explores their contribution to the control required to permit smooth motion and the proper stabilization needed to promote smooth movement and prevent excessive strain. The muscles and related connective tissues of the lumbar spine are described much in the same way that they might be encountered in a dissection of the lumbopelvic region. After reviewing the posterior spinal musculature, the musculature of both the abdominal wall and the hip is reviewed, since they have a profound influence on lumbopelvic mechanics.

The Three Musculofascial Systems of the Lumbopelvic Region

Lumbopelvic stability and mobility are dependent upon three musculofascial systems: the thoracolumbar fascia, fascia lata, and abdominal fascia systems. It is through these fascial systems that forces are transferred through from the upper extremity to the lower extremity, or from the lower extremity to the upper extremity through the low back. Each fascial system features two important similarities: muscles attached to the fascia can exert a tensile force by "pulling" on the

Table 3–1. Thoracolumbar Fascia

Muscle "pull"	Muscle "push"
Latissimus dorsi	Superficial erector spinae
Internal abdominal oblique	Deep erector spinae
Transversus abdominus	Multifidus
Gluteus maximus	

Table 3–3. Abdominal Muscle Actions

EXTERNAL ABDOMINAL OBLIQUE
Flex the vertebral column by bringing the thorax closer to the pelvis
Flex the lumbosacral junction by posteriorly rotating the pelvis
Compress the abdominal viscera
Increases tensile force to abdominal fascia
Rotate thorax to contralateral side

INTERNAL ABDOMINAL OBLIQUE
Compress the abdominal contents
Increase tension to thoracolumbar fascia and abdominal fascia
Flex vertebral column by bringing thorax closer to pelvis
Rotate thorax in same direction as opposite external oblique

TRANSVERSUS ABDOMINIS
Compress the abdominal contents
Increase tension to thoracolumbar and abdominal fascia

RECTUS ABDOMINIS
Flexes the thorax on the pelvis
Upward tilt of pelvis
Fills rectus sheath

fascia, and muscles encased within the fascial envelope can exert a "pushing" force due to the broadening effect of the muscle within the fascial envelope acting to also increase tension on the fascial walls (Tables 3–1 to 3–5). In addition to detailing these fascial elements, the following sections will also examine the relationships of individual muscles to these fascial networks.

THORACOLUMBAR FASCIAL SYSTEM AND ASSOCIATED MUSCULATURE

Thoracolumbar fascia

The first structure encountered when the skin and subcutaneous fat are removed from the posterior aspect of the lumbar spine is the thoracolumbar fascia (Fig. 3–9). The thoracolumbar fascia forms a network of noncontractile tissue that plays an essential role in the function of the lumbar spine due to its attachment and relationship to several powerful muscles of the lumbopelvic region. Its highly organized morphology is consistent with fascia that has significant mechanical tension imparted to it.[3]

In the lumbar region the fascia can be divided into posterior, middle, and anterior layers. The most important of these three fascial layers are the posterior and middle, and for that reason, descriptions of the thoracolumbar fascia often simply refer to the posterior layer as the superficial layer of thoracolumbar fascia, and the middle layer as the deep layer of thoracolumbar fascia. From the standpoint of understand-

Table 3–2. Abdominal Fascia

Muscle "pull"	Muscle "push"
External oblique	Rectus abdominus
Internal oblique	
Transversus abdominus	
Pectoralis major	
Serratus anterior	

Table 3–4. Abdominal Wall Functions

Provide anterior and anterolateral structure to trunk cylinder
Increase tension in throacolumbar and abdominal fascia
Check anterior shear via control of pelvis in sagittal plane
Control rate and amplitude of torsion to lumbar spine
Control relationship of abdominal wall to thorax
Increase compression at sacroiliac joints and pubic symphysis

Table 3–5. Fascia Lata

Muscle "pull"	Muscle "push"
Gluteus maximus	Quadriceps
Tensor fascia latae	Hamstrings
	Hip adductors

ing lumbopelvic mechanics, the superficial and deep layers of the thoracolumbar fascia are the important ones to consider, and it is this terminology that will be used throughout this chapter.

The superficial layer of thoracolumbar fascia is a thick, fibrous covering that can be further subdivided into two lamellae.[6, 55] This layer is attached to the spinous processes and the supraspinous ligament, from which points it courses laterally over the erector spinae muscle. At the lateral aspect of the erector spinae it forms the lateral raphe, a region of muscle origin for the internal abdominal oblique and transversus abdominus muscles (Fig. 3–10). From this juncture the fascia then courses medially to gain the anterior surface of the erector spinae muscles and ultimately attaches to the lumbar transverse processes and intertransverse ligaments. This portion of the fascia that is directly anterior to the erector spinae muscle is the deep layer of thoracolumbar fascia. Note that the bony attachments of the thoracolumbar fascia to the lumbar spine (spinous processes and transverse processes) compartmentalize the primary spinal extensor muscle mass.

The superficial layer of thoracolumbar fascia also courses inferiorly and inferolaterally where it is attached

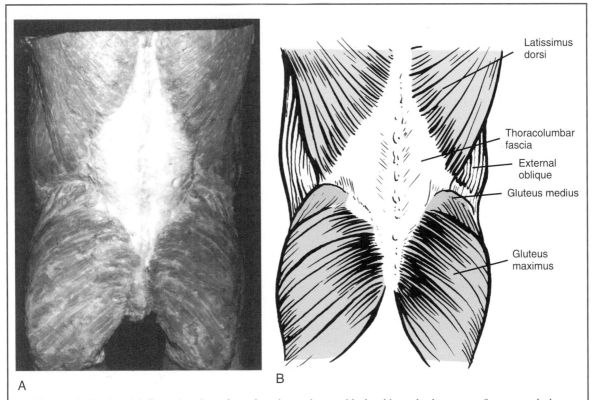

A   B

Figure 3–9. *A* and *B*, Posterior view of a cadaveric specimen with the skin and subcutaneus fat removed, showing the latissimus dorsi, and the gluteus maximus muscles as they attach to the posterior layer of the thoracolumbar fascia. The relationship of the posterior extent of the abdominal muscles and the gluteus medius muscles is also seen.

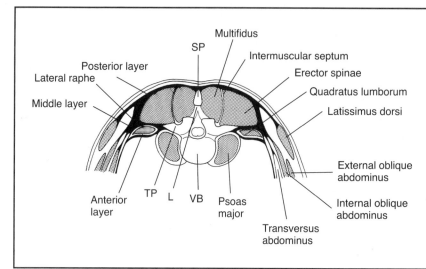

Figure 3–10. Transverse (cross) section of the lumbar spine showing the layers of thoracolumbar fascia (posterior, middle, and anterior) and the muscles attached to it and contained within it. Also labeled are the spinous process (SP), transverse process (TP), vertebral body (VB), and lamina (L). The juncture of the posterior and middle layers is the lateral raphe.

to the sacrum and ilium (Fig. 3–11), and blends with the fascia of the contralateral gluteus maximus. Superolaterally, the superficial layer of thoracolumbar fascia blends with the latissimus dorsi muscle. The latissimus dorsi and contralateral gluteus maximus muscles are thus "mechanically linked" through the superficial layer of the thoracolumbar fascia (Fig. 3–12). It has been suggested that such a mechanical linkage is important in increasing the stability of the sacroiliac joints.[55] The coupled action of the latissimus dorsi and the contralateral gluteus maximus muscles has a line of force that acts perpendicular to the plane of the sacroiliac joints, and thus increases the compressive force between the sacrum and ilium. This increased compressive force increases the stability of the sacroiliac joint. Such a line of force also crosses the lumbosacral and lumbar articulations and potentially afford stability in the same manner. Note the relevance of exercise training for the latissimus dorsi and gluteus maximus muscles, and the potential benefit of reciprocal upper and lower extremity exercises that focus the training effect to these muscles (see Chapter 6).

The thoracolumbar fascia is directly attached to the lumbar vertebrae and pelvis, and therefore spans the lumbar, lumbosacral, and sacroiliac articulations. When a connective tissue structure spans any articulation, an increase in tension of the collagenous framework of such tissue potentially minimizes aberrational motion between the adjacent bony segments. The tension in the thoracolumbar fascia, although a noncon-

tractile tissue, can be engaged dynamically as a result of the contractile tissues attached to it and contained within it (Fig. 3–13).[10, 42] Tension of the fascia can be increased by contraction of the muscles housed within the thoracolumbar fascia "envelope," namely the superficial and deep erector spinae and the multifidus muscles (detailed below). The dynamics of the thoracolumbar tissue network relative to these spinal extensors can be compared to the stabilization of a tent. The central pole of the tent compares to the superficial and deep erector spinae and multifidus muscles. These muscles are contained within the fascia or "tent," and their contraction results in broadening of the muscle and subsequent "pushing" force on the fascia (Table 3–1, see Figure 3-13c).[16]

The latissimus dorsi, gluteus maximus, transversus abdominis, and internal oblique muscles are similar to the guy wires of a tent that are used to tighten and secure the structure. Just as the guy wires of the tent are pulled tight and secured, the tent assumes its shape and becomes stable enough to perform its function because there is increased tension in tent walls. The latissimus dorsi, transversus abdominis, internal abdominal oblique, and gluteus maximus serve in a similar manner—pulling on the fascial network by pulling superolaterally, laterally, and inferolaterally, respectively (Fig. 3–13b). Therefore, as the body moves, muscular forces internal and external to the thoracolumbar fascia potentially afford this same type of stabilizing function.

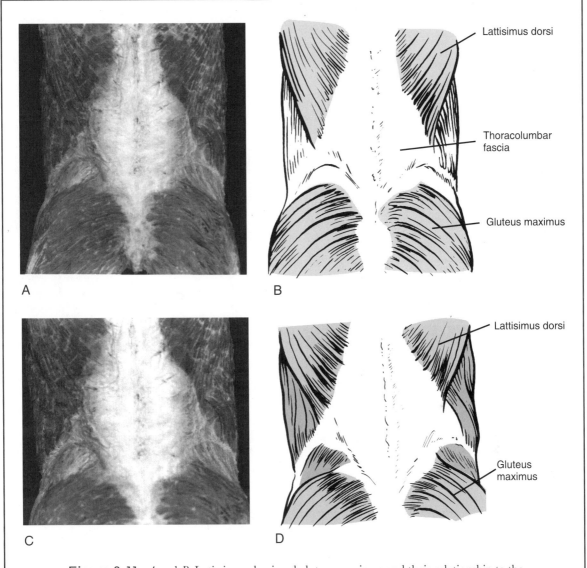

Figure 3–11. *A* and *B*, Latissimus dorsi and gluteus maximus and their relationship to the thoracolumbar fascia. *C* and *D:* Close-up view showing the inferior and inferolateral aspects of thoracolumbar fascia as it courses over the sacrum and blends with the fascia of the contralateral gluteus.

In Chapter 6 such mechanics are emphasized, and serve as a basis for developing resistance exercises for muscles related to the spine. Tension generating ability—strength—is important to develop in muscles pulling on fascia (latissimus dorsi, gluteus maximus, internal abdominal oblique, and transversus abdom-

inis), while therapeutic exercise to stimulate relative hypertrophy is essential for muscles encased within the fascia (erector spinae and multifidus).

Lastly, tension can also be imparted to the thoracolumbar fascia indirectly as a result of movement of the lumbar spine or pelvis.[49] Contraction of the pos-

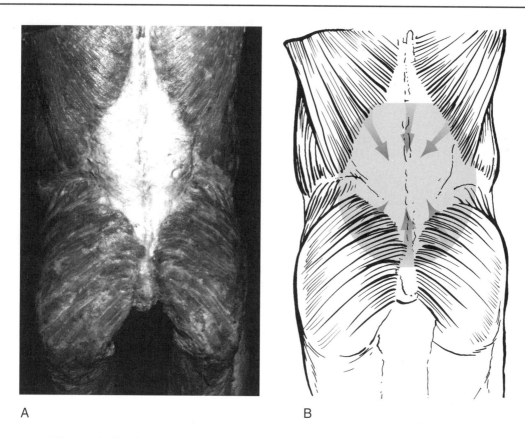

A

B

Figure 3–12. *A* and *B*, The mechanical coupling of the contralateral latissimus dorsi and gluteus maximus muscles provides a line of force over the lumbar spine, sacroiliac articulation, and hip joints that "cinches" the lumbopelvic unit together by increasing compression between the articulations and enhancing stability.

terior hip (gluteus maximus or hamstring) muscles, or the abdominal muscles results in a posterior rotation of the pelvis. Posterior rotation of the pelvis is essentially a flexion moment at the lumbosacral junction which increases the tension of the thoracolumbar fascia (Fig. 3–14). Flexion of the lumbar spine on the pelvis, as in forward bending, similarly results in tightening of the fascia. In both these instances, tension is placed on the fascia because of the lumbar flexion motion, which results in passive engagement of the fascia. It has been suggested that one of the reasons that competitive weight-lifters engaged in the Olympic deadlift event "round out" their lumbar spines is to

take advantage of the stabilization afforded to their lumbar spine by increased tension in the thoracolumbar fascia and the posterior ligamentous complex.[12, 13]

Latissimus Dorsi Muscle

At first inspection it would not appear that the latissimus dorsi muscle, usually described as an extensor, adductor, and medial rotator of the humerus, has a significant effect on lumbopelvic mechanics. However, its attachments warrant its consideration as a muscle

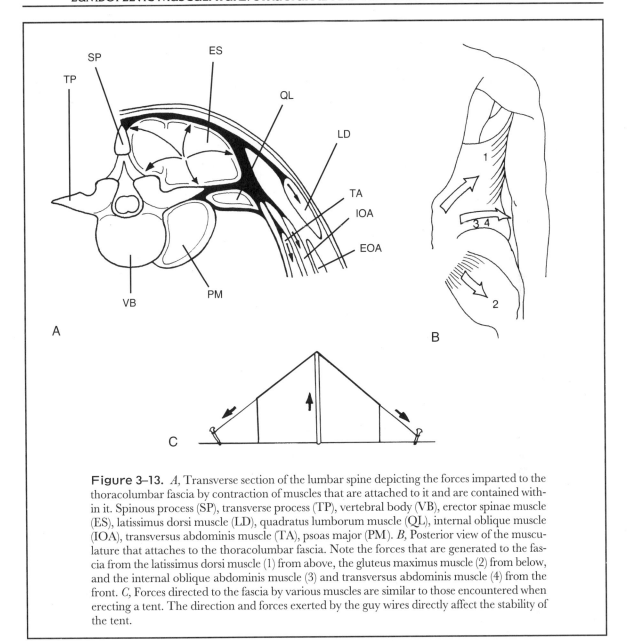

Figure 3–13. *A,* Transverse section of the lumbar spine depicting the forces imparted to the thoracolumbar fascia by contraction of muscles that are attached to it and are contained within it. Spinous process (SP), transverse process (TP), vertebral body (VB), erector spinae muscle (ES), latissimus dorsi muscle (LD), quadratus lumborum muscle (QL), internal oblique muscle (IOA), transversus abdominis muscle (TA), psoas major (PM). *B,* Posterior view of the musculature that attaches to the thoracolumbar fascia. Note the forces that are generated to the fascia from the latissimus dorsi muscle (1) from above, the gluteus maximus muscle (2) from below, and the internal oblique abdominis muscle (3) and transversus abdominis muscle (4) from the front. *C,* Forces directed to the fascia by various muscles are similar to those encountered when erecting a tent. The direction and forces exerted by the guy wires directly affect the stability of the tent.

that has significant force generating potential over the low back region.

The latissimus dorsi muscle is attached to the lower six thoracic spinous processes and all of the spinous processes of the lumbar vertebrae and sacrum through the fascial network of the thoracolumbar fascia (Fig. 3–15). The inferior attachment of the latissimus dorsi muscle continues laterally along the iliac crest toward the point of attachment of the lateral raphe of the thoracolumbar fascia and very often the latissimus dorsi is attached directly to the iliac crest. From these points of attachment the muscle converges superiorly and laterally to attach to the lesser tubercle of the humerus and the floor of the intertubercular groove.

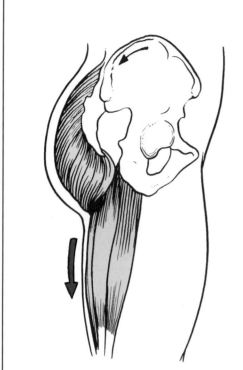

Figure 3–14. Posterior rotation of the pelvis can be accomplished by contraction of the gluteus maximus and hamstrings, which increases tension of the thoracolumbar fascia, and hence stability of the spine.

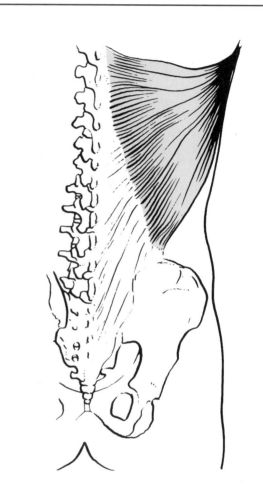

Figure 3–15. Illustration of spine and pelvic attachments of the latissimus dorsi. The muscle is attached to the thoracic spinous processes, the lumbosacral spinous processes through the thoracolumbar fascia, and the iliac crest. The lumbar and pelvic attachments suggest an influence on spinal mechanics.

Because the lumbopelvic attachment of the latissimus dorsi muscle is by way of the thoracolumbar fascia, the influence to spine mechanics can be readily appreciated. McGill and Norman[34] note that when all of the posterior trunk tissues are considered, the latissimus dorsi muscle has the greatest moment arm length. This implies that the latissimus dorsi muscle potentially influences lumbopelvic mechanics with less effort than do other tissues because of this mechanical advantage.

Before considering the force vector that this muscle exerts on the thoracolumbar fascia, it should be noted that the position of the humerus influences tension through the thoracolumbar fascia. If the humerus is in an abducted and flexed position, as is typical for a person reaching for an object to lift or pull toward the body, the latissimus dorsi muscle is stretched. As a result, there is increased tension through the thoracolumbar fascia. If there is concurrent posterior rotation of the pelvis, the tensile force to the fascia is further enhanced. If the latissimus dorsi muscle is now called on to contract, then an active tensile force is also imparted to the fascia (Fig. 3–16). Tension to the

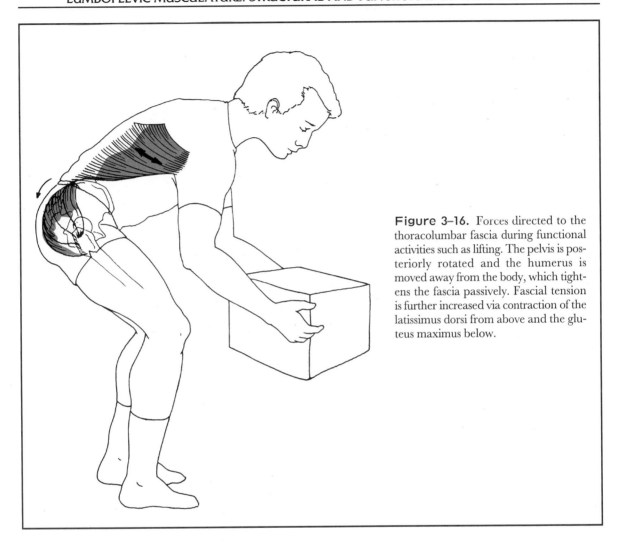

Figure 3–16. Forces directed to the thoracolumbar fascia during functional activities such as lifting. The pelvis is posteriorly rotated and the humerus is moved away from the body, which tightens the fascia passively. Fascial tension is further increased via contraction of the latissimus dorsi from above and the gluteus maximus below.

thoracolumbar fascia is a summation of passive tension from humerus and pelvic positioning, and active tension from contraction of the latissimus dorsi muscle. As will be seen later, the active tension in the thoracolumbar fascia can be further increased via contraction of the gluteus maximus muscle.

The latissimus dorsi muscle is not typically viewed as a muscle intimately involved in lifting. A kinematic analysis of the lifting task suggests that the latissimus dorsi muscle is capable of helping to overcome the inertia of the object in order to move it closer to the body. When functional lift tasks are scrutinized, it is apparent that the latissimus dorsi muscle assists in moving the center of gravity of a load closer to the subject's

center of gravity. As the lift continues, the angle between the humerus and the body changes. Note that it is also possible to lift or move the weight toward the body without significant latissimus dorsi contribution. With only a strong spinal extensor contraction and the subject's hands firmly grasping the object, the weight can be accelerated by spinal extensor muscle action, which can also overcome the inertia of the stationary object. The upper limbs then move toward the subject's trunk while the weight is held. Without latissimus dorsi activity to pull the object closer, there is increased demand on the spinal extensor muscles. It is reasonable to conclude that the latissimus dorsi muscle contributes to equalizing forces over lumbopelvic region.

Stabilization of the spine and pelvis is enhanced by muscle contraction which increases fascial tension. A pull bilaterally on the fascia by both latissimus dorsi muscles has the effect of pulling on both sides of the spinous and transverse process attachments of the thoracolumbar fascia, which assists in checking rotation and flexion of the lumbar spine. A contraction of the ipsilateral latissimus dorsi muscle requires a counterforce by the musculature on the contralateral side to minimize aberrant motion in the lumbar spine. The oblique and transverse abdominal muscles, for example, by virtue of their attachments and fiber direction, appear capable of providing this counterforce.[50] As previously mentioned, the important mechanical link between the ipsilateral latissimus dorsi muscle and contralateral gluteus maximus muscle also applies such a counterforce.

Erector Spinae Muscles: The Superficial and Deep Erector Spinae Muscles

The term erector spinae is used in reference to the paraspinal muscles innervated by branches of the dorsal rami (see Chapter 2). Although the erector spinae muscles traverse the complete length of the spine, this discussion will be limited to the superficial and deep erector spinae related to the lumbopelvic region. Both the superficial and the deep erector spinae muscles can be further subdivided into a lateral iliocostalis and medial longissimus group, but for the ease of description the muscles will simply be referred to as the superficial and the deep erector spinae muscles.

Superficial Erector Spinae Muscles

The superficial erector spinae muscles are attached to the undersurface of a broad, flat aponeurotic tendon referred to as the erector spinae aponeurosis (ESA) and the iliac crest (Fig. 3–17). The ESA attachments have a broad medial–lateral expanse from the spinous processes of the lumbar and sacral regions to the ilium. The superficial erector spinae muscles arise from the anterior aspect of this thick aponeurosis and ascend to attach to the ribs.

Since palpation of the spine is an integral part of the examination process for the patient with low back pain, one should recognize the extent of the ESA, and

where superficial erector spinae is muscular or tendinous. Note that the muscular elements of the superficial erector spinae are at distance laterally from the spinous processes, and only in the mid to upper lumbar region (Fig. 3–18). When one is palpating the back in the lower lumbar region or over the dorsal aspect of the sacrum, the tissues encountered are skin, superficial fat, posterior layer of thoracolumbar fascia, and the thick ESA. Deep to these significant connective tissue structures will be the deep erector spinae and multifidus muscles which are detailed in the next section. Therefore, in using palpation techniques to assess areas of increased muscle tension or trigger point pain, one must realize that the prominent muscle belly of the superficial erector spinae is at a significant distance lateral to the spinous processes and in the upper lumbar and lower thoracic spine toward the ribs.

Figure 3-19 provides a view of the orientation of the superficial erector spinae muscle when viewed in the sagittal plane. The position of the rib cage relative to the pelvis suggests that the muscle courses superiorly and posteriorly from its point of origin at the pelvis to its attachment to the ribs. Clinicians utilizing spray and stretch techniques or muscle shortening or lengthening techniques such as strain–counterstrain or muscle energy might consider that elongation of the muscle occurs when the thorax (on the same side as the superficial erector spinae being examined) is brought even further posterior, or the iliac crest on that side is brought forward. Such rotary movements of the thorax or pelvis take advantage of the superior-to-posterior inclination of the superficial erector spinae muscle. Shortening of the superficial erector spinae occurs with thorax or pelvis movement opposite those just described.

Even though the superficial erector spinae muscles do not attach directly to the lumbar spine, they have an optimal lever arm for lumbar extension by virtue of their attachments. By pulling the thorax posteriorly, they create an extension moment over the lumbar spine. In addition, they function eccentrically to control the descent of the spine during forward bending, and isometrically to control the position of the lower thorax with respect to the pelvis during functional movements.[14, 19, 35, 39, 46, 47]

The erector spinae muscles enter into a period of electromyographic silence toward the end of forward bending.[19, 29, 41, 59] It has been proposed that at this point the stabilization of the spine has been relinquished or passed on to the noncontractile structures of the back

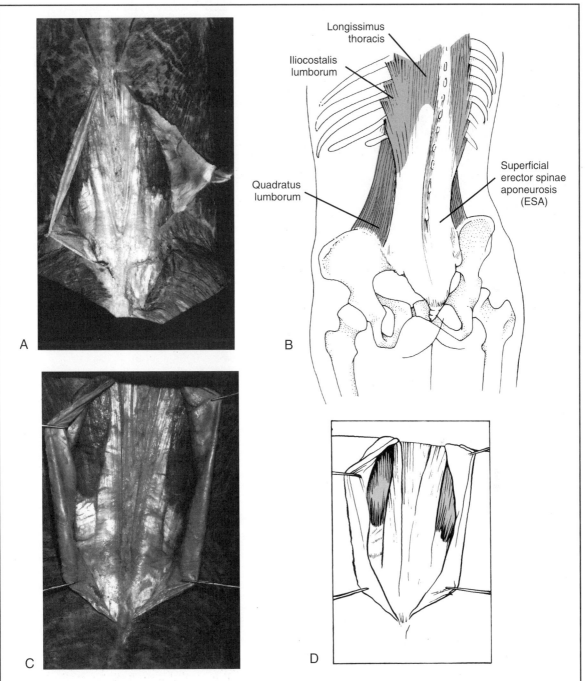

Figure 3–17. *A* and B, Posterior view with thoracolumbar fascia reflected revealing the erector spinae aponeurosis (ESA) which serves as the lumbar and pelvic attachment for the superficial erector spinae muscles. The cranial attachment of the superficial erector spinae is the ribs. The superficial erector spinae can be subdivided into a lateral iliocostalis group and a medial longissimus group. *C* and *D*, With the thoracolumbar fascia reflected, the strong tendons constituting the erector spinae aponeurosis can be readily appreciated.

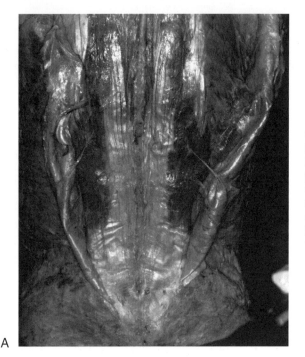

A

Figure 3–18. *A* and *B,* The superficial erector spinae muscle is largely tendinous at the region of the spinous processes and over the lower lumbar spine and sacrum. One must palpate in the upper lumbar spine and well lateral to the spinous processes to be over muscle tissue. (A from DeRosa C: Integration as the Objectives of Treatment for Low Back Pain with Lumbar Spine Anatomy. Ph.D. Thesis Cincinnati, Union Institute, 1993.)

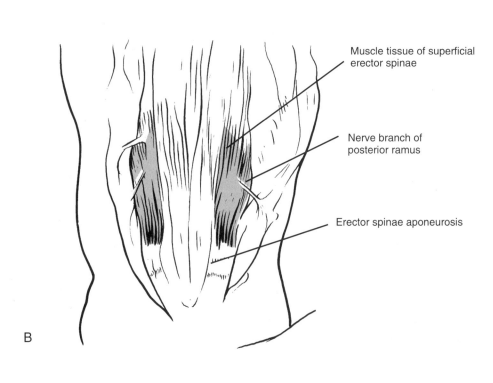

Muscle tissue of superficial erector spinae

Nerve branch of posterior ramus

Erector spinae aponeurosis

B

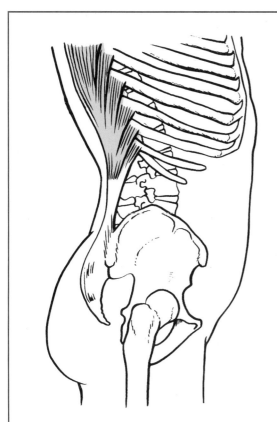

Figure 3–19. When viewed from a lateral perspective, the superficial erector spinae can be seen to course superiorly and posteriorly from its pelvic attachment to the ribs owing to the convexity of the thoracic cage. Note that movement of the right side of the pelvis forward (rotation), or the right thoracic cage backward (rotation), lengthens the superficial erector spinae, while the opposite motions place it in a shortened position.

such as the fascial and ligamentous elements, and that the muscle has been stretched to a length that minimizes its ability to contract.[17] The concept of an electrically silent muscle should be interpreted with caution, however. It may be incorrect to assume that the electrically silent muscle is inactive. A muscle at rest still maintains a resting tension or tone. Thus, even in this lengthened state the musculature contributes to limiting further forward bending.

The attachment of the superficial erector spinae muscle also has an influence on sacroiliac joint mechanics (Fig. 3–20). Due to the attachment of the erector spinae aponeurosis to the sacrum, the pull of the erector spinae tendon on the dorsal aspect of the sacrum induces a flexions (nutation) moment of the sacrum on the ilium. As will be detailed in Chapter 4, flexion (nutation) is a movement that helps ligamentously lock the pelvis because it increases the tension of the sacrotuberous and interosseous ligaments. Thus, strong contraction of the superficial erector spinae muscle contributes to stability of the sacroiliac joint articulation due to the induced flexion moment and illustrates the importance of maintaining the strength of the superficial erector spinae muscles.

Deep Erector Spinae Muscles

Bogduk[5, 7] has described a significant deeper division of the erector spinae muscles that is distinct from the previously described superficial component. This deep, lumbar division originates from the ilium above and just lateral to the posterior superior iliac spine, and also from the undersurface of the erector spinae aponeurosis. From these points, the deep erector spinae courses superiorly, anteriorly, and medially to attach to the lumbar transverse processes (Fig. 3–21).[8] Like its analog muscle in the neck, the levator scapula—which also has a superior, medial, and anterior inclination as it courses toward the transverse processes—the muscle is "twisted" on itself so that the superlateral fibers originating on the ilium have the lowest insertion on the lower lumbar transverse processes, and the inferomedial fibers on the ilium have the highest insertion on the upper lumbar transverse processes.

The attachments of the deep portion of the erector spinae imply important functional and clinical considerations. Figure 3-22 shows the orientation of the muscle fibers of the deep erector spinae. Note that the inclination and direction of pull of the muscle can be illustrated as the hypotenuse of a triangle. The other two sides of the triangle represent a compressive force and a posterior shear force. Since the axis of motion for the lumbar spine is located in the posterocentral aspect of the intervertebral disc, it is clear that an attachment to the transverse process results in the deep erector spinae muscle having a poor lever arm for lumbar extension. However, the muscle is aligned to exert a posterior shear force, or perhaps more accurately, provide a dynamic counterforce to the anterior shear force imparted to the lumbar spine due to the gravitational force.

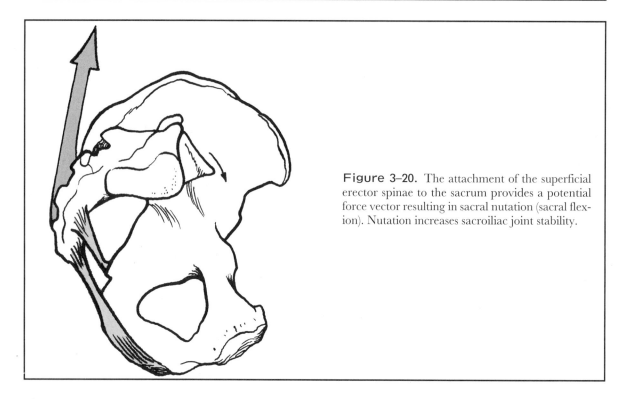

Figure 3–20. The attachment of the superficial erector spinae to the sacrum provides a potential force vector resulting in sacral nutation (sacral flexion). Nutation increases sacroiliac joint stability.

The importance of a dynamic restraint to anterior shear is essential to understand when considering the mechanics of the lumbosacral and lumbar articulations. There are several connective tissue restraints to anterior shear (detailed in Chapter 4) that include such structures as the iliolumbar ligament, fibers of the annulus fibrosus, and frontal plane of the apophyseal joints. As a result of injury to these connective tissue restraints, or as a sequelae of the aging process, the specialized connective tissues offering restraint to anterior shear lose their effectiveness, and neuromuscular strategies to dynamically minimize anterior shear force in painful syndromes are initiated at a reflexive, central nervous system level. The strategy is to increase motor activity or increase muscle tension in the associated muscles. In this case, one of the associated muscles would be the deep erector spinae muscles. This is a functional example of the increased setpoint concept introduced earlier in the chapter. An example of this in the peripheral joints is the increased muscle tension of the hamstrings in the knee with anterior cruciate insufficiency in order to minimize anterior shear of the tibia.

This discussion is especially noteworthy when considering palpation findings in a low back examination.

An interesting aspect of the deep erector spinae muscle is that when one is palpating the iliac crest region just above and immediately lateral to the posterior superior iliac spine, the only muscle belly encountered is in fact the deep erector spinae muscle, because overlying it is the erector spinae aponeurosis and the superficial layer of thoracolumbar fascia—two connective tissue structures. When palpating this region above and lateral to the posterior superior iliac spine, and noting increased tissue tension of the muscle (deep erector spinae) or muscle discomfort, it is essential to determine whether in fact this state of muscle contraction is appropriate and essential neuromuscular strategy for dynamically stabilizing spinal segments that cannot withstand the anterior shear stress. This is analogous to observing the increased muscle tension sense in the hamstrings in the knee with an anterior cruciate ligament injury. The treatment strategy in both instances is not to decrease the increased muscle activity with stretching techniques, manual techniques, or modalities, but rather to consider strengthening the muscle tissue.

The deep erector spinae muscle thus affords stability of the lumbar spine and lumbosacral articulation in the sagittal plane. An anteroposterior (sagittal plane)

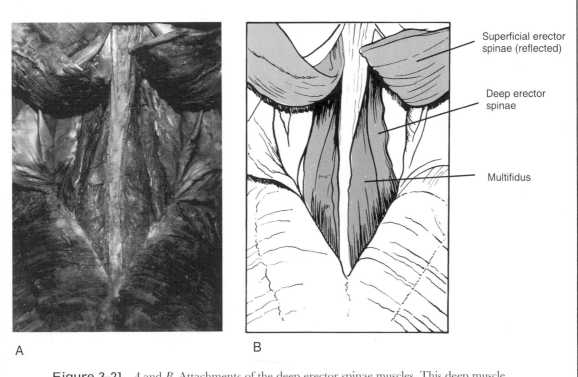

A   B

Superficial erector
spinae (reflected)

Deep erector
spinae

Multifidus

Figure 3–21. *A* and *B*, Attachments of the deep erector spinae muscles. This deep muscle, located just lateral to the multifidus muscle at the region of the posterior superior iliac spine, helps anchor the lumbar vertebrae to the ilium. Note the attachment of the deep erector spinae at the region of, and superolateral to, the posterior superior iliac spine. This should be appreciated during palpation as the superficial structures to the deep erector spinae are connective tissues (ESA and thoracolumbar fascia).

guy wire or check system is available when considering the combined vectors of the psoas major and deep erector spinae muscle. Contraction of the psoas major muscle can cause an anterior shear force on the lumbar vertebrae while the deep erector spinae exerts a posterior shear force. The deep erector spinae perhaps works with the contralateral psoas major muscle to create a sagittal plane check-and-balance system for lumbar stability (Fig. 3–23).

Multifidus Muscles

The multifidus muscles are typically referred to as "transversospinalis muscles" in most textbooks of anatomy. This name is used to represent muscles coursing in a lateral to medial direction from the transverse processes to the spinous processes of the vertebrae. Unfortunately, this description is inadequate for the multifidus muscles in the lumbopelvic region, especially at the lower lumbar, lumbosacral, and sacral regions.

In the lumbopelvic region the multifidus arises from the dorsal surface of the sacrum, sacrotuberous ligament, aponeurosis of the erector spinae muscle, medial surface of the posterior superior iliac spine, and the posterior sacroiliac ligaments (Fig. 3–24). The muscle also originates from the mammillary processes of the lumbar vertebrae.[7, 40] From these caudal attachments the muscle runs superiorly and medially to attach to the

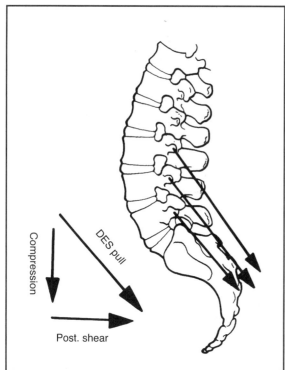

Compression

DES pull

Post. shear

Figure 3–22. Line of pull due to orientation of the deep erector spinae (DES) muscle. Since it attaches close to the axis of lumbar motion, it provides a dynamic posterior shear force and a compression force.

spinous processes of the lumbar and sacral vertebrae. Because of the posterior concavity of the lumbar spine and the convexity of the sacral kyphosis, the muscle also has a slight anterior inclination as it travels to attach to the lumbar spinous processes at the apex of the lordosis. Since it spans several spinal segments it plays a major role as a prime mover and stabilizer of the lumbar spine.[11]

The multifidus musculature is large and prominent in the lumbopelvic region. It fills the extensive channel bordered by the lumbar transverse and spinous processes and covers the dorsal surface of the sacrum. The cross-section of the multifidus muscle in the lumbosacral region is quite impressive over the dorsal surface of the sacrum. This cross-section is more significant than the multifidus muscle in other areas of the spine. The gross structure, particularly the expanse

and the cross-section of the multifidus is markedly different in the lumbopelvic region when compared in the cervical and thoracic spine. It becomes much more compact as it is closely attached to the sides of the progressively smaller spinous processes as one moves up the spine.

The extensive attachment of the multifidus muscle to the dorsal surface of the sacrum and surrounding ligaments makes it the major tissue mass filling the deep sulcus formed by the overlapping ilium and the sacrum. This sulcus is directly medial to the posterior superior iliac spine. When palpating the region of the spine immediately medial to the posterior superior iliac spine, the examiner should realize that the palpation includes skin, superficial fat, superficial layer of thoracolumbar fascia, erector spinae aponeurosis (ESA) and the extensive muscle belly of the multifidus (Fig. 3–25).

Injury to any of the tissues in the lumbopelvic region may lead to excessive muscle activity or muscle guarding, which is initiated to protect the injury site from further movement. The increased tissue tension that is often felt over the dorsal surface of the sacrum is most likely the resting state of muscle contraction for the multifidus as it is the only muscle belly under the palpating hand in this region. The extensive direct attachment of the multifidus muscle to the lumbar spine makes it a prime candidate for reflex muscle guarding due to low back injury. Note also that just deep to the multifidus muscle belly lies the posterior capsular ligaments of the sacroiliac joint.

The attachment of the multifidus muscles to the spinous processes results in an effective lever arm for lumbar extension (Fig. 3–26). Because the axis of rotation for flexion and extension in the lumbar spine is located in the posterior region of the intervertebral disc, the distance from the spinous processes to this axis is longer than the lever arm of the deep portions of the erector spinae, which attaches to the transverse processes. The multifidus muscle is therefore more effective in creating an extension moment over the lumbar vertebral segments.[18, 31] From the standing position, the action of the muscle might be considered as "antiflexion" (controlled eccentric lengthening of the multifidus muscle as the spine is forward bent) and "antishear." This refers to multifidus muscle contraction helping to control the rate and magnitude of these two forces (flexion and anterior shear) during forward bending.

The multifidus muscle also has an oblique orientation in the frontal plane. Most anatomy textbooks state

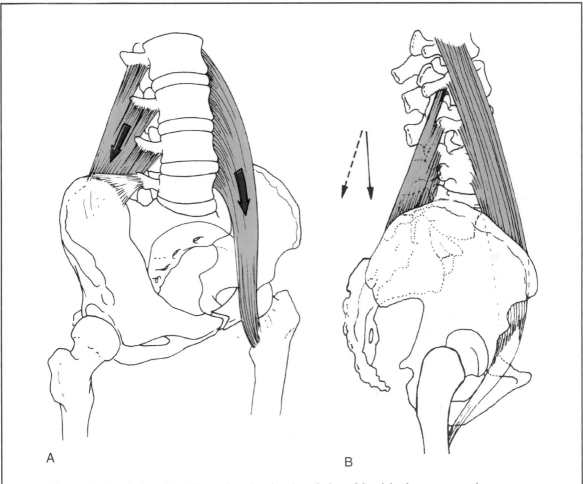

Figure 3–23. *A,* Anterior oblique view showing the relation of the right deep erector spinae muscle and the left psoas major muscle as they function together contralaterally to stabilize the lumbar spine by way of the anteroposterior guy wire check system. The arrows depict the direction of the muscular forces imparted to the lumbar spine. *B,* Sagittal view showing the stabilizing relation of the deep erector spinae muscle and psoas major muscle.

that contraction of the muscle causes rotation to the opposite side. Although the potential for such action exists, the lever arm for this activity is not optimal, the facets of the lumbar spine are not oriented for rotation, and the muscle appears mechanically inefficient for this activity. The multifidus is active in nearly all anti-gravity activities however, and its contribution to rotation is more likely as a result of countering the flexion

moment that results as the abdominal oblique muscles rotate the trunk.[52]

Like the superficial and deep erector spinae muscles, contraction of the multifidus muscles exerts a compressive force between each lumbar vertebrae and between L5 and the sacrum. Stability of the lumbar spine increases when compressive forces are placed on it. When loaded in compression, the lumbopelvic unit

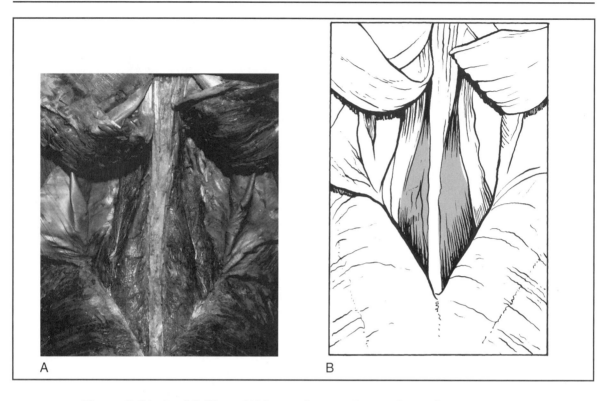

Figure 3–24. *A* and *B*, The multifidus muscle covers the complete surface of the sacrum and courses superior and medial to attach to the spinous processes of the lumbar and sacral vertebrae.

is much more resistant to torsional forces which enhance the potential for damage to the outer annular rings and the lumbar zygapophyseal joint.[16] Therefore, the multifidus muscle may contribute to spinal stability by "squeezing" the vertebrae together and locking or engaging the vertebral assembly.

There appears to be a greater percentage of type I than type II fibers in the multifidus muscles of the lumbar spine, which suggests that this muscle has an important stabilizing function.[48] Histologic analysis of the multifidus muscles in patients with chronic low back pain reveals marked degenerative changes. These changes include selective type II muscle fiber atrophy, moth-eaten appearance to type I fibers, and an increase in the amount of adipose tissue between the muscle fibers.[45] Recruitment of the multifidus muscle for hyperextension of the lumbar spine is also markedly different in patients with chronic low back pain than in persons without low back pain.[18]

In addition to its important functions over the lumbar spine, the multifidus is mechanically linked to the lower extremity via closer relationship to the gluteus maximus. Figure 3-27 illustrates the location in which the gluteus maximus and multifidus muscle show their interconnection. In essence, this linkage connects the powerful extensor muscle of the lumbar spine to the powerful extensor of the hip. The linkage establishes the multifidus–gluteus maximus as an exceptionally powerful extensor unit of the lumbopelvic region.

The multifidus muscle also contributes dynamically to the stability of the sacroiliac joint. Since it is attached to the sacrotuberous ligament, tension to the ligament imparted as a result of multifidus muscle contraction potentially increases the ligamentous stabilizing mechanism of the sacroiliac joint (Fig. 3–28). In addition, since the gluteus maximus crosses the sacroiliac joint and is mechanically linked to the multifidus muscle, contraction of the multifidus–gluteus max-

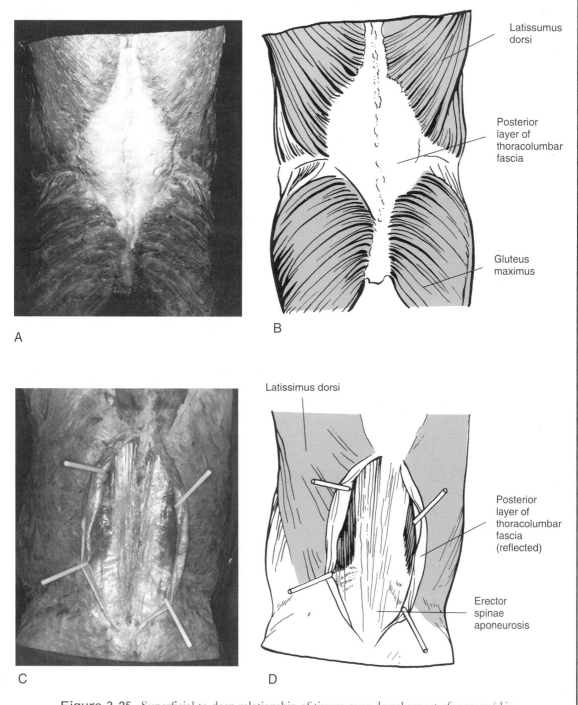

Figure 3–25. Superficial to deep relationship of tissues over dorsal aspect of sacrum (skin removed). *A* and B, Thoracolumbar fascia. *C* and *D*, Erector spinae aponeurosis.

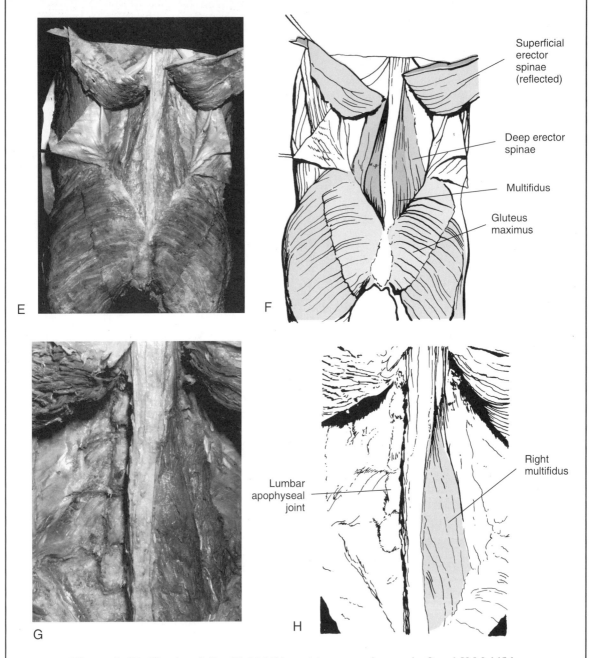

Figure 3–25. (Continued) *E and* F, *Multifidus and deep erector spinae muscles*. G and *H*, Multifidus removed on left side revealing apophyseal joints, multifidus left intact on right.

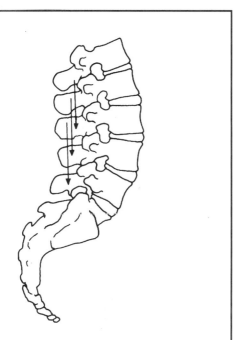

Figure 3–26. Sagittal view revealing the vector or line of pull of the multifidus muscle that makes it a strong spinal extensor. (Adapted from Bogduk N, Twomey LT: Clinical Anatomy of the Lumbar Spine. Churchill Livingstone, New York, 1987.)

imus complex increases the compressive force to the sacroiliac articulation thereby enhancing joint stability (see Chapter 4).

It should be evident from the above discussion that optimizing the strength and girth of the multifidus muscle (as well as the erector spinae muscles) is essential for successful spine rehabilitation programs. It has been suggested that intensive spine exercises, particularly those focused on resistance exercises to the extensor muscles, are of benefit to patients with low back pain.[32] The necessity for overload stimulus to these muscles must not be underestimated. The multifidus and erector spinae muscles must fill the thoracolumbar fascial envelope, be capable of moving and controlling the body weight, and assist the lumbopelvic region in attenuating ground and trunk forces. The clinician must design resistance exercise programs (Chapter 6) that are of sufficient intensity to stimulate muscle growth (hypertrophy) and tension-generating

ability based on the results of the functional assessment (Chapter 5).

Intersegmental Muscles

There is a series of small muscles of the lumbopelvic region that connect one intervertebral segment with another. These muscles are typically named for the portions of the bone to which they attach. Many of their functions can only be presumed from observation of their anatomical position. They are the interspinales, which are located on either side of the interspinous ligament, and the intertransversarii muscles, which attach to adjacent mammillary and transverse processes (Fig. 3–29A and B).

The interspinales muscles are considered to be extensors of the lumbar segments, while the intertransversarii participate in extension and lateral flexion. The cross-sectional area of these muscles is small, and therefore the magnitude of their contribution is small. However, because of their attachment to each vertebra, they may be responsible for providing proprioceptive input to the central nervous system, as they are continually placed under a variety of tensile or compressive forces with activity.

Quadratus Lumborum Muscle and Iliolumbar Ligament Complex

The superficial and deep erector spinae and multifidus muscles fill the thoracolumbar fascial envelope and the deep layer of thoracolumbar fascia is anterior to these spinal extensors. If this deep layer of thoracolumbar fascia is removed, the quadratus lumborum muscle is exposed (Figs. 3-10 and 3-30). Typically, the quadratus lumborum muscle is studied with the posterior abdominal wall, but when viewed in this manner its influence on lumbopelvic mechanics is seldom appreciated. However, its attachment to the lumbar spine and pelvis warrants its study as a muscle of the lumbopelvic region.

The quadratus lumborum muscle is a thin, flat muscle consisting of fibers that are oriented in several directions.[27] The muscle can be divided into a component that extends from the iliac crest to the lumbar transverse processes (iliotransverse), another part that extends from the lumbar transverse processes to the

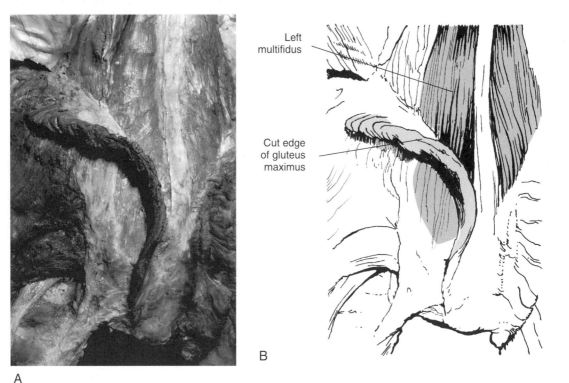

Left multifidus

Cut edge of gluteus maximus

A

B

Figure 3–27. *A* and *B*, The multifidus muscle can be seen blending in with the superior medial aspect of the gluteus maximus, forming a mechanical linkage between the two powerful extensors of the lumbar spine and hip. In this photo, the gluteus maximus has been completely removed except for its most proximal sweeping attachment to the sacrum and ilium. The cut end of the gluteus maximus is seen in the photo directly over the multifidus muscle. The most distal aspect of the erector spinae aponeurosis, often thin, has been reflected in order to demonstrate this gluteus maximus—multifidus linkage between the two powerful extensors of the hip and lumbar spine.

lower ribs (costotransverse), and still another part that originates from the iliac crest and proceeds to the lower ribs (iliocostal). The costotransverse portion is very small and often not discernible; therefore, will not be considered in this discussion.

The quadratus lumborum occupies the region over the iliac crest deep to the erector spinae muscles. It is located deep to the thoracolumbar fascia (both the superficial and deep aspects), the erector spinae aponeurosis and a portion of the superficial erector spinae, and the deep erector spinae muscle. Its cross-sectional area is much less than the superficial and

deep erector spinae muscles. Although clinicians sometimes speak of palpating the resting muscle tension in the quadratus lumborum, it is questionable whether it would be possible to discern this muscle from the overlying larger erector spinae muscles.

From the iliac crest, the iliocostal portion of the quadratus lumborum muscle ascends superiorly and medially under cover of this thick component of the erector spinae muscle to attach to the lower ribs. The ileotransverse portion travels superiorly and medially to attach to the lateral aspect of the transverse process of the lumbar vertebrae. The latter portion is not

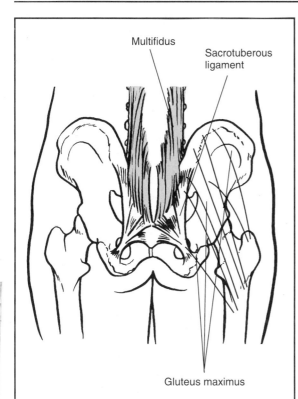

Multifidus

Sacrotuberous
ligament

Gluteus maximus

Figure 3–28. Anatomical relationship of multi-fidus over sacroiliac articulation as it is attached to the sacrotuberous ligament, and is mechanically linked to the gluteus maximus muscle.

under cover of any thick musculature, but is deep to the thoracolumbar fascia and the muscular attachments to this fascia—the internal oblique, transversus abdominis, and latissimus dorsi muscles. This anatomical relation should be considered when palpating areas of tenderness, especially in relation to the muscle's attachment on the iliac crest.

The action of the quadratus lumborum muscle is often described as "hiking the hip." It seldom functions in this manner unless we are attempting to compensate for a relatively longer limb during gait. The muscle has perhaps more important functions relative to moving and stabilizing the pelvis and lumbar spine in the frontal plane and horizontal planes.

For example, during a side-bending motion of the trunk from the standing position, the quadratus lum-

borum muscle on the convex side of the curve eccentrically contracts to help control the rate of descent. The return to an upright position requires a concentric contraction by the same muscle. In the upright standing posture, lateral trunk movements require synchronized contractions, using both eccentric and concentric contractions between the right and left quadratus lumborum muscles as well as other lumbopelvic muscles to assure postural stability. Just as the deep erector spinae and multifidus work in concert with the psoas major in establishing a guy wire function for stability in the sagittal plane, frontal plane guy wires might include the quadratus lumborum and the hip abductors and adductors during the swing phase of the gait (Fig. 3–31).

Another example of mechanical stresses imparted to this muscle occurs as the upper extremities are elevated from the side and the lower ribs away from the iliac crest. If the individual now forward bends, there is marked increase in the tensile stress to the quadratus lumborum muscle from both the flexed trunk and the upper extremities elevation. The two motions are often combined in daily activities, resulting in a near maximal elongation of the quadratus lumborum muscle. If a person is forward bending and side bending to the left in order to pull an object toward him, the right quadratus lumborum muscle is placed in a position of stretch by virtue of the elevation of the rib cage in forward bending and left lateral flexion. It is reasonable to postulate that this stretch, if excessive, or the initial concentric burst of activity as the person returns to the upright position, can potentially strain the muscle.

The quadratus lumborum muscle also has a role in controlling lumbar spine motion in the horizontal plane. The attachments to the lumbar transverse processes give the muscle a reasonable lever arm in attempting to control torsion of the lumbar spine. We can again view the quadratus lumborum muscle as participating with the deep erector spinae and psoas major muscles in preparing the lumbar spine for force transference.

Immediately inferior and medial to the quadratus lumborum muscle is the iliolumbar ligament, spanning the region between the fourth and fifth transverse processes of the lumbar vertebrae and the iliac crest (Fig. 3–32). Luk and colleagues[30] have suggested that the iliolumbar ligament has developed as a result of metaplasia of the inferior most aspect of the quadratus lumborum muscle. This, however, has been chal-

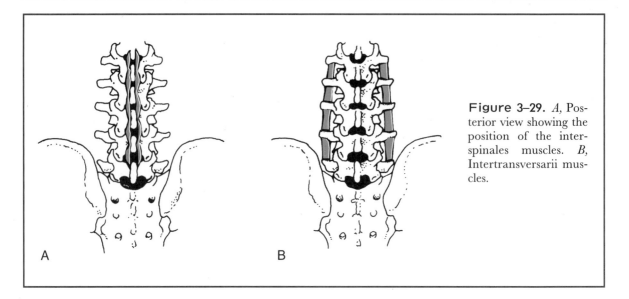

Figure 3–29. *A*, Posterior view showing the position of the interspinales muscles. *B*, Intertransversarii muscles.

lenged in more comprehensive studies demonstrating the presence of the ligament at gestational ages of 15–16 weeks.[23, 51]

The iliolumbar ligament is extremely broad and variable in its expanse. The fibers typically blend with the intertransverse ligaments of the lumbar spine as well as the anterior sacroiliac ligaments. The ligament has segments that are designed to stabilize the anterior aspect of the sacroiliac joint and the. L5–S1 segment, particularly the action of lateral bending and the force of anterior shear of the fifth lumbar vertebrae on the sacrum. Following bilateral transaction of the iliolumbar ligaments, lateral bending of the spinal segment increases nearly 30 percent, flexion and extension approximately 20 percent, and rotation 18 percent.[61] The iliolumbar ligament is therefore an extremely important structure that stabilizes the lumbar spine on the sacrum.

The quadratus lumborum, working with such structures as the iliolumbar ligament and deep portion of the erector spinae, psoas major, and hip muscles, helps maintain stability of the lumbar spine and pelvis in the frontal, horizontal, and sagittal planes. The iliolumbar ligament "squares" or anchors the L5 vertebra down onto the S1 vertebral body[30] while muscles such as the quadratus lumborum dynamically contribute to stabilization This compressive force of the L5 vertebra is counteracted by the hydrophilic pressure of the L5–S1 intervertebral disk (Fig. 3–33).

Lumbar Musculature: Summary

The thoracolumbar fascia and attached latissimus dorsi, gluteus maximus, internal abdominal oblique, and transversus abdominis are superficially located over the posterior aspect of the lumbopelvic region. The prominent bilateral muscular ridges on the back correspond to the erector spinae and multifidus muscle groups. Just lateral to these ridges, above the level of the iliac crest is the location of the lateral raphe which is the attachment site for the abdominal muscles. Medially, the quadratus lumborum is under cover of the deep erector spinae and multifidus muscles. At the lumbosacral segment the quadratus lumborum muscle is replaced by the iliolumbar ligament. The relations of these structures must be considered when functionally assessing the lumbopelvic region, and exercise programs designed for these muscles must take into account their relationship to the fascia and their actions over the spine and pelvis.

Iliopsoas: Psoas Major and Iliacus Muscles

The psoas major muscle is attached to the anterolateral surfaces of the vertebral bodies and their respective transverse processes, and the lumbar intervertebral discs. The muscle then passes inferiorly and

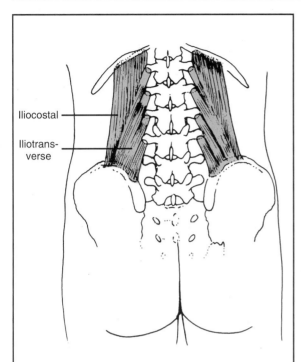

Figure 3–30. Posterior view showing the quadratus lumborum muscle. This muscle has three portions, iliocostal, iliotransverse, and costotransverse. This figure does not show the costotransverse portion because it is often insignificant in its size and function and, if present, lies on the anterior aspect of the muscle. These muscles produce lateral guy wire forces to the lumbar spine.

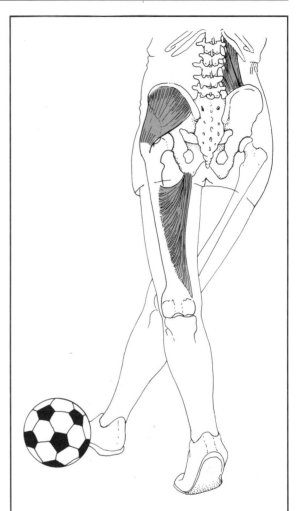

Figure 3–31. Right quadratus lumborum muscle, left gluteus medius muscle, and left femoral adductor muscles working together to stabilize the frontal plane of the pelvis while kicking a soccer ball with the right foot. These muscular forces are necessary to assure nondestructive weight-bearing of the lumbopelvic bone and joint structures.

laterally to merge with the tendon of the iliacus muscle. The iliacus is attached superiorly to the iliac fossa and the inner lip of the iliac crest. The combined tendons then track over the superior lateral aspect of the pubic ramus and attach to the lesser trochanter of the femur (Fig. 3–34). Both the iliacus and the psoas major muscles are normally considered together, thus the term iliopsoas. This discussion reviews the muscles as a synergistic group, and then each muscle is considered individually.

The iliopsoas muscle is a flexor of the femur on the pelvis when the foot is off the ground. This action can occur when the lumbar attachment of the psoas major muscle and the pelvic attachment of the iliacus are fixed or stabilized. By keeping the lumbar spine and

pelvis in a stable, nonmovable position, the femur then becomes the movable segment and flexion of the hip occurs.

The iliopsoas muscle is also a lateral rotator of the femur when the foot is free of the ground. This action can be appreciated by recognizing that in the frontal

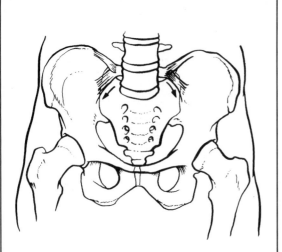

Figure 3–32. Anterior view, iliolumbar ligament. The ligament spans the distance between the transverse processes of the lower lumbar spine and the pelvis. The ligament "pulls" the L5 vertebrae down on the sacrum helping to stabilize the fifth lumbar segment against anterior shear. It is broad enough to also reinforce the anterior aspect of the sacroiliac joint.

plane, the lesser trochanter is positioned posteriorly on the medial surface of the femur. Contraction of this muscle directs a force to the lesser trochanter, pulling it forward, which results in lateral rotation of the femur.

Although these actions are important, the actions of the muscles when the foot is fixed on the ground have greater importance in a discussion of lumbopelvic mechanics. Under these closed kinetic chain conditions the insertion at the lesser trochanter becomes the fixed end, and force occurs at the pelvis in the case of the iliacus muscle, and at the lumbar spine in the case of the psoas major muscle.

For example, when the foot is fixed on the ground and contraction of the iliacus muscle occurs, the resultant force to the ilium produces an anterior torsion of the ilium and extension of the lumbosacral zygapophyseal joints (Fig. 3–34). Anterior torsion of the ilium represents a forward and downward movement of the anterior superior iliac spines. Extension to the lumbosacral joints occurs as a result of the anterior pelvic rotation, which causes the superior articular process of S1 to move up on the inferior articular process of the L5 vertebrae.

If there is decreased length of the muscle due to adaptive shortening, or if there is increased efferent

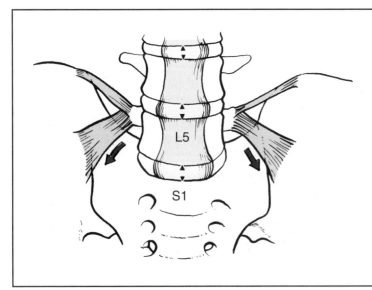

Figure 3–33. The compressive force between the fifth lumbar vertebrae and sacrum—due to ligamentous pre-stress (such as that exerted by the iliolumbar ligament and longitudinal ligaments)—and the force of muscle contraction, is countered by the hydrophilic pressure of the L5–S1 intervertebral disc and the articular cartilages of the facets.

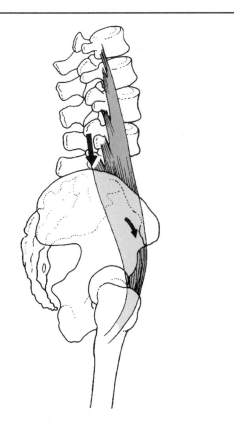

Figure 3–34. Anterior view showing the iliopsoas muscle complex. It is directed inferiorly and anteriorly above the pubic ramus, and inferiorly and posteriorly below the pubic ramus; eventually attaching to the lesser trochanter of the femur. This results in an anterior shear at the lumbar spine and a downward and forward tilt of the pelvis.

lumbar extension), and flexion of the lumbopelvic unit on the femur.

Consider for example the pregnant female in her second or third trimester. The weight of the fetus and the increased lever arm length at which this weight acts from the axis of the lumbar spine results in a much greater shear and extension stress to the lumbar spine. One compensation to minimize shear stress to the lumbar spine is to laterally rotate the femurs and walk with a toe-out gait pattern. Such a gait pattern decreases the tension in the psoas major (internal rotation of the hip would stretch the psoas major and increase tension), and this decreased muscle tension over the lumbar spine lessens the anterior shear imparted by the psoas major (Fig. 3–35). It is also common to note the patient

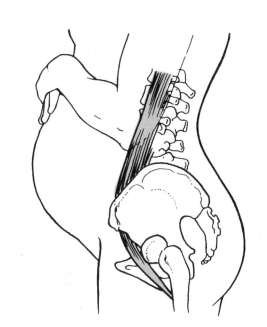

Figure 3–35. During the last trimester, the female's center of gravity lies more anterior increasing the shear over the lumbar spine. By externally rotating the hips during gait, tension is lessened in the psoas major (and hip capsule), which lessens the anterior shear. In the standing position, internal rotation would tighten the psoas and hip capsules, increasing shear stress at the lumbar spine.

neural input into the muscle, then a downwardly tilted or anteriorly rotated position of the complete pelvis results. This increases the compressive and anterior shear stress on the lumbosacral and lumbar zygapophyseal joints because they move toward increased extension (see Chapter 4).

The psoas major muscle has different actions than the iliacus by virtue of its lumbar attachments when the foot is fixed to the ground. The force at the lumbar spine is one of anterior shear which potentially increases the lumbar lordosis (increased

with a pendulous abdomen, weakened abdominal wall, and tight hip flexors walking with a toe-out gait for the same reason. They are attempting to minimize the compression and anterior shear stress to the lumbar spine (Fig. 3–36).

It has been noted that the psoas major muscle is electromyographically active in many different postures and movements, and that psoas activity adds a compressive effect on the lumbar body–intervertebral disc interface resulting in increased intradiscal pressure.[37] Since the muscle directly crosses the vertebral body and intervertebral disc, it is easy to ascertain how compression occurs. The increased compression occurring as a result of muscle contraction increases the stability of the lumbar in antigravity postures.

It is interesting to note that the psoas major muscle is more consistently active than other trunk muscles when a person assumes different positions. When the importance of stability of the lumbar spine rather than actual movement is appreciated, the stabilization role of the psoas major muscle becomes important to consider. An example is the theoretical guy wire action of the psoas muscle as it works with the deep portion of the erector spinae, multifidus, and quadratus lumborum muscles for stability in the sagittal, frontal, and horizontal planes. The guy wire stabilization concept, coupled with the compression of the vertebral bodies in the weight-bearing postures, results in securing the interlocking assembly of the lower lumbar articulations. This in turn renders the lumbar joints more resistant to various forces and motions. In both stabilization and movement roles the iliopsoas muscle presumably contracts to counterbalance the forces of the posterior lumbar muscles creating equilibrium. The balance, most likely occurring as a result of central mediated motor control mechanisms, helps optimize force attenuation through lumbar vertebral tissues.

Depending on the side to which the spine is laterally bent and rotated, both psoas major muscles must respond appropriately. Gracovetsky and Farfan[21] present a mathematical model describing the function of the psoas major muscle in lifting and walking. The iliopsoas muscle appears to have a significant function in the three cardinal planes of motion; thus the importance of adequate strength and coordination of the iliopsoas muscle in stabilization and movement of the lumbar spine.

A consideration of the adequacy of muscle length is equally important. When the normal postural positions of the adult are analyzed, it is apparent that a sit-

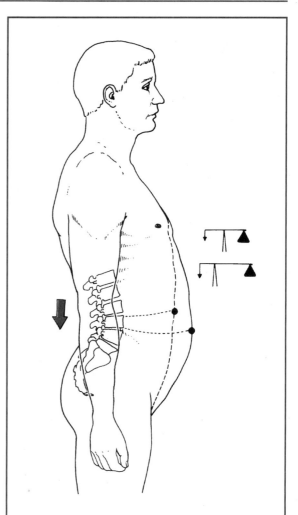

Figure 3–36. A pendulous abdomen renders the lumbar spine vulnerable to increased weight-bearing demands. In the example of the abdomen (1) the distance from the center of the spine and the abdominal wall is X, and the muscle force to counterbalance the lever arm is Y. In example (2), the distance from the center of the spine and the abdominal wall is X+ and the muscle force to counteract the lever arm is Y+. This increased muscular force results in elevated lumbar vertebral weight-bearing and increased shear stress. (Adapted from White AA, Panjabi MM: Clinical Biomechanics of the Spine. J. B. Lippincott, Philadelphia, 1978).

ting position is common in both work and rest. The effect of these prolonged postures coupled with an inadequate abdominal mechanism might result in adaptive shortening of the iliopsoas muscle as well as other hip flexors. When the person now assumes the upright position, or an attempt is made to place the hip into hyperextension, the pelvis is pulled into anterior rotation, the lumbar spine is pulled forward and downward, and an extension moment and compressive force on the lumbar zygapophyseal joints is generated. This potentially results in prolonged and excessive compressive loading to the bony elements of the posterior arch of the lumbar vertebrae. The question that needs to be asked is whether this type of loading begins to exceed the optimal loading capacity of the tissues, potentially resulting in injury or adaption such as lamina thickening.

If this posture is further compounded by a pendulous abdomen and in particular weakness of the abdominal muscles and hip degeneration, it is readily apparent that such mechanics may be injurious because they result in excessive loads to the tissues. To maintain the upright posture and counterbalance the pendulous abdomen, the person must further extend the trunk, increasing the weight-bearing demands on the lumbar tissues under compression (Fig. 3–36). Posterior lumbar tissues, such as the zygapophyseal joints, may be the source of pain, but the cause is probably altered postural mechanics.

The function of the psoas major muscle must, therefore, be looked at in terms of strength, coordination, and adequate length. Because it is strategically placed, it has numerous control functions related to lumbar spine motions, and shortness or altered contraction patterns of the muscle jeopardize the normal biomechanical relation between the intervertebral discs and zygapophyseal joints.

THE ABDOMINAL MUSCULATURE AND ITS RELATED FASCIAL SYSTEM

The vertebrae, intervertebral disc, zygapophyseal joints, and intervening soft tissues of the vertebral column are subjected to significant forces during work, athletics, and daily activities. In its simplest description, the spine can be considered to be an elastic rod that must respond in many ways to forces placed on it. One of the key muscle units contributing to mobility and stability of the lumbar spine and pelvis is the abdominal wall mechanism.

The abdominal wall consists of the external abdominal oblique, internal abdominal oblique, transversus abdominis, and rectus abdominis muscles, and the fascial contributions of these muscles that form their respective aponeurosis and contribute to the rectus sheath. The abdominal wall musculature has been extensively studied both experimentally and through mathematical modeling.[2, 22, 36, 39, 47, 50] Various roles have been attributed to the musculature related to the spine and most authorities agree that this muscle group is extremely important in offering stability to the vertebral column.

Just as the muscles of the low back were largely described around their relationship to the thoracolumbar fascia, the abdominal muscles will be described in relationship to the abdominal fascia.

Abdominal Fascia

There are several layers of superficial fascia (fatty layer, membranous layer, and deep layer) which lie above the anterior abdominal wall. They are connected to the superficial fascias of the thigh and perineum, and will not be detailed in this text.

The fascia that will be detailed is directly related to the abdominal muscles, and presents as *the aponeuroses* of the external and internal abdominal oblique and transverse abdominis muscles, and the *rectus sheath* related to the rectus abdominus muscle (Fig. 3–37). The aponeuroses and the rectus sheath are directly related (Table 3-2). As the aponeuroses of the three muscles course anteriorly, they enclose the rectus abdominis from the rectus sheath. However, the formation of the rectus sheath by the different layers of aponeuroses is different in the region above the umbilicus, and below the umbilicus (Fig. 3–38). The anteriorly placed latticework arrangement of the abdominal fascia is similar to the lattice-work of the thoracolumbar fascia posteriorly. These fascial sheaths will now be discussed in relationship to the specific abdominal muscles.

External Abdominal Oblique

The external abdominal oblique muscle originates by way of fleshy digitations to the last eight ribs and extends inferiorly to insert into the iliac crest, and inferiorly and medially to blend with the abdominal

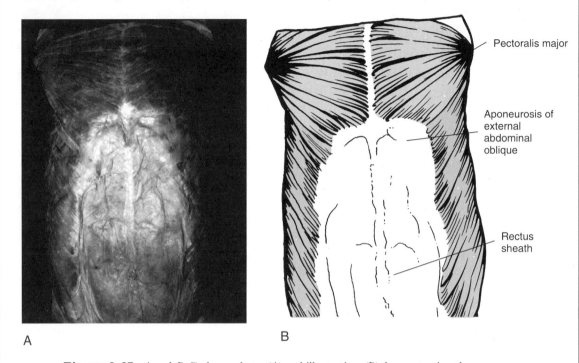

Pectoralis major

Aponeurosis of
external
abdominal
oblique

Rectus
sheath

A

B

Figure 3–37. *A* and *B*, Cadaver photo *(A)* and illustration *(B)* demonstrating the aponeurosis of the external oblique and the rectus sheath. Note the relationship of the pectoralis muscle with the rectus sheath. Both the external abdominal oblique and the pectoralis are mechanically linked to the rectus sheath.

aponeurosis, which in turn attaches to the linea alba (Fig. 3–39). It is the largest and most superficial anterolateral muscle.[58] Between the anterior superior iliac spine and pubic tubercle it forms a thick, inrolled band known as the inguinal ligament. Close inspection of the external abdominal oblique reveals that it interdigitates and is typically fused with the serratus anterior muscle (Fig. 3–40). In addition, the pectoralis major muscle and its fascial elements blend into the aponeurosis of the abdominal muscles and often cross the midline to blend with the abdominal fascia on the opposite side and the superficial aspect of the rectus sheath (Fig. 3–41). These "linkages" between shoulder girdle muscles and the abdominal musculature should be appreciated when analyzing or designing exercises to train the abdominal mechanism. Chapter 6 illustrates several exercises taking advantage of this anatomical arrangement, such as pullover exercises

with a free weight, standing "crunch" type of exercise, and pressing activities with free weights to simultaneously recruit the serratus anterior and pectoralis major as protractors of the scapula, and external abdominal oblique muscles as a trunk flexor.

The functions of the external abdominal oblique include flexing the vertebral column by bringing the thorax closer to the pelvis, flexing the lumbosacral junction by posteriorly rotating the pelvis, compressing the abdominal viscera posteriorly against the spine, increasing tension on the abdominal fascia, and rotating the thorax to the contralateral side (Table 3–3). Note that for the right external abdominal oblique muscle to rotate the thorax to the left, a synergistic contraction by multifidus muscles to cancel the flexion vector of the external oblique and allow the thorax to move in pure rotation is necessary. The inferior and medial direction of the fibers of the external abdom-

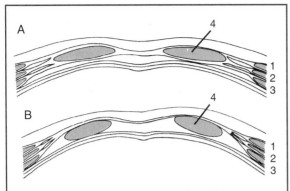

Figure 3–38. Transverse section of the rectus sheath seen at two levels. *A*, Between the costal margin and the level of the anterior superior iliac spine (above the umbilicus), and *B*, below the level of the anterior superior iliac spine (below the umbilicus).

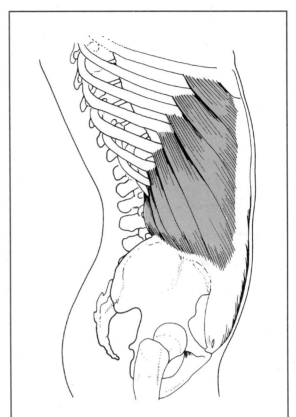

Figure 3–39. The attachments of the external abdominal oblique muscle from the ribs to the iliac crest. This muscle helps check the downward and forward motion of the pelvis, i.e., check the anterior tilt of the pelvis and extension of the lumbosacral joints.

inal oblique muscle are positioned to help check the downward and forward motion of the pelvis.[28]

Internal Abdominal Oblique

The internal abdominal oblique muscle lies deep to the external abdominal oblique muscle (Fig. 3–42). This muscle is attached to the lateral half of the inguinal ligament, the iliac crest, and the inferior portion of the lateral raphe of the thoracolumbar fascia. From these attachments the muscle extends superiorly and medially to insert into the cartilaginous border of the last three or four ribs, the abdominal aponeurosis, and the linea alba (Fig. 3–43). Above the umbilicus the aponeurosis splits at the lateral border of the rectus abdominis and courses anterior and posterior to the rectus abdominis (Fig. 3–38). Below the umbilicus, however, the aponeurosis stays "double walled" and courses in front of the rectus abdominis. Note that this region (below the umbilicus) where a "double wall" of fascial aponeurosis is placed corresponds to the region of maximal anterior shear stress at the lumbar spine.

Actions of the internal abdominal obliques include compressing the abdominal contents posteriorly against the spine, increasing tension through the thoracolumbar and abdominal fascia, flexing the spine by bringing the thorax closer to the pelvis, and rotating the thorax on the pelvis (Table 3-3).

Transversus Abdominis

The transversus abdominis muscle is located deep to the internal abdominal oblique muscle (Fig. 3–44). It is attached to the lateral one-third of the inguinal ligament, the inner lip of the iliac crest, and the thoracolumbar fascia in a common attachment shared with the internal abdominal oblique muscle. The fiber direction is more horizontal than that of the internal oblique muscle as it travels to attach to the abdominal aponeurosis and the linea alba. The transversus abdominis aponeurosis courses anteriorly to the rectus abdomin-

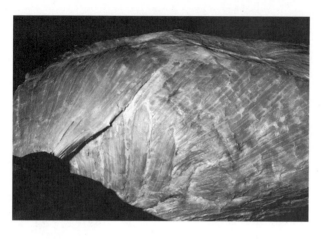

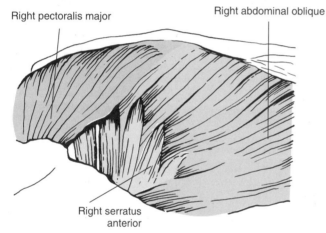

Right pectoralis major

Right abdominal oblique

Right serratus anterior

Figure 3–40. *A* and *B*, The serratus anterior muscle interdigitates and is often fused to the external abdominal oblique muscle. There is a strong mechanical linkage between the pectoralis major, serratus anterior, and abdominal muscles as can be seen in this view.

is below the level of the umbilicus, further reinforcing the anterior fascial support at the level of the lumbar spine subject to maximal anterior shear. Actions of the transversus abdominis include compressing the abdominal contents and increasing tension to the thoracolumbar and abdominal fascia such as would occur when one attempts to "pull their abdomen in" away from their beltline (Table 3-3).

Rectus Abdominus

The last component of the abdominal wall is the rectus abdominis muscle. This muscle extends vertically from the pubic tubercles to attach to the lower rib cage on either side of the sternum. The rectus abdominis muscle is long and straplike, and divided by intermuscular connective tissue bands (Fig. 3–45). The oblique muscles attach to the rectus sheath at the level of these tendinous intersections, thereby exerting a laterally directed force to the rectus sheath and anchoring these tendinous intersections (Fig. 3–46). Note how such an attachment affords a mechanical link between the pull of the obliques and the pull of the rectus abdominis. A lateral pull at the intermuscular septa stabilizes the rectus attachments and in essence results in the rectus abdominis functioning segmentally rather than simply as one long strap muscle. The rectus abdominis muscles lie on either side of the linea alba and fill the rectus sheath,

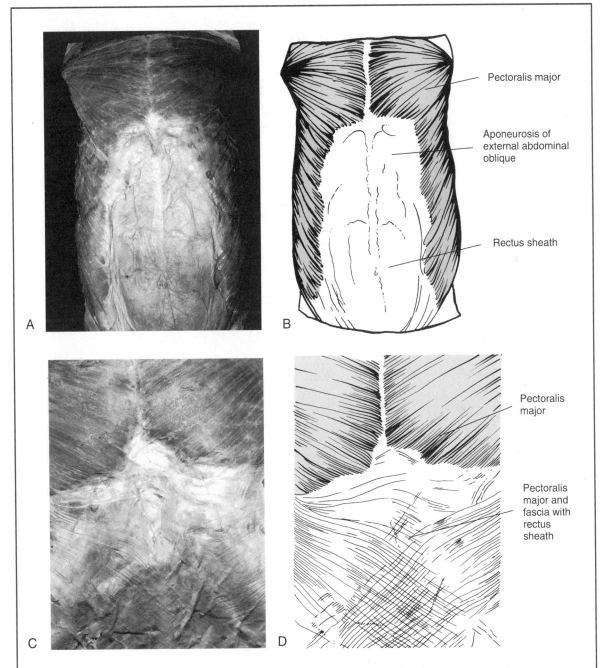

Figure 3–41. *A* and *B*, Pectoralis major and external abdominal oblique and their relationship to the rectus sheath. *C* and *D*, Close-up view of fibers of the pectoralis attachment crossing midline and blending with rectus sheath. The pectoralis major muscle and its fascial elements blend into the aponeurosis of the abdominal muscles and often cross the midline to blend with the aponeurosis of the opposite side.

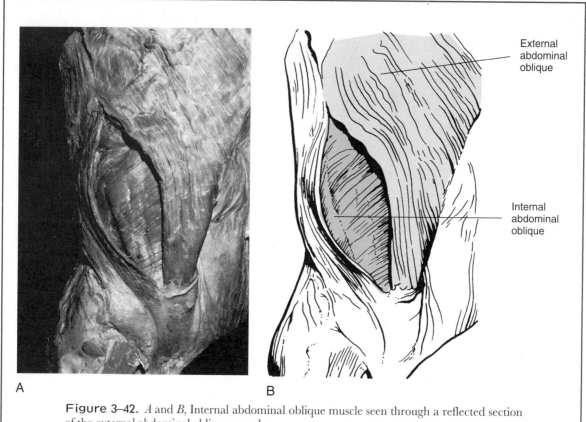

A   B

Figure 3–42. *A* and *B*, Internal abdominal oblique muscle seen through a reflected section of the external abdominal oblique muscle.

and are positioned to flex the trunk check anterior shear as well as to help contain the abdominal contents (Table 3-3).

As noted above, the rectus abdominis muscle is surrounded by its own fascial layer (the rectus sheath), formed by the individual aponeurotic contributions of the transversus abdominis, external oblique, and internal oblique muscles as they converge toward the linea alba (Fig. 3–38). Above the umbilicus the external oblique muscle sends its aponeurosis anterior to the rectus abdominis. The aponeurosis of the internal abdominal oblique muscle splits at the lateral border of the rectus abdominis, and the aponeurosis passes anterior and posterior to it. The aponeurosis of the transversus abdominis muscle travels behind the rectus abdominis muscle.

Below the umbilicus, all three lateral abdominal muscles pass aponeurotic expansions anterior to the rectus abdominis muscle. One explanation for such an arrangement might be that below the umbilicus the added aponeurosis anterior to the rectus abdominis offers additional connective tissue support to counter the anterior shear stress of the lumbar spine and abdominal viscera in this region. The extra fascial support is perhaps a response to the forces generated from the lordotic angle at the corresponding level in the lumbar spine (i.e., the L4–L5 and L5–S1 region). In this region of the lumbar spine, the rate of curvature is greater than the rate of curvature for the upper lumbar spine. Accompanying this lordotic curve is the increased inferiorly and anteriorly directed force of the abdominal contents, which

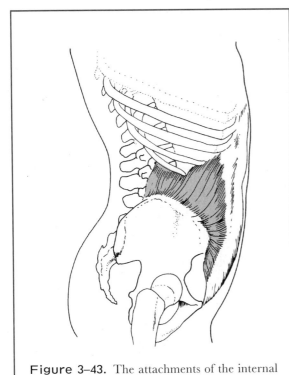

Figure 3–43. The attachments of the internal abdominal oblique muscle.

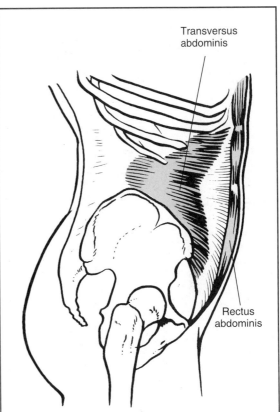

Figure 3–44. Attachments of the transversus abdominis muscle. Note how the fiber direction of this muscle compresses the abdominal contents, as if one is attempting to pull their abdomen in, away from the beltline.

helps create the need for the additional connective tissue support.

Functions of the Abdominal Mechanism

Table 3-4 lists the essential functions of the abdominal wall mechanism. Each will now be briefly discussed relative to the mechanics of the lumbopelvic regions.

Provide anterior and anterolateral support to the spine

One of the classic theories of the role of the abdominal mechanism considers the trunk as a cylinder, with the walls of the cylinder being the abdominal muscles and their associated aponeuroses.[36] As walls of the cylinder, the abdominal mechanism works with the pelvic floor, diaphragm, and epiglottis, to convert the thoracic and abdominal chambers, that are filled with air and semisolid contents, into rigid cylinders. These cylinders theoretically help unload the spine by actually transmitting part of the forces applied. The cavities become pressurized cylinders that help absorb forces. This is one of the basic principles behind the use of abdominal binders, lumbar supports, and weight belts.

Gracovetsky and Farfan[22] have taken this concept of increased intra-abdominal pressure one step further. Rather than consider that the intra-abdominal pressure unloads the spine, they suggest that the oblique direction of the abdominal muscle fibers contract around a pressurized cylinder instead of simply

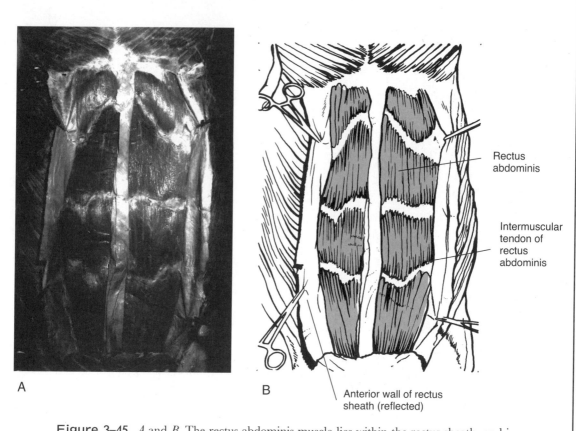

A   B

Rectus
abdominis

Intermuscular
tendon of
rectus
abdominis

Anterior wall of rectus
sheath (reflected)

Figure 3–45. *A* and *B,* The rectus abdominis muscle lies within the rectus sheath, and is divided by intermuscular connective tissue strands.

contracting and collapsing toward the center. They theorize that the internal oblique and transversus abdominis muscles exert a lateral and posteriorly directed pull to their attachment at the lateral raphe of the thoracolumbar fascia. As previously described, the lateral raphe lies posterior and lateral to the transverse process of the vertebrae.

By containing the abdominal contents within this walled cylinder, anterior shear of the lumbar lordosis is countered by the force of the abdominal wall as it lifts and pushes the abdominal contents back against the anterior aspect of the lumbar spine (Fig. 3–47). This mechanism is illustrated by the simple exercise of standing and pulling the abdomen in and away from one's beltline.

Increase tension to the thoracolumbar and abdominal fascia

Connective tissues such as ligaments, joint capsules, and fascia require tension to stabilize bone segments. Tesh and associates[50] suggest that the transversus abdominis muscle and the internal abdominal oblique muscle attach by way of the deep layer of the thoracolumbar fascia in a direct line to the transverse process, and consequently contribute to the stability of the spine by a laterally directed pull on the vertebrae (Fig. 3–13). The controlled contraction of the abdominal wall would minimize lumbar movement in the frontal and horizontal planes and also minimize aberrational translation movements between each vertebrae. Like-

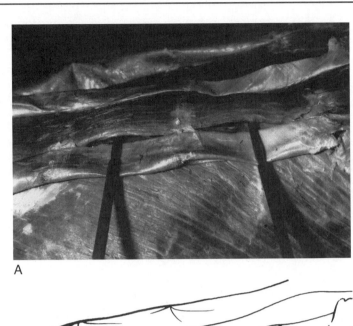

A

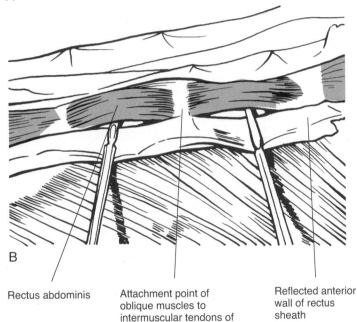

B

| Rectus abdominis | Attachment point of oblique muscles to intermuscular tendons of rectus abdominis | Reflected anterior wall of rectus sheath |

Figure 3–46. *A* and *B*, Attachment of the oblique muscles to the rectus sheath, which helps anchor the tendinous intersections. The attachment affords a mechanical link between the abdominal obliques and the rectus abdominis.

wise, the attachment of the external oblique to the ribs and the iliac crest provides efficient leverage, relative to the lumbopelvic joints, to offer a resistance to axial rotation and lateral motions.

Because the abdominal muscles blend with the abdominal aponeuroses anteriorly, contraction of the muscles increases tension on this important anterior strut of the abdomen. In addition, contraction of the rectus abdominis creates a broadening effect within the rectus sheath, further increasing tension in the aponeurosis (Table 3-4). The oblique muscles are also mechanically linked to the rectus sheath at the regions

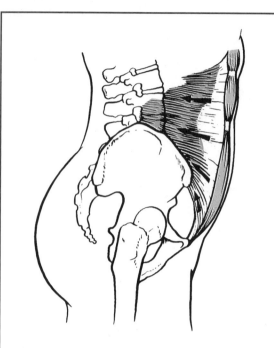

Figure 3–47. Contraction of the abdominal muscles helps contain the abdominal contents within the cavity by "pushing" the abdominal contents up and back against the spine. This force helps counter the anterior shear of the lumbar spine that results from the gravitational force on the abdominal contents.

decreases the lumbosacral angle and as the lumbosacral angle is decreased, there is less anterior shear of the fifth lumbar vertebrae on the sacrum owing to the more horizontal positioning of the sacrum (Fig. 3–48). The flexion moment on the lumbosacral junction results in less compression at the apophyseal joints and increased compression at the bone–intervertebral disc interface.[1, 15] Only a few degrees of flexion are actually needed to relieve the apophyseal joints of this compressive loading, and a moderately flexed posture optimally loads the bone–intervertebral disc–bone interface, and the apophyseal joints.[13] The moderately flexed posture is a preferred posture for lifting as it minimizes anterior shear, properly distributes compressive stresses across the vertebral body and apophyseal joints, and allows the specialized connective tissues posterior to the axis of motion to store strain

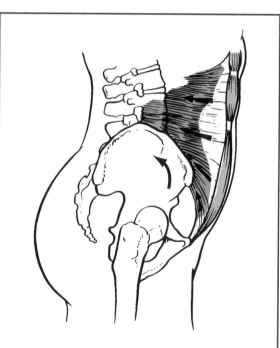

Figure 3–48. Contraction of the abdominal muscles results in posterior tilt of the pelvis, which decreases the lumbosacral angle. A decrease in the lumbosacral angle results in decreased anterior shear at the lumbosacral junction and decreased compression at the apophyseal joints.

of the tendinous insertions of the rectus abdominis. Figure 3-46 illustrates the mechanical linkage between the abdominal muscles, and key muscles of the shoulder girdle, the pectoralis major and serratus anterior muscles. Contraction of these muscles against resistance exerts increased tensile stress in the abdominal fascia through the abdominal muscles, much in the same way the latissimus dorsi muscle transmits increased tension to the thoracolumbar fascia.

Check anterior shear via control of pelvis in sagittal plane

The rectus abdominus, external oblique, and internal oblique exert a flexion moment over the lumbosacral junction by posteriorly rotating ("upwardly tilting") the pelvis. This posterior rotation of the pelvis

energy and generate significant extensor moments across the lumbar spine. Trained subjects average 57 percent lumbar flexion when lifting weights from a floor even if they try their best to "keep a lordosis while lifting."[13] Thus, although individuals are often given the instruction "keep your back hollow or arched" the reality is that the lumbar spine flexes during any lift. The abdominal muscles minimize compressive loading at the vertebral arch and the resultant shear that accompanies such lifting postures.

Control the rate and amplitude of torsion to lumbar spine

Because of their attachments to the rib cage and the pelvis, the abdominal muscles are effective rotators of the spine. However, there is only a small degree of rotary motion available at each lumbar zygapophyseal joint (see Chapter 4). High torsional stresses increase compressive loads between the facets of the apophyseal joints on the side opposite the direction of rotation in the lumbar spine. In addition, torsion increases tension to the collagen framework of the annulus fibrosus of the intervertebral disc. Although there are restraints to excessive torsion from the passive, inert tissues, the abdominal muscles offer one of the dynamic restraints. Rather than considering the abdominal muscles as flexors and rotators of the trunk—for which they certainly have the capacity—their function might be better viewed as antirotators and antilateral flexors of the trunk, illustrated by stabilization of the trunk against excessive rotary forces that accompany upper and lower extremity motions.

As mentioned previously, the degree of curvature in the lower lumbar spine is greater than that in the upper lumbar spine. This is of interest because the majority of zygapophyseal joint and disc degeneration problems are usually greater in the lower lumbar region. Many activities require motion of the lumbar spine. Recognizing that only small amounts of lateral bend or axial rotation cause obligatory coupled motion, a muscular design that decreases the chance for destructive forces to reach the lower lumbar spine is essential.

Control relationship of abdominal wall to thorax

By "pushing" the abdominal contents posteriorly against the spine, and simultaneously upward against the diaphragm, the abdominal muscles assist in maintaining the spatial relationship between the thorax, abdomen, and pelvis (Fig. 3–49). Patients with upper-quarter pain often present with a rounded shoulder and forward head postures. One of the contributing factors to this posture is a weakened abdominal wall that results in the sternum and chest being carried more caudally. The change in thorax posture results in the scapulae assuming a more protracted and elevated position and the head and neck brought forward over the thorax.[44] Strength of the abdominal mechanism is important because it controls not only the position of the pelvis in the sagittal plane but the relationship of the shoulder girdle and thorax to the abdominal cavity and pelvis. The abdominal mechanism should be assessed in all patients complaining of upper-quarter pain and having a forward head posture in sitting or standing.

Increase compression at sacroiliac joints and pubic symphysis

The sacroiliac joint is subject to significant shear stresses as a result of ground forces and trunk forces converging into the pelvis. Although the joint has an exceptional degree of ligamentous support, muscle action contributes significantly to the stability of the sacroiliac joint. This is especially true for muscle–fascial units, which cross perpendicular to the joint plane and thus have the effect of increasing joint compression. Compression of the joint surfaces increases friction between the sacrum and ilium and the result is to contribute to stability of the sacroiliac joint.

The obliquely directed fibers of the external and internal abdominal oblique muscles tie into an abdominal fascial network that decussates across the midline. The resultant abdominal oblique muscle activity increases the compressive force between the two pubic bones at the pubic symphysis. Even more significantly, however, contraction of the abdominal muscles also increases the compression at the sacroiliac joint (Fig. 3–50). The interosseous ligament of the sacroiliac joint lies posterior to the sacroiliac joint cavity and is essentially nonyielding to tensile stress. The abdominal muscles pull the iliac crests medially via their contraction in a manner similar to the mechanics of a nutcracker. In this case, the hinge of the nutcracker is represented by the interosseous ligament, and compression of a nut just in front of this hinge represents the location of the

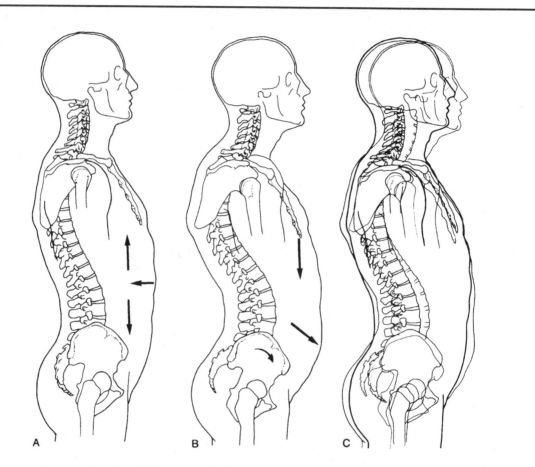

Figure 3–49. The abdominal wall helps maintain the spatial rdelationships between the thorax, abdomen, and pelvis. Loss of this relationship results in the forward head, rounded shoulder posture.

synovial joint cavity. Just as one might squeeze the two handles of a nutcracker together to apply a compressive force to the nut, contraction of the abdominal muscles over the "handles" of the ilium increases the compressive force and stability at the sacroiliac joint.

Abdominal Muscle Summary

The muscular design of the abdominal wall illustrates the concept of dynamic stabilization and the importance of muscle strength in helping attenuate trunk and ground forces. This section also illustrates the intimate relationship the abdominal muscles have with the thoracolumbar and abdominal facial systems. In addition, it is important to note the connections between the powerful latissimus dorsi, pectoralis major, serratus anterior, and the abdominal muscles that create a mechanical linkage between the shoulder girdle and the abdominal musculature. The abdominal muscles make extremely important contributions to the mobility and stability requirements of the lumbopelvic region, and minimize excessive loading of the specialized connective tissues.

Abdominal wall musculature without adequate endurance, strength, and coordination is more likely

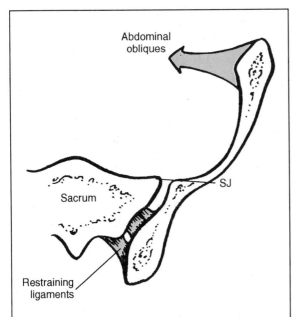

Figure 3–50. Contraction of the abdominal oblique muscles, acting over the fulcrum of the interosseous ligament, increase sacroiliac joint (SJ) and pubic symphysis compression.

to permit other lumbar-stabilizing and weight-bearing tissues to be taken past their physiologic limit, such as excessive tensile forces on the annulus fibrosus or excessive compressive forces on the zygapophyseal joints. Thus, the musculature of the abdominal wall plays a considerable role in the maintenance of a healthy lumbopelvic region.

HIP AND THIGH MUSCULATURE AND ITS RELATED FASCIA LATA SYSTEM

Fascia Lata

The final fascial complex to be discussed relative to the musculature of the lumbopelvic region is the fascia lata system of the thigh. As with the thoracolumbar fascia and abdominal fascia, muscles attach directly to the fascia lata and can increase fascial tension via

contraction, and since they are also encased within the fascia, the broadening effect of contraction will also increase tension. This suggests that muscle hypertrophy results in increased fascia lata tension (see Table 3–5).

The fascia lata is the deep fascia of the thigh, as opposed to the superficial fascia which is the layer immediately under the skin largely impregnated with fat. The fascia lata splits to enclose the gluteus maximus muscle. Above the gluteus maximus it is a single layer covering the gluteus medius muscle and attached posteriorly to the iliac crest, sacrum, coccyx, and sacrotuberous ligament, and anteriorly to the pubic rami. Distally, the fascia lata is attached to all bony prominences of the knee such as the condyles of the femur and tibia, but it has an especially strong attachment to the lateral tibial condyle where it is blended with an aponeurotic expansion from the vastus lateralis. The subcutaneous ridge seen on the lateral side of the fully extended knee is the iliotibial tract portion of the fascia lata.

Two septa subdivide the fascia lata, and ultimately form three compartments within the thigh (Fig. 3–51). The compartments house the adductor muscles posteromedially, the hamstrings posterolaterally, and the quadriceps anteriorly, anteromedially, and anterolaterally.

Muscles of the Hip

The psoas major muscles have been previously described with the muscles of the lumbar spine, since the psoas major has significant attachments to the lumbar spine. A review of the remaining musculature and fascia of the hip is essential to appreciate the influence of lower extremity muscle actions over the lumbopelvic region.

There are 29 muscles that originate or insert into the pelvis. Twenty of these muscles link the pelvis with the femur, and the remainder link the pelvis with the spine. This implies that significant forces can be generated through the pelvis and subsequently into the lumbar spine by various combinations of hip and knee muscle activity and is most likely the reason why it is easier to stabilize the pelvis from the standing position than sitting. It is not just the muscles above the pelvis (lumbar spine and abdominal wall musculature) but also the muscles from below (muscles of the hip and knee joints) that work synergistically to assure proper attenuation of forces through the lumbar spine. When

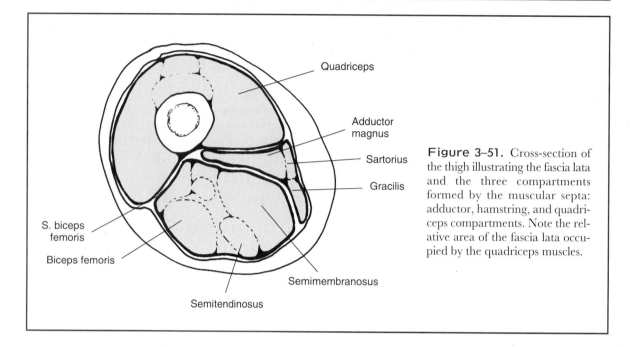

Quadriceps

Adductor magnus

Sartorius

Gracilis

S. biceps femoris

Biceps femoris

Semimembranosus

Semitendinosus

Figure 3–51. Cross-section of the thigh illustrating the fascia lata and the three compartments formed by the muscular septa: adductor, hamstring, and quadriceps compartments. Note the relative area of the fascia lata occupied by the quadriceps muscles.

the foot is fixed on the ground and the individual is weight-bearing through the lower extremity, a closed kinetic chain is established. Contraction of the hip musculature does not necessarily move the femur on the pelvis; instead, the pelvis is made to move on the lumbar spine. In addition, several of the powerful hip muscles cross the sacroiliac joint and are mechanically linked to the musculature of the lumbar spine, significantly influencing lumbopelvic mechanics.

Gluteus Maximus

The gluteus maximus muscles are a large and powerful muscle group with distinctive attachments and function. From a sweeping attachment at the iliac crest, gluteal raphe, thoracolumbar fascia, sacrum, coccyx, and sacrotuberous ligament, the muscle courses inferolaterally to attach to the fascia lata of the thigh and the gluteal tuberosity of the femur (Fig. 3–52, 3–53, and 3–54).

There are several important considerations relative to these attachments. The connection to the thoracolumbar fascia effectively links this powerful muscle to the contralateral latissimus dorsi (Fig. 3–11). Contraction of the gluteus maximus increases tension to the thoracolumbar fascia, which increases lumbar stabil-

ity. Simultaneous contraction of the gluteus maximus and contralateral latissimus dorsi has an even more pronounced effect over the thoracolumbar fascia. In addition, the linkage between the gluteus maximus and the contralateral latissimus dorsi spans the sacroiliac articulation, and contraction increases compression between the joint surfaces, which increases joint stability.[55]

The gluteal raphe is a unique region over the posteromedial aspect of the pelvis that links the gluteus maximus with the multifidus muscles and the erector spinae aponeurosis (Fig. 3–53). Located at the superomedial aspect of the gluteus maximus, the raphe can be seen as a connective tissue junction blending the gluteus maximus with the superficial erector spinae and the multifidus muscles. This essentially converts the three most powerful extensors on the posterior aspect of the body into an extensive extensor muscle assemblage spanning the lumbar spine, pelvis, and hip.

The attachment of the gluteus maximus to the sacrotuberous ligament also contributes to the dynamic stabilization of the sacroiliac joint (Fig. 3–54). Tension to the sacrotuberous ligament is increased by pull of the gluteus maximus. With increased tension to the sacrotuberous ligament, motion between the sacrum and ilium is minimized, resulting in increased stability of the sacroiliac joint (see Chapter 4).[56]

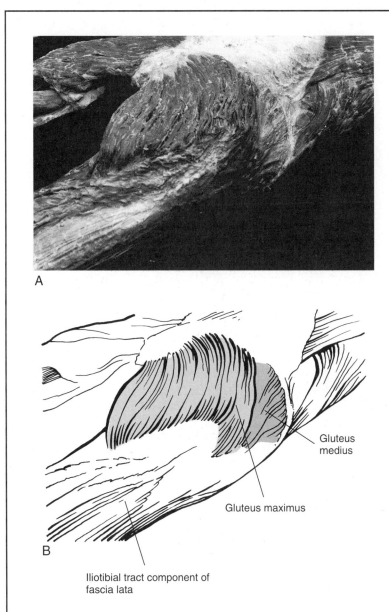

Figure 3–52. *A* and *B,* The broad attachments of the gluteus maximus include the iliac crest, gluteal raphe, thoracolumbar fascia, sacrum, coccyx, and sacrotuberous ligament. From these points, the muscle courses inferolaterally to attach to the fascia lata of the thigh and the gluteal tuberosity of the femur.

As the gluteus maximus courses inferolaterally, it has an expansive attachment to the fascia lata of the thigh, especially to the specialized thickening of the lateral aspect of this fascia, the fascia lata. The majority of the gluteus maximus inserts into this fascia, and the remaining part inserts into the gluteal tuberosity of the femur. That the largest muscle in the human

body inserts primarily into fascia rather than bone suggests complex mechanical functions. The fascia lata spans the hip and knee joints, and contraction of the gluteus maximus increases tension of this extensive fascial system. Increased tissue tension of the fascia lata system potentially enhances stability at the hip and the knee.

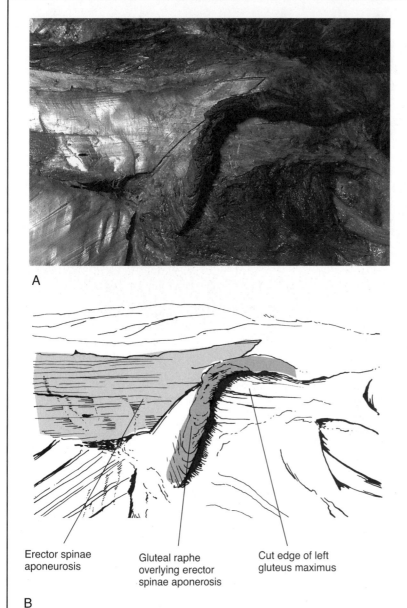

A

B

Erector spinae
aponeurosis

Gluteal raphe
overlying erector
spinae aponerosis

Cut edge of left
gluteus maximus

Figure 3–53. The gluteal raphe provides a mechanical link between the multifidus muscle and erector spinae aponeurosis. *A* and *B*, It is located at the superomedial aspect of the gluteus maximus and serves as a connective tissue junction between this muscle and the powerful spine extensors.

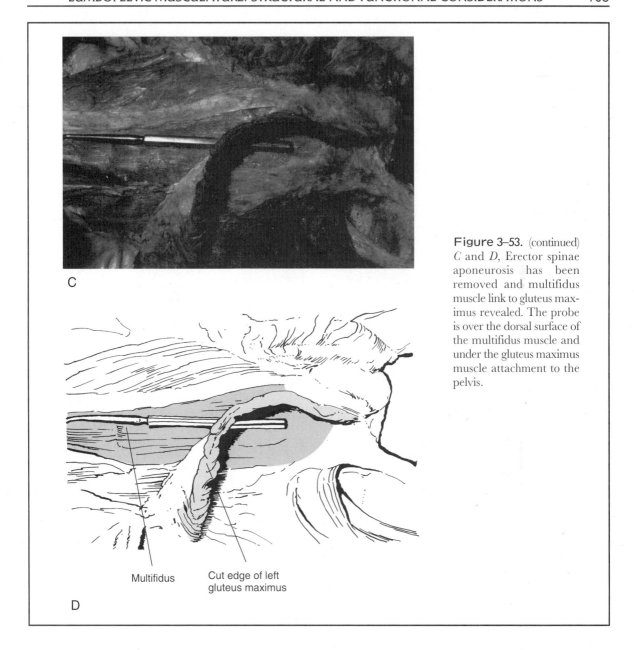

C

Figure 3–53. (continued) *C* and *D*, Erector spinae aponeurosis has been removed and multifidus muscle link to gluteus maximus revealed. The probe is over the dorsal surface of the multifidus muscle and under the gluteus maximus muscle attachment to the pelvis.

Multifidus   Cut edge of left
                gluteus maximus

D

In addition to the above functions, the gluteus maximus is a powerful influence on the postural position of the pelvis in the sagittal plane. With the foot on the ground, contraction of the gluteus maximus in this closed kinetic chain results in a posterior rotary moment of the pelvis. This posterior rotation creates a flexion moment at the lumbosacral junction (Fig. 3–14). By flexing the lumbosacral articulation, the lumbosacral angle is decreased and the anterior shear stress between the fifth lumbar vertebrae and the sacrum is lessened. The lumbosacral flexion moment also minimizes the compressive force between the apophyseal joints. This type of postural positioning is often seen in the patient with central

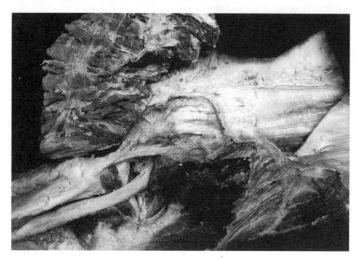

A

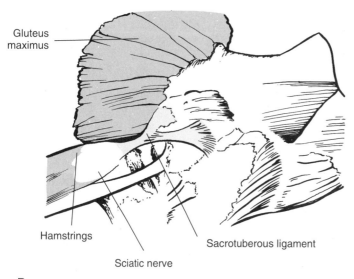

Gluteus
maximus

Hamstrings

Sciatic nerve

Sacrotuberous ligament

B

Figure 3–54. Several muscles attached to the sacrotuberous ligament potentially increase ligamentous tension via contraction as a result of their attachment and line of force. They include the gluteus maximus, biceps femoris, and piriformis muscles. *A* and *B,* This lateral view shows the right gluteus maximus reflected from its origins on the pelvis, allowing the undersurface of the muscle to be seen. When the gluteus maximus is followed in this manner, its attachment to the sacrotuberous ligament complex can be probed. The biceps femoris–sacrotuberous ligament linkage can be seen as well, along with the sciatic nerve.

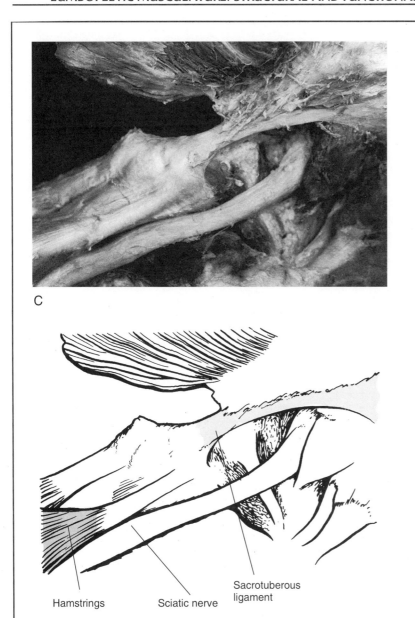

C

D

Hamstrings   Sciatic nerve   Sacrotuberous ligament

Figure 3–54. (continued) *C* and *D*, Close-up view of relationship between the hamstrings and sacrotuberous ligament.

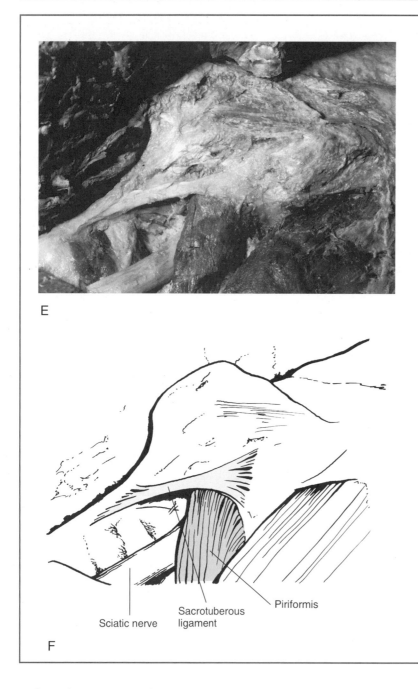

E

F

Sciatic nerve   Sacrotuberous ligament   Piriformis

Figure 3–54. (continued) *E* and *F*, The piriformis muscle can be seen coursing anterior to, and attaching to the anterior surface of the sacrotuberous ligament.

or lateral recess stenosis or apophyseal joint degeneration. To minimize the compression and shear at the lumbosacral articulation and the lower lumbar spine, the pelvis is often "rolled posteriorly," effectively "tucking" the buttock under the spinal column. This sagittal plane posture utilizes the gluteus maximus and hamstrings to position the pelvis in the sagittal plane to decrease the compression and shear load at the lumbar apophyseal joints.

Quadriceps

The quadriceps muscles are also intimately related to the fascia lata because they are essentially encased within this fascial envelope (Fig. 3–55). Contraction of the quadriceps results in broadening of the muscle with a consequent "pushing" effect on the fascia lata walls (Fig. 3–56). This action results in an increase in fascia lata tissue tension contributing to stability at the hip and knee. One can feel this broadening effect of the quadriceps simply by palpating the muscle at heel-strike in the gait cycle.

The strength and hypertrophy of these two extremely powerful muscles, the gluteus maximus and the quadriceps, is essential to consider in any low back rehabilitation program. Hypertrophy is especially important to consider with respect to the quadriceps. Like the erector spinae and multifidus muscles within the thoracolumbar fascia envelope, the quadriceps must be of sufficient girth in order to exert this "pushing" effect to amplify tension within the fascia lata envelope. Atrophy due to disuse or prolonged rest results in a less efficient mechanical interaction between the quadriceps and fascia lata.

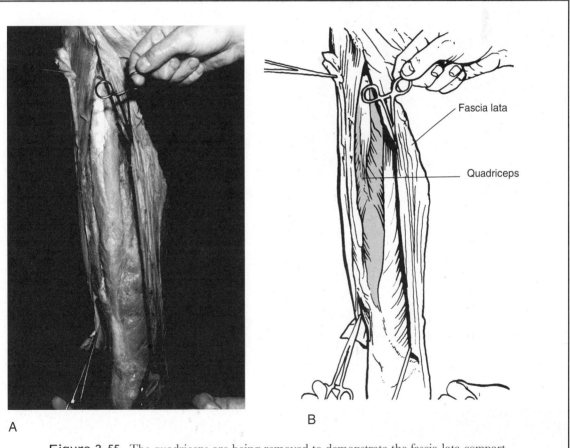

A

B

Fascia lata

Quadriceps

Figure 3–55. The quadriceps are being removed to demonstrate the fascia lata compartment. *A* and *B*, The compartment is opened anteriorly. The tensor fascia lata muscle can be seen inserting into the inner wall of the fascia lata, and the tendinous origin of the rectus femoris is seen.

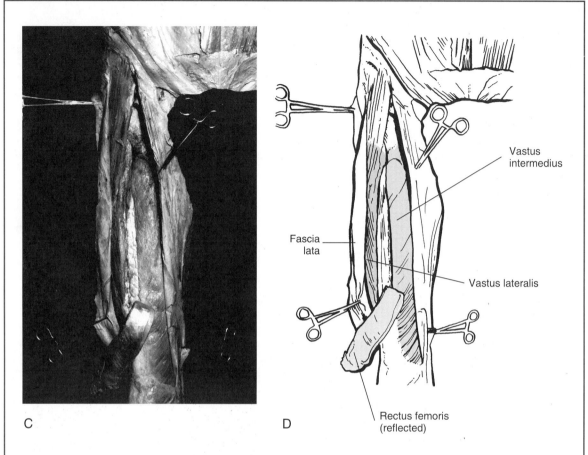

Vastus intermedius

Fascia lata

Vastus lateralis

Rectus femoris (reflected)

C

D

Figure 3–55. (continued) *C* and *D*, The rectus femoris has been cut from its proximal attachments and reflected distally.

Because the rectus femoris crosses the hip joint, it can have a direct effect in positioning the pelvis in the sagittal plane (Fig. 3–57). Contraction of the rectus femoris with the foot fixed (closed kinetic chain) results in an anterior rotary moment of the pelvis. The anterior rotary moment increases the lumbosacral angle with results in increased extension at the lumbosacral joint.

Hamstrings

The hamstrings are composed of the semimembranosus and semitendinosus on the posteromedial side of the thigh, and the short and long head of the biceps femoris on the lateral side. All of the hamstrings with the exception of the short head of the biceps femoris cross the hip and the knee joint. Because the hamstrings are attached to the pelvis at the ischial tuberosity, they control the rate and amount that the pelvis rotates over the hip joints when one bends forward from a standing position. Changes in hamstring stiffness constrain the rotation of the pelvis during forward bending, resulting in increased lumbar flexion. The hamstrings are thus a very important contributor to lumbo-pelvic rhythm. Training the hamstrings through resistive exercises from the standing position mimics this function and is one of the best exercises for

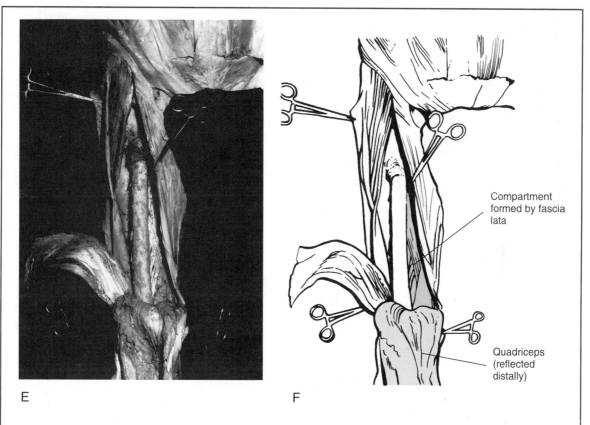

E

F

Compartment
formed by fascia
lata

Quadriceps
(reflected
distally)

Figure 3–55. (continued) *E* and *F*, The remaining three heads of the quadriceps have been detached from the femoral origins and reflected distally, out of the fascia lata envelope, illustrating the extent of this compartment.

improving hamstring strength and dynamic flexibility (see Chapter 6).

In addition to the attachment to the ischial tuberosity, the long head of the biceps femoris is attached to the sacrotuberous ligament (Fig. 3–54). Contraction of the biceps femoris increases the tension of the sacrotuberous ligament and pulls the sacrum against the ilium, effectively increasing the stability of the sacroiliac joint.[53, 56, 57]

Deep Hip Rotators

The deep hip rotators lie immediately beneath the gluteus maximus muscle. From cranial to caudal they are the piriformis, obturator internus with the associated superior and inferior gemelli, and the quadratus femoris muscles (Fig. 3–58). The quadratus femoris typically has the largest cross-sectional area of this group. When these muscles are removed, the tendon of the obturator externus is uncovered and can be seen blending in with the posterior aspect of the hip joint capsule. All of these deep rotators externally rotate the hip joint when the foot is free of the ground, but perhaps more importantly, they stabilize the head of the femur in the acetabulum during weight-bearing.

The piriformis muscle attaches to the sacrum, the anterior surface of the sacrotuberous ligament, and the medial edge of the sacroiliac joint capsule. From this attachment it extends laterally to insert into the trochanteric fossa. Contraction of the piriformis

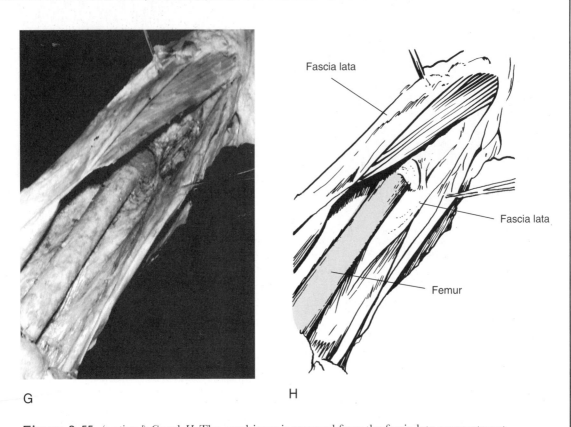

G   H

Figure 3–55. (*continued*) *G* and *H,* The quadriceps is removed from the fascia lata compartment, leaving the compartment medial, lateral, and posterior walls intact.

increases tension to the sacroiliac joint capsule and the sacrotuberous ligament, which enhances sacroiliac joint stability by pulling the sacrum against the ilium.

Anterior Hip Musculature

Since the iliacus and psoas major muscles have already been discussed, actions of the remaining anterior hip muscles influencing lumbopelvic mechanics are briefly noted. The sartorius and rectus femoris muscles attach to the anterior pelvis and proceed inferiorly to cross the knee joint. These muscles have well-recognized actions at the hip and knee joints, but they can also play a role in the generation of forces to the pelvis. For example, if either has increased tension due to an increased efferent motor response, or tightness as

a result of adaptive shortening, an increased anterior moment to the ilium can result as tension in the muscle increases.

As previously mentioned, this anterior movement to the ilium can increase the extension forces to the tissues of the lumbar spine. These muscles, coupled with a tight iliopsoas muscle and a tight hip joint capsule on the ipsilateral side, render the lumbopelvic articulations vulnerable to injury. Because the sagittal plane mechanics of the lumbopelvic tissue are now altered, increased contractile states of muscles to accommodate new tissue stresses are inevitable. The L5–S1 zygapophyseal joints, for example, must endure increased vertical forces. Recognition of the influence of the sartorius and rectus femoris muscles on sagittal plane mechanics warrants their attention during lumbopelvic evaluation.

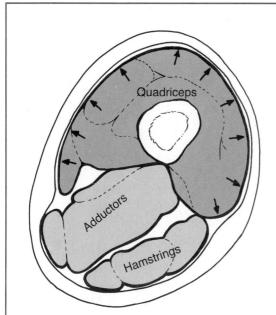

Figure 3–56. Contraction of the quadriceps within the fascia lata envelope increases fascial tension due to the broadening effect of the muscle contraction.

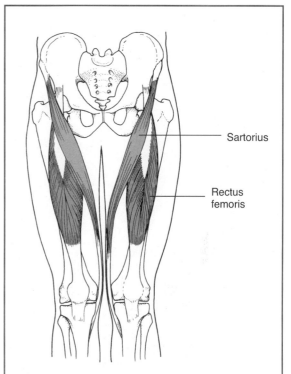

Figure 3–57. The relation of the rectus femoris muscle and the sartorius muscle to the lumbopelvic region. Contraction of these muscles imparts forces to the pelvis and hip joint that affect weight-bearing of the lumbopelvic region.

Medial Thigh Musculature

The pectineus, adductor brevis, adductor longus, anterior aspect of the adductor magnus, and gracilis muscles attach to the pubic and ischial rami, and extend inferiorly and laterally to attach to the femur. These muscles are considered to be adductors and external rotators of the femur in the open kinetic chain. The first three muscles are also femoral flexors.

However, when the foot is fixed on the ground, contraction of these muscles imparts a force to the pelvis that influences the frontal and sagittal plane positions of the lumbopelvic unit. This ultimately affects the weight-bearing positions of the lumbar spine, sacroiliac, and hip joints. Note how these muscles must work with the contralateral quadratus lumborum, gluteus medius, and ipsilateral psoas major muscles to control the frontal plane position of the spine and pelvis (Fig. 3–59). Like the anterior muscles of the thigh, the adductor muscles exert an inferior and anterior rotary moment at the pelvis, increas-

ing lumbosacral extension when the foot is on the ground. This force can be due to the extended position of the femur or to the contraction of these muscles when the femur is fixed.

The functions of these muscles when the opposite limb is in swing phase of gait should be realized. They work with the abductors on the same side to create a weight-bearing posture of the hip joint to assure the proper transference of forces. These muscle groups probably contract together not only to balance the pelvis and stabilize the joints of the spine but to properly secure the acetabulum onto the femoral head. This demonstrates the importance of evaluating function in the weight-bearing position and performing close inspection of gait during the functional assessment (see Chapter 5).

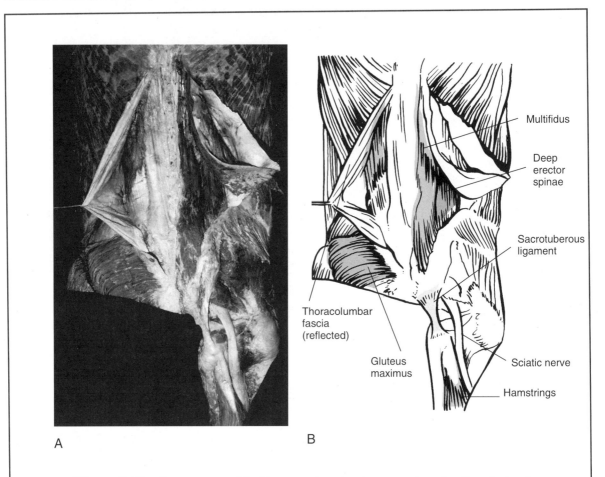

A   B

Figure 3–58.   Deep rotators of the hip, seen when the gluteus maximus is reflected. *A* and *B*, On the cadaver's left side, the gluteus maximus is left in situ and the thoracolumbar fascia is reflected to reveal the superficial erector spinae muscle. On the right, the gluteus maximus has been removed showing the sciatic nerve and deep rotators of the thigh. The hamstring attachment to the sacrotuberous ligament can also be seen. The superficial erector spinae has also been reflected revealing the multifidus and deep erector spinae muscles.

Lateral Thigh Musculature

The muscles of the lateral thigh include the gluteus medius and minimis and the tensor fascia latae. They play an important role in the frontal plane stability of the lumbopelvic unit. Therefore, it is important that they work in a synergistic manner with the medial thigh muscles and lateral trunk muscles to assure that nondestructive weight-bearing patterns occur.

It is especially important to examine these hip abductors when weakness of the L4 or L5 nerve roots is found during the low back examination. Since the large hip abductors (including the gluteus maximus) are primarily innervated by the fourth and fifth lum-

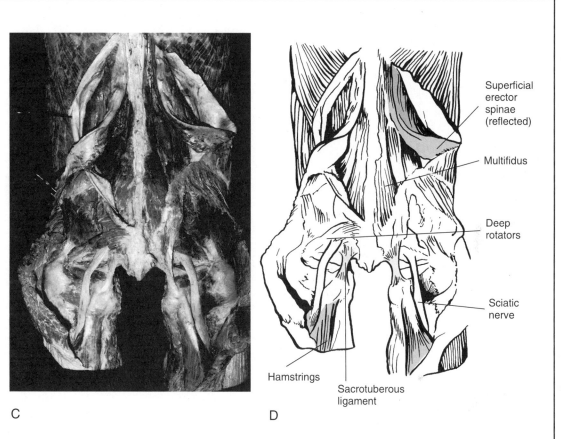

Superficial
erector
spinae
(reflected)

Multifidus

Deep
rotators

Sciatic
nerve

Hamstrings

Sacrotuberous
ligament

C

D

Figure 3–58. *(continued) C* and *D,* The gluteus maximus and superficial erector spinae muscles have been reflected on both sides showing the deep hip rotators and sciatic nerve, and the multifidus and deep erector spinae muscles. Note the relationship of the hamstrings to the sacrotuberous ligament.

bar segments, a frontal plane Trendelenburg gait, or forward bending of the trunk at heel strike, may be evident due to nerve root involvement. Although these nerve roots are typically assessed at the foot and ankle (i.e., anterior tibialis and extensor hallucis longus muscles), during the low back examination, it is important to consider the effects of weakness of any muscles supplied by these nerve roots.

If there is a difference in strength of the right and left hip abductor muscles, then the amount of frontal plane motion during stance phase of gait will be different on the two sides. One side of the pelvis drops further in the frontal plane than the other because of the inability of the hip abductors to stabilize the pelvis. This excessive frontal plane motion of the pelvis

results in increased compressive forces to the apophyseal joints of the lumbar spine on the opposite side of the drop, and increased varus load to the lower extremity.

Because the weight-bearing line is shifted to either side owing to hip abductor weakness, the forces on the femoral head are also altered. In the example above the right femur is now relatively adducted when compared with the left. This results in increased compressive force on the right femoral head when compared with the loading pattern on the left femoral head. Friberg[20] has noted that a relatively adducted femur leaves the lower extremity in a varus position. The varus position also increases compressive forces to the lateral aspect of the greater trochanter owing to the stretched

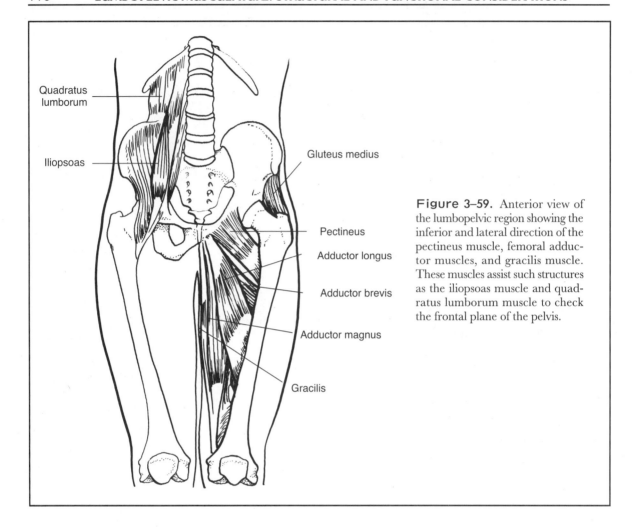

Quadratus
lumborum

Iliopsoas

Gluteus medius

Pectineus

Adductor longus

Adductor brevis

Adductor magnus

Gracilis

Figure 3–59. Anterior view of the lumbopelvic region showing the inferior and lateral direction of the pectineus muscle, femoral adductor muscles, and gracilis muscle. These muscles assist such structures as the iliopsoas muscle and quadratus lumborum muscle to check the frontal plane of the pelvis.

lateral hip musculature (Fig. 3–60). This compressive force, if prolonged or excessive, may result in inflammation to the bursa that lies beneath the gluteus maximus. Greater trochanteric bursitis may be a result of altered frontal plane biomechanics. Treatment of the irritated bursa tissue is most successful when the forces that are responsible for its irritation are minimized.

SUMMARY

The musculature of the lumbopelvic region is designed to initiate and control multiplanar movements and to assist in the attenuation of forces reach-ing the lumbopelvic region. The central nervous system ultimately controls the motor behavior of these tissues. As in the extremities, a balance of muscle strength, neuromuscular coordination, and tissue length must be maintained to avoid injury. Although the intervertebral discs are often considered to be shock absorbers for the spine, it is actually the lumbopelvic musculature that is responsible for shock absorption. The physiology of passive and active muscle tension is therefore an important consideration.

As the musculoskeletal tissues adaptively change with age, and tissues are repaired from previous injuries, the force absorption and transference capabilities of this hub of weight-bearing diminish. Painful

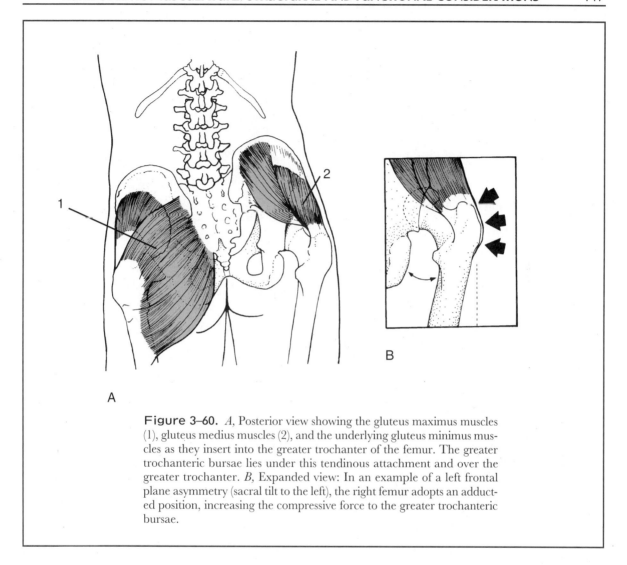

Figure 3–60. *A,* Posterior view showing the gluteus maximus muscles (1), gluteus medius muscles (2), and the underlying gluteus minimus muscles as they insert into the greater trochanter of the femur. The greater trochanteric bursae lies under this tendinous attachment and over the greater trochanter. *B,* Expanded view: In an example of a left frontal plane asymmetry (sacral tilt to the left), the right femur adopts an adducted position, increasing the compressive force to the greater trochanteric bursae.

mechanical syndromes often result. The lumbopelvic musculature is anatomically and mechanically linked through the fascial systems. Three key musculofascial systems are related to the lumbopelvic region: the thoracolumbar, abdominal, and fascia lata. These systems and the muscles attaching to them and encased within are detailed to assist the reader in functional assessment and to provide a foundation from which to build therapeutic exercise programs. Without an appreciation of the structure and function of the lumbopelvic musculature, successful long-term management and prevention programs are difficult to achieve.

REFERENCES

1. Adams MA, Dolan P, Hutton WC: The lumbar spine in backward bending. Spine 13:1019, 1988.
2. Banff ADP, Furling J: Electromyographic study of the rectus abdominis and external oblique muscles during exercises. Electromyogr Clin Neurophysiol 24:501, 1984.
3. Bednar DA, Orr FW, Simon GT: Observations on the pathomorphology of the thoracolumbar fascia in chronic mechanical back pain. Spine 20:1161, 1995.
4. Bigland-Ritchie B: Muscle fatigue and the influence of changing neural drive. Symposium on Exercise: Physiology and Clinical Application. Clin Chest Med 5:21, 1984.
5. Bogduk N: A reappraisal of the anatomy of the human erector spinae. J Anat 131:525, 1980.

6. Bogduk N, Macintosh JE: The applied anatomy of the tho-racolumbar fascia. Spine 9:164, 1984.
7. Bogduk N, Twomey LT: Clinical Anatomy of the Lumbar Spine. London, Churchill Livingstone, 1987.
8. Bustami FMF: A new description of the lumbar erector spinae in man. J Anat 144:81, 1986.
9. Carew TJ, Ghez C: Muscles and muscle receptors. In Kandel ER, Schwartz JS (eds): Principles of Neural Science, 2nd ed. New York, Elsevier, 1985, p. 443.
10. Carr D, Gilbertson L, Frymoyer J, et al: Lumbar paraspinal compartment syndrome: A case report with physiologic and anatomic studies. Spine 10:816, 1985.
11. Crisco JJ, Panjabi MM: The intersegmental and multisegmental muscles of the lumbar spine: A biomechanical model comparing lateral stabilizing potential. Spine 16:793, 1991.
12. Dolan P, Earley M, Adams MA: Bending and compressive stresses acting on the lumbar spine during lifting activities. J Biomech 27:1237, 1994.
13. Dolan P, Mannion AF, Adams MA: Passive tissues help the back muscles to generate extensor moments during lifting. J Biomech 27:1077, 1994.
14. Donisch EW, Basmajian JV: Electromyography of deep back muscles in man. Am J Anat 133:25, 1972.
15. Dunlop RB, Adams MA, Hutton WC: Disc space narrowing and the lumbar facet joints. J Bone Joint Surg Br 66:706, 1984.
16. Farfan HF: Mechanical Disorders of the Low Back. Philadelphia, Lea & Febiger, 1973.
17. Farfan HF: Muscular mechanism of the lumbar spine and the position of power and efficiency. Orthop Clin North Am 6:135, 1975.
18. Flicker PL, Fleckenstein J, Ferry K, et al: Lumbar muscle usage in chronic low back pain. Spine 18:582, 1993.
19. Floyd WF, Silver PHS: The function of erector spine muscles in certain movements and postures in man. J Physiol 129:184, 1955.
20. Friberg O: Clinical symptoms and biomechanics of lumbar spine and hip joint in leg length inequality. Spine 8:643, 1983.
21. Gracovetsky S, Farfan H: The optimum spine. Spine 11:543, 1986.
22. Gracovetsky S, Farfan HF, Helleur C: The abdominal mechanism. Spine 10:317, 1985.
23. Hanson P, Sonesson B: The anatomy of the iliolumbar ligament. Arch Phys Med Rehabil 75:1245, 1994.
24. Hukins DWL: Disc structure and function. In Ghosh P (ed): The Biology of the Intervertebral Disc, vol 1. Boca Raton, FL, CRC Press, 1988, p. 1.
25. Huxley HE, Hanson J: The structure and function of muscle. vol 1, Bourne GH (ed), New York, Academic Press, 1960.
26. Kandel ER: Factors controlling transmitter release. In Kandel ER, Swartz JH (eds): Principles of Neurosciences. New York, Elsevier, 1985, p. 120.
27. Kapandji IA: The Physiology of the Joints, vol 3. Edinburgh, Churchill Livingstone, 1974.
28. Kendall F, McCreary EK, Provance PG: Muscles: Testing and Function, 4th ed. Baltimore, Williams & Wilkins, 1993.
29. Kippers V, Parker AW: Posture related to myoelectric silence of erector spinae during trunk flexion. Spine 9:740, 1984.
30. Luk KDK, Ho HC, Leong JCY: The iliolumbar ligament: A study of its anatomy, development, and clinical significance. J Bone Joint Surg 68:197, 1986.
31. Macintosh J, Bogduk N: The biomechanics of the lumbar multifidus. Clin Biomech 1:205, 1986.
32. Manniche C, Asmussen K, Lauritsen B, et al: Intensive dynamic back exercises without hyperextension in chronic back pain after surgery for lumbar disc protrusion. Spine: 18:560, 1993.
33. McArdle WD, Katch FI, Katch VL: Skeletal muscle: Structure and function. In Exercise Physiology: Energy, Nutrition, and Human Performance. Philadelphia, Lea & Febiger, 1986, p. 289.
34. McGill SM, Norman RW: Partitioning of the L4-L5 dynamic moment into disc, ligamentous, and muscular components during lifting. Spine 11:566, 1986.
35. Morris JM, Benner G, Lucas DB: An electromyographic study of the intrinsic muscles of the back in man. J Anat 96:509, 1962.
36. Morris JM, Lucas DB, Bresler B: The role of the trunk in stability of the spine. J Bone Joint Surg 43A:327, 1961.
37. Nachemson A: Electromyographic studies of the vertebral portion of the psoas muscle. Acta Orthop Scand 37:177, 1966.
38. Nordin M, Frankel VH: Biomechanics of tendons and ligaments. In Frankel VH, Nordin M: Basic Biomechanics of the Skeletal System. Philadelphia, Lea & Febiger, 1989, p. 59.
39. Ortengren R, Andersson GBJ: Electromyographic studies of trunk muscles with special reference to the functional anatomy of the lumbar spine. Spine 2:44, 1977.
40. Paris SV: Anatomy as related to function and pain. Orthop Clin North Am 14:475, 1983.
41. Pauly J E: An electromyographic analysis of certain movements and exercises in some deep back muscles. Anat Rec 155:223, 1966.
42. Peck D, Nicholls PJ, Beard C, Allen JR: Are there compartment syndromes in some patients with idiopathic back pain? Spine 11:468, 1986.
43. Porterfield JA: Dynamic stabilization of the trunk. J Orthop Sports Phys Ther 6:271, 1985.
44. Porterfield JA, DeRosa C: Mechanical Neck Pain: Perspectives in Functional Anatomy. Philadelphia, W.B. Saunders, 1995, p. 62.
45. Rantanen J, Hurme M, Falck B, et al: The lumbar multifidus muscle five years after surgery for a lumbar intervertebral disc herniation. Spine 18:568, 1993.
46. Schultz A, Anderson GBJ, Ortengren R, et al: Analysis and quantitative myoelectric measurements of loads on the lumbar spine when holding weights in standing postures. Spine 7:390, 1982.
47. Seroussi RE, Pope MH: The relationship between trunk muscle electromyography and lifting movements in the sagittal and frontal planes. J Biomech 20:135, 1987.
48. Sirca A, Kostevc V: The fibre type composition of thoracic and lumbar paravertebral muscles in man. J Anat 141:131, 1985.

49. Sullivan MS: Back support mechanisms during manual lifting. Phys Ther 69:38, 1989.
50. Tesh KM, Dunn JS, Evans JH: The abdominal muscles and vertebral stability. Spine 12:501, 1987.
51. Uhthoff K: Prenatal development of the iliolumbar ligament. J Bone Joint Surg (Br) 75:93, 1993.
52. Valencia FP, Munro RR: An electromyographic study of the lumbar multifidus in man. Electromyogr Clin Neurophysiol 25:205, 1985.
53. van Wingarden JP, Vleeming A, Snidjers CJ, Stoeckart R: A functional–anatomical approach to the spine–pelvis mechanism: Interaction between the biceps femoris muscle and the sacrotuberous ligament. Eur Spine J 2:140, 1993.
54. Vander AJ, Sherman JH, Luciano DS: Biological control systems: Muscle. In Human Physiology: The Mechanism of Body Function. New York, McGraw-Hill, 1976, p. 34.
55. Vieeming A, Pool-Goudzwaard AL, Stoeckart R, van Windergarden JP, Snijders CJ: The posterior layer of the thoracolumbar fascia: Its function in load transfer from spine to legs. Spine 20:753, 1995.
56. Vleeming A, Stoeckart R, Snidjers CJ: The sacrotuberous ligament: A conceptual approach to its dynamic role in stabilizing the sacroiliac joint. Clin Biomech 4:201, 1989.
57. Vleeming A, Stoeckart R, Snidjers CJ, Stoeckart R, Stijnen T: Load application to the sacrotuberous ligament: influences on sacroiliac joint mechanics. Clin Biomech 4:204, 1989.
58. Warwick R, Williams P (eds): Gray's Anatomy, 35th ed. London, Longmans, 1980.
59. Wolf SL, Basmajian JV, Russe CTC, Kutner M: Normative data on low back mobility and activity levels. Am J Phys Med 58:217, 1979.
60. Woo SL-Y, Buckwalter JA: Injury and Repair of the Musculoskeletal Soft Tissues. Park Ridge, IL, American Academy of Orthopedic Surgeons, 1988.
61. Yamamoto I, Panjabi MM, Oxiand TR, Crisco JJ: The role of the iliolumbar ligaments in the lumbosacral junction. Spine 15:1138, 1990.

CHAPTER 4

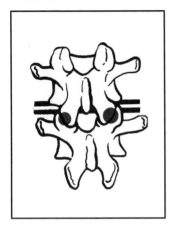

ARTICULATIONS OF THE LUMBOPELVIC REGION

A separate chapter regarding the articulations of the lumbopelvic region is provided to detail their structure and function and to discuss their relevance to painful syndromes of the low back. The articulations that will be discussed include the L4–L5 and lumbosacral (L5–S1) zygapophyseal joints, the intervertebral discs, especially the intervertebral discs between the fourth and fifth lumbar vertebrae and the lumbosacral junction, the sacroiliac joints, symphysis pubis, and the hips (Fig. 4–1). These articulations define the lumbopelvic articulations for the purposes of this chapter, and are selected to detail because of the contribution each makes to the transference of trunk and ground forces and their involvement with low back pain.

A great deal of experimental study and observation by engineers, anatomists, and orthopedic specialists regarding the lumbopelvic articulations has been documented in the literature, and these investigations have helped form the rationale for many orthopedic therapeutic interventions. Facet joint syndrome, degenerative disc disease, and sacroiliac joint dysfunction are such common clinical terms that an understanding of their individual and collaborative function is essential to provide a framework for logical evaluation and treatment processes.

The articulations feature highly specialized connective tissues such as bone, hyaline and fibrous car-tilage, and ligaments, and the highly organized connective tissue framework of the intervertebral disc. Although many of the specialized connective tissues are considered to be a source of pain, it is often not possible to distinguish between the normal aging process and those degenerative changes that might be considered pathologic. Such uncertainty often results in a dilemma regarding the interpretation of evaluation findings and choices of intervention.

As with all articulations of the musculoskeletal system, there is significant interplay between all of the articulating components (bones with their hyaline cartilage surfaces) and their connective tissue stabilizers and associated muscles. The efficiency by which smooth movement and shock attenuation occurs is dependent on these specialized connective tissues as well as on the strategies used by the central nervous system as a result of the afferent input from the receptors located in the connective tissues and muscles.

Because low back pain remains a major concern to society in terms of cost, work loss, and suffering, the articulations of this area have been subject to a great deal of analysis. It is the purpose of this chapter to describe the anatomy and function of the various articulations of the lumbopelvic region to better understand their synergistic relationship with one another and with the neuromuscular systems.

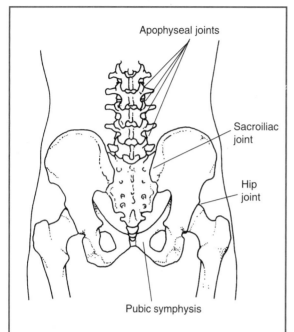

Figure 4–1. The lumbopelvic region defined. This region consists of the L4–L5 and lumbosacral zygapophyseal joints, the sacroiliac joints, pubic symphysis, and the hips.

THE FUNCTIONAL SPINAL UNIT

Although subsequent sections of this chapter will examine the zygapophyseal joints and intervertebral discs as separate entities, to consider the zygapophyseal joints independent from the intervertebral disc–vertebral body interface disregards the true movement pattern of the lumbar spine. Loads placed upon the spine occur as a result of weight-bearing, movement, and muscle contraction, and do not selectively affect the zygapophyseal joints or disc but ultimately affect all tissues of the spine. The zygapophyseal joints, intervertebral disc, and surrounding tissues work together as a functional unit that allows these forces to be transferred through the lumbar spine.

The concept of a "functional spinal unit" was first proposed by Schmorl and Junghans.[105] The functional spinal unit is the smallest segment of the spine that contains all of the components of the complete spine and demonstrates the characteristics of the complete spine (Fig. 4–2).[90] It consists of two vertebrae, the zygapophyseal joints, intervertebral discs, and all soft tissue structures such as muscles, ligaments, joint capsules, neural structures, and vasculature. The functional spinal unit is an important concept because it stresses the interdependence of the articulations, muscles, and the architecture and contents of the spinal canal and intervertebral foramen. The clinical relevance is that no pathological process, whether congenital or acquired, can exist which does not affect the function of other aspects of the functional spinal unit. Degenerative or pathological changes of the intervertebral disc, for example, have the effect of altering spinal kinematics above and below that level, which in turn leads to asymmetrical movements and loading at the lumbar zygapophyseal joints (Fig. 4–3). Because of this interplay between all spine tissues, injury, adaptive changes, aging, and the degenerative process of individual components of the functional spinal unit alter the function of associated tissues.

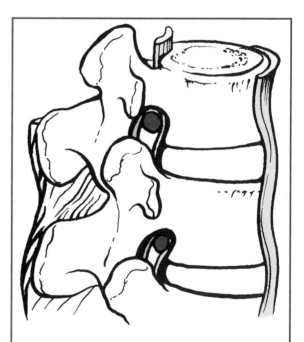

Figure 4–2. The functional spinal unit is the smallest structure of the spine that contains all spinal components, namely two vertebrae, joints, disc, muscles and ligaments, neural and vascular elements.

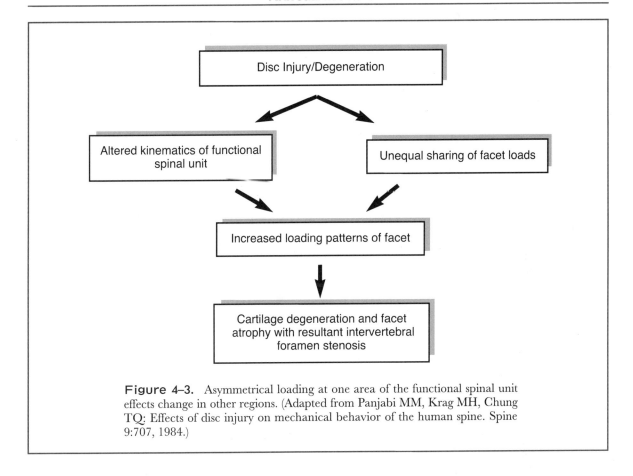

Figure 4–3. Asymmetrical loading at one area of the functional spinal unit effects change in other regions. (Adapted from Panjabi MM, Krag MH, Chung TQ: Effects of disc injury on mechanical behavior of the human spine. Spine 9:707, 1984.)

Loads on the lumbar spine are primarily produced by muscle contraction, body weight, and gravitational and external forces. Muscle contraction imparts especially significant forces to the lumbopelvic articulations (see Chapter 3). Forces are distributed and redirected, and as a result imposed loads are shared by all components of the functional spinal unit. This is especially true for torque loads placed over the spine. Compressive and shear loads are primarily borne by the bony and soft tissue components of the ligamentous spine (Fig. 4–4).

Excessive or asymmetrical loading patterns to the articulations result in connective tissue changes, which are typically followed by structural adaptations. In the zygapophyseal joints, the response of the facets (which are the articulating surfaces of the zygapophyseal joints) to abnormal loading patterns or direct injury might be cartilage degeneration, facet atrophy, and, if excessive forces are maintained over a long period,

bony adaptation in the form of sclerosis or osteophyte formation (Fig. 4–5).[115] Changes in joint structure ultimately alter joint function which affects intervertebral disc mechanics. Likewise, intervertebral disc injury alters the manner in which the zygapophyseal joints function. This helps underscore the significance of the synergistic roles played by the constituents of the functional spinal unit during force attenuation.

INSTABILITY OF THE FUNCTIONAL SPINAL UNIT

Although the term "spinal instability" is commonly used in clinical discussions, there is little uniform agreement on a single definition. A wide range of opinions prevail regarding both the etiology and injury mechanisms that result in clinically significant seg-

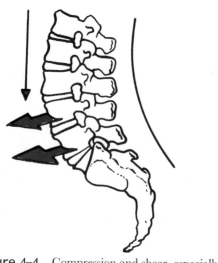

Figure 4–4. Compression and shear, especially anterior shear due to the lumbar lordosis, are two loads to which the elements of the functional spinal unit are subjected.

mental instability, and the clinically relevant signs and symptoms associated with instability. The simplest definition of instability is "loss of stiffness."[95] A definition with more clinical implications is "an abnormal response to applied loads, characterized by movements in the motion segment beyond normal constraints".[7] Stiffness of the spinal column is provided passively by the specialized connective tissues of the spinal column itself, and actively by the neuromuscular system. The loss of this stiffness and the resultant spinal instability can be due to injury, age-related degenerative changes of the specialized connective tissues, muscle insufficiency, or a combination of all three of these factors.

Kirkaldy-Willis and Farfan advanced a model of instability that attempted to correlate the pathology with the clinical presentation.[61] The model defined the spectrum of degeneration over three distinct phases: *dysfunction*, followed by *instability*, and then *restabilization* (Fig. 4–6). In the first phase, normal function of the functional spinal unit is compromised due to injury. It is during the next phase, the unstable phase, that the disc and zygapophyseal joints have degenerated to such an extent that they are unable to

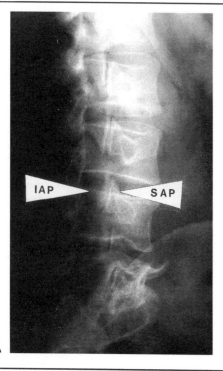

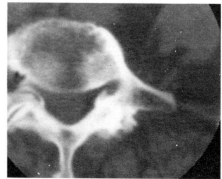

Figure 4–5. *A*, Oblique lateral radiograph showing the sclerotic and osteophytic changes of the zygapophyseal joint. The inferior articulating process (IAP) and superior articulating process (SAP) are labeled to identify the degenerative apophyseal joints above and below. *B*, CT scan revealing severe degeneration of the right lumbar apophyseal joint.

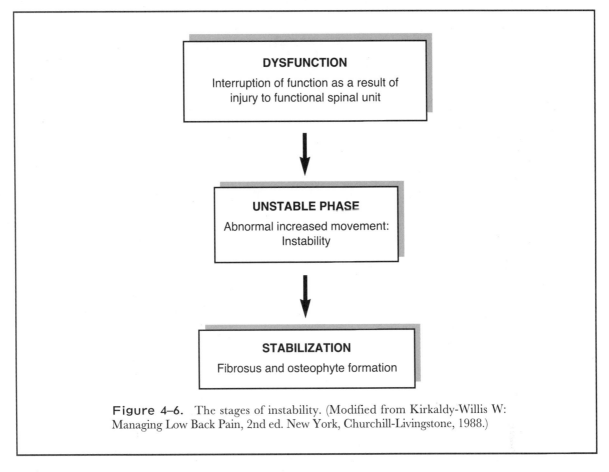

Figure 4–6. The stages of instability. (Modified from Kirkaldy-Willis W: Managing Low Back Pain, 2nd ed. New York, Churchill-Livingstone, 1988.)

adequately bear loads and ligamentous laxity results. This phase is characterized by abnormal, increased movement.

In addition to the degenerative processes, cyclic loading of the spine can also result in the anatomical changes suggestive of instability, depending on the magnitude and number of cycles of the applied loads. These changes include annular tears, distortions of the lamellae of the annulus fibrosus, facet fracture, and disc herniations.[135] Anatomical changes in the functional spinal unit resulting in segmental instability might include decreased disc height and joint capsule laxity. As a result of the aberrational segmental motion and loading patterns, osteophytes and traction bone spurs often develop at the margins of the annulus fibrosus and vertebral body (Fig. 4–7). In the final phase, the degenerative stage is more advanced but the unstable segment regains its stability because of increased fibrosus and the presence of osteophytes in the region of the zygapophyseal joints and intervertebral disc.

It is important to note that the peak incidence of disabling symptoms in the low back occurs between the ages of 35 and 55.[60] This suggests that the last stage of degeneration, the stabilization phase, has a protective effect to the functional spinal unit, while the stage of instability is correlated with the age in which symptoms, pain, and disability in the low back pain population predominate.

THE ZYGAPOPHYSEAL JOINTS

Regional Anatomy

The zygapophyseal joints of the lumbar spine are synovial joints formed by the articulation between the

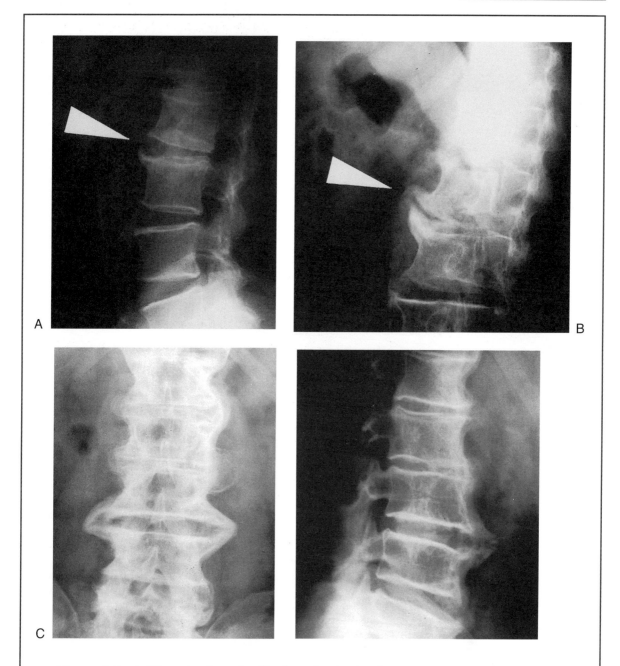

Figure 4–7. *A–C,* Lateral radiographs of lumbar spine showing three examples of traction spurs and osteophytes at the region of the bone–disc interface. The last example *(C)* shows a frontal (left) and sagittal (right) view. These are excellent examples of how the bone responds to overload—Wolff's law. In the frontal view, note the progression toward physiologic fusion.

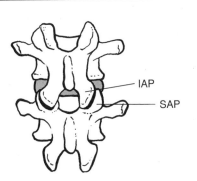

Figure 4–8. Posterior view of two lumbar vertebrae. Note that the inferior articular process (IAP) of the superior vertebrae is medial to the superior articular process (SAP) of the subjacent vertebrae.

inferior articular process of one vertebra and the superior articular process of the subjacent vertebra. In the lumbar spine, the inferior articular process lies medial to the superior articular process (Fig. 4–8). These joints feature all components typical of synovial joints, including articular cartilage, synovial lining, synovial fluid, and a joint capsule.

Each articular process is covered with hyaline cartilage with a thickness typically ranging from 2 to 4 mm.[80, 81] This thickness of the cartilage contributes to load-bearing in these lumbar joints. When compressive forces are applied to the joint surfaces, the approximation of the facet surfaces results in water being expressed from the hyaline cartilage. When the compressive forces are removed, fluid seeps back into the hyaline cartilage. Although this behavior typifies the normal behavior of healthy articular cartilage of any synovial joint to compressive forces, it is mentioned in reference to the zygapophyseal joints to illustrate their role in weight-bearing and accepting compressive loads. Different load-bearing functions also occur when the lumbar spine assumes various postures and moves through different planes. Cartilage deformation followed by the restoration of its thickness is important not only for nutritive functions but also in transference of the forces of gravity and movement.

The fetal and infant zygapophyseal joints of the lumbar joints are initially oriented in the frontal plane. As the lordotic posture develops during childhood, a curved and biplanar shape of the facet surfaces develops with the posterior aspect of the joint assuming an orientation in the sagittal plane and the anterior aspect of the facet retaining the original frontal plane orientation (Fig. 4–9). The shape of the adult joints is not a flat, planar surface as implied in some mechanical models but rather demonstrates a concave–convex relationship. The inferior articulating process of the superior vertebrae displays the convex surface while the superior articulating process of the subjacent vertebrae is relatively concave. Such an orientation refers to a compound joint surface since it faces in more than one plane.

The concavity of the superior articular process is also functionally deepened by the posterior aspect of the ligamentum flavum (Fig. 4–10). Serving as the anterior wall of the zygapophyseal joint capsule, the location of the ligamentum flavum allows for the inferior facet to make contact with the posterior aspect of the ligament. The inferior articular process can "ride" on the posterolateral surface of the ligamentum flavum during movement. Some cadaver specimens show the development of fibrous cartilage on this posterolateral corner of the ligamentum flavum, perhaps due to the response of the ligament to the various stresses placed on it. In addition, hypertrophy of the ligamentum flavum is often seen in imaging studies showing advanced degenerative changes of the zygapophyseal joints and spinal stenosis of the lumbar spine since the ligamentum flavum is a component of the zygapophyseal joint complex (Fig. 4–11).

The articulations between the inferior and superior articular processes of adjacent lumbar vertebrae are not true ball-and-socket articulations, but rather a structural arrangement that allows the facet of the zygapophyseal joint to face in at least two planes. The two planes of alignment seen with facet orientation of the L4–L5 and lumbosacral articulations are the frontal and sagittal (Fig. 4–9). The importance of these planes is addressed later when function is discussed, but it is important to note that there are varying degrees of sagittal and frontal plane orientation at all levels of the lumbar spine. There is also asymmetry between two sides of the same vertebra. These variations contribute to the differences between the joints of the upper and lower lumbar spine.[33, 72, 133] Asymmetry is the rule rather than the exception, and therefore palpation for bony position and comparison of movement patterns at different segmental levels is of questionable value and reliability.

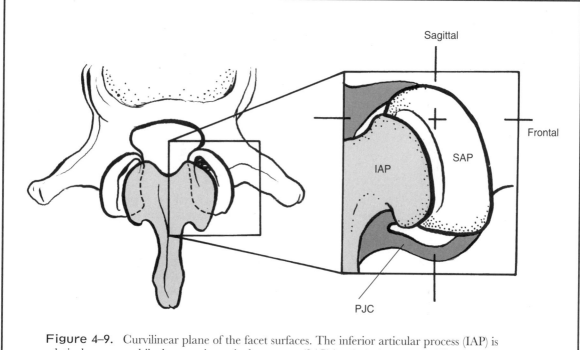

Figure 4–9. Curvilinear plane of the facet surfaces. The inferior articular process (IAP) is relatively convex while the superior articular process (SAP) is relatively concave. The anterior aspect of the joint surface is oriented in the frontal plane, while the posterior aspect is oriented in the sagittal plane. Posterior Joint Capsule (PJC).

Engagement by the two articulating partners of the joint occurs when the inferior articulating process of the superior vertebra of the functional spinal unit translates forward (due to anterior shear of the superior vertebra) on the subjacent vertebra (Fig. 4–12). This anterior shear force is greatest at the lower lumbar levels (L4–L5 and L5–S1) because the curve of the lower lumbar spine is more pronounced than the curve in the upper lumbar spine. The anterior shear force is also greater in the standing position than in the sitting position because of the different degree of lordosis that results with the two postures (Fig. 4–13).

Therefore, the erect posture results in engagement of the frontal plane component of the zygapophyseal joint. An anterior shear stress occurs during weight-bearing at the last two lumbar levels, and these segments are designed to counter this force. Note that an anterior shear force occurs perpendicular to the frontal plane. Only the portion of the inferior articular process that is oriented in the frontal plane engages with the portion of the superior articular process that is also oriented in the frontal plane, and together they minimize the tendency of the fourth lumbar vertebra to slide forward on the fifth lumbar vertebra. The articulation of the fifth lumbar vertebra on the sacrum is stabilized in much the same manner. However, engagement by the joint surfaces is not the only restraint to anterior shear. Table 4–1 lists other structures also oriented to stabilize the lumbar spine against anterior shear.

The Zygapophyseal Joint Capsule

If the concave surface of the superior articular facet is followed medially, the posterolateral aspect of the ligamentum flavum is reached. As mentioned previously, this ligament further increases the surface area

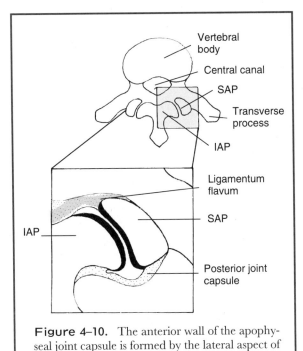

Figure 4–10. The anterior wall of the apophyseal joint capsule is formed by the lateral aspect of the ligamentum flavum.

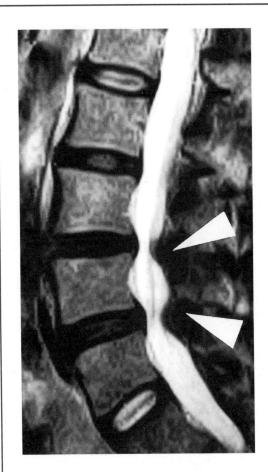

Figure 4–11. Lateral view of a magnetic resonance image of the lumbar spine showing hypertrophic ligamentum flavum at L3–L4 and L4–L5 and how such degenerative change results in stenosis of the spinal canal.

of the concave superior articular surface, and a small region on the posterior aspect of the ligamentum can function as an articular surface for the inferior facet. It is a highly elastic structure that blends with the extensive fibrous joint capsule.

The fibers of the zygapophyseal joint capsule are oriented perpendicular to the joint plane. Resistance to joint motion occurs as a result of increased facet contact as well as stretching of the capsular ligaments. As with any joint capsule, the direction of the fibers allows movement in some directions more than in others. When combined with the orientation of joint surfaces, the potential for various combinations of motion can be inferred. In the case of the lumbar zygapophyseal joints, the capsular arrangement and joint design are oriented to favor flexion and extension (sagittal plane) motion.

The capsules of the zygapophyseal joints of the lumbar spine are innervated by the medial branch of the dorsal primary rami. Input to the central nervous system from the capsules is presumed to include both nociceptive and proprioceptive afferent nerve fibers.[139] As with other synovial joints, the zygapophyseal joints are subject to pathologic changes resulting from injury, degeneration, or disease process; and the capsular ligament, subchondral bone, and reinforcing connective tissue are recognized as sources of back pain and have the potential to refer pain into the lower extremity. The prevalence of facet joint syndrome and the clinical signs and symptoms predicting facet involvement have not been fully elucidated, however.[55, 83, 99, 106]

The joints are also important for the contribution to joint position and movement sense. Afferent informa-

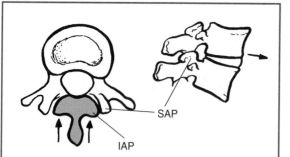

Figure 4–12. Anterior shear of the superior vertebrae results in engagement between the inferior articular process (IAP) and this vertebrae, and the superior articulating process (SAP) of the subjacent vertebrae.

tion is relayed from the joints to the central nervous system, triggering reflex motor responses that have yet to be fully understood. Deeper muscles such as the multifidus have direct attachments to the joint capsule, and the tension they exert on the capsular walls may provide an additional stimulus to the proprioceptors located in the joint capsule.

Zygapophyseal Joint Motion

The plane of the zygapophyseal joints and the orientation of the fibers of the joint capsule and reinforcing ligaments contribute to the plane of motion for the lumbar spine. As mentioned above, the greatest movement capabilities of the lumbar spine are in the sagittal plane, while the least amount of move-

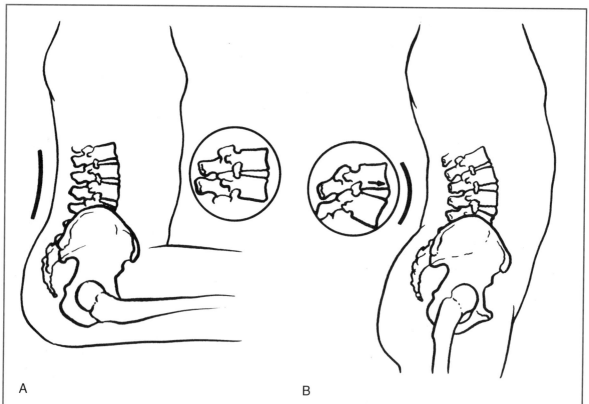

A   B

Figure 4–13. In the sitting position the anterior shear is decreased because the lumbar lordosis is decreased *(A)* as compared with the standing position in which the increased lordosis results in greater anterior shear *(B)*.

Table 4–1. Structures That Check Anterior Shear of the Lumbar Spine

Anterior longitudinal ligament
Wedge shape of intervertebral disc
Rings of annular fibrosus
Iliolumbar ligament
Frontal plane aspect of zygapophyseal joint
Deep erector spinae muscles
Oblique fibers of multifidus
Abdominal muscles
Posterior hip muscles (gluteus maximus, hamstrings)

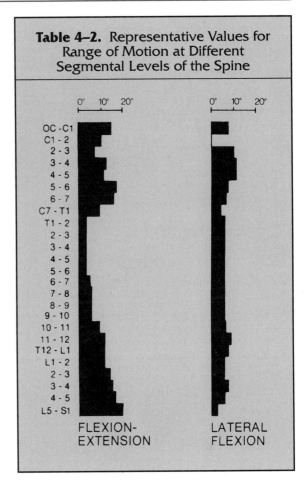

Table 4–2. Representative Values for Range of Motion at Different Segmental Levels of the Spine

ment is in the frontal and horizontal planes. Sagittal plane motion has been quantified by numerous investigators demonstrating the large range of movement possible in flexion and extension (Table 4–2). Taylor and Twomey[115, 118] note that it is the frontal plane orientation of the articular processes and the fibrous joint capsule that limit anterior shear and forward bending, respectively, during forward bending (Fig. 4–14).

The L4–L5 and lumbosacral segments are designed to move in the direction of flexion and extension and are not especially designed for rotation. Because these lower lumbar segments are the region in which the majority of segmental degeneration and low back pain occurs, the clinician should be aware of primary movement patterns in this region. There are approximately 20–25 degrees of sagittal plane movement between the L4 and L5 vertebrae and the same amount for the L5–S1 segment.[133] This results in these last two segments accounting for nearly 40–50 degrees of sagittal plane motion.

By comparison, the lower lumbar intervertebral joints have only 3–5 degrees of motion in the horizontal plane (rotation) at each zygapophyseal joint. Although some rotation is available, a rotational maneuver, if carried to an extreme, has the potential to result in tissue damage. During rotation the facet surfaces on one side are placed under compression, whereas on the contralateral side there is a distraction force at the joints (Fig. 4–15). If the torque is continued even though the limits of rotation have been reached, an abrupt change in the location of the axis of motion for the lumbar spine ensues. Normally, the axis of motion for the lumbar spine is located in the posterocentral of the intervertebral disc. However, by engaging the inferior and superior articular processes on one side with the rotational maneuver, the axis shifts

posterior to the engaged facets (Fig. 4–15). With increased torque and further rotation, the vertebral body now pivots around this new axis formed by the engaged joints. Instead of an axial torque between the bone–disc interface, there is now a shear stress to the disc.[12] The end range rotary motion thus places a compressive force on the engaged facets, a shear force on the intervertebral disc–vertebral body interface, and a distractive force on the capsular structures on the contralateral side.

Recognizing the minimal amount of rotation available at the lumbar spine, it would be extremely difficult for the clinician to have a high degree of accuracy in quantifying horizontal plane (rotation) hypomobility. This is especially true since 23 percent of the apophyseal joints are asymmetrical in the lower lumbar region.[33] In addition, ballistic rotary torso exercises (motion in the horizontal plane) with the pelvis fix-

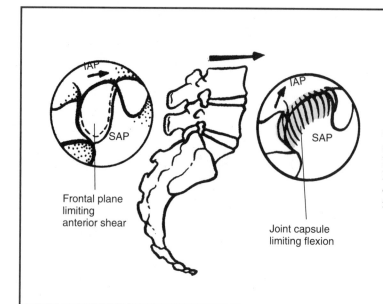

Figure 4–14. Forward bending of the lumbar spine is resisted by several elements of the functional spinal unit, but the frontal plant aspect of the joint helps limit anterior shear, and the joint capsule helps limit the degree of lumbar flexion.

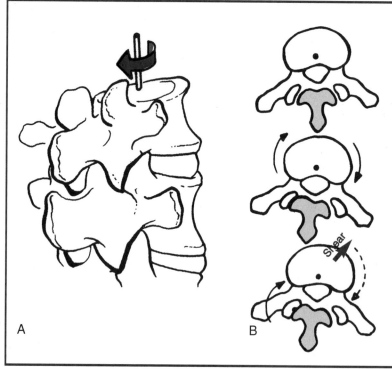

Figure 4–15. *A,* During rotation there is a compressive load between the two facets on one side and a distraction force on the opposite side. *B,* If the torsional force is continued after the facets are already engaged, the axis of motion is shifted to the joint under compressive load, which results in shear stresses at the bone–disc interface.

ated may place an excessive load on the lumbar joints and disc.

The analysis of rotation of the lower lumbar joints is interesting from another perspective. Damage to the zygapophyseal joints and the intervertebral disc with excessive torsional forces has been previously documented.[4, 32] The torsional force potentially places a large compressive load between the articular cartilage surfaces of the joint. Although there are several connective tissue restraints to excessive torsion, one mechanism opposing these torsional forces is the dynamic contribution of the internal and external abdominal obliques muscles. In addition to the abdominal obliques, several other muscles, such as the multifidus, deep erector spinae, quadratus lumborum, and psoas major muscles, potentially provide an antitorsion or counterrotation effect in order to counter the torsional force, but they do not have the same lever arm as the abdominal obliques.[97, 116]

The potential for spinal injury is illustrated by the person attempting to lift an object or move an object overhead. Various combinations of sagittal, frontal, and horizontal plane motions are demanded of the zygapophyseal joints. The weight that is being lifted significantly increases the torque acting at the joints because of the length of the lever arm that the weight is now acting over, and there is increased potential for large torque to reach these joints. Adams and Hutton[5] suggest that only a small additional torque to a fully rotated lumbar spine produces damage. The zygapophyseal joint in compression is the first structure to fail at torsional limits, since it is this articulation that offers the primary resistance. Trunk musculature offers a measure of protection if contraction can be elicited to minimize the torsional forces.

In summary, the zygapophyseal joints and the intervertebral discs contribute to the limitations of segmental motion. However, the intervertebral disc allows movement in many planes owing to the oblique orientation of the collagen fibers of the annular rings (see below), whereas the zygapophyseal joints allow a disproportionate amount of movement in one plane—the sagittal—compared with the other planes.

Weight-bearing by the Zygapophyseal Joints

The facets of the zygapophyseal joints provide a mechanism for load-bearing (Fig. 4–16). The inferi-

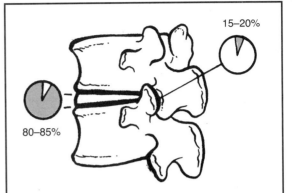

Figure 4–16. In the upright standing posture, compressive loads of the lumbar spine are borne primarily by the bone–disc interface (approximately 80–85 percent) and by the facets and lamina (approximately 15–20 percent).

or facet of the superior vertebrae engages with the superior facet and pars interarticular is of the inferior vertebrae. These facets carry between 10 and 20 percent of the compressive load and more than 50 percent of the anterior shear load on the lumbar spine when an individual is standing.[4, 39, 71] With torsional stresses, a significant compressive load is placed between the two facet surfaces. During the early stages of lumbar flexion, the compressive load to the facets is decreased while the compressive load to the intervertebral disc is increased. However, as the flexion motion continues, there is increased anterior shear that loads the frontal plane aspect of the facets in compression (Fig. 4–17A).

As the lumbar spine is extended, weight-bearing by the zygapophyseal joints increases (Fig. 4–17B). Instead of the compressive force being primarily distributed to the bone–disc interface, the posteriorly placed zygapophyseal joints and lamina are subject to increased compressive load. As extension increases, the inferior articulating process impacts against the lamina and lower aspect of the superior articular process. Because of the sagittal plane orientation of the superior facet surface, less weight-bearing occurs between the two sagittal surfaces, since the inferior articular process glides by the superior articular process. More compressive force occurs between the inferior articular process and the lamina in this case. However,

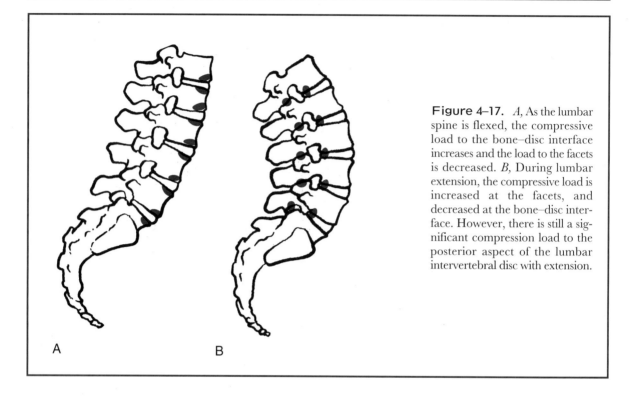

Figure 4–17. *A*, As the lumbar spine is flexed, the compressive load to the bone–disc interface increases and the load to the facets is decreased. *B*, During lumbar extension, the compressive load is increased at the facets, and decreased at the bone–disc interface. However, there is still a significant compression load to the posterior aspect of the lumbar intervertebral disc with extension.

A   B

if the superior articular process has a more concave shape, the inferior articular process is compressed into this concave partner.

It has been suggested that the lumbar spine is best able to resist compression stresses when it is flexed approximately 60–80 percent of the range of motion between erect standing and full lumbar flexion.[3] This lumbar flexion allows the connective tissues, which are located posterior to the axis of lumbar motion, to generate extensor moments.[27] True lordotic postures, which are sometimes advocated in lifting, potentially increase the compressive stresses to the zygapophyseal joints and posterior aspect of the annulus. However, maintenance of a true lordotic posture during lifting rarely occurs. Individuals attempting to lift with the lumbar spine maintained in lordosis actually flex their lumbar spine this 60–80 percent of full lumbar range because of the posterior rotary moment of the pelvis at the lumbosacral articulation as well as the flexion motion between the lumbar vertebrae themselves.[26] Bending the knees and lifting with the lumbar spine flexed 60–80 percent of its full range distributes the compressive stresses over the intervertebral disc and

helps unload the zygapophyseal joints.[26] In practical terms, the command to keep one's back straight during a lift probably results in the lumbar spine positioned in the optimal range of flexion. Practical points to consider with regard to safe lifting strategies are noted in Table 4–3.

As with other synovial joints in the body, the zygapophyseal joints have limits in their ability to accept compressive load. Degeneration of the hyaline cartilage of the facet is a sequelae of intervertebral disc degen-

Table 4–3. Practical Strategies to Consider for Lifting
Maintain symmetric, relatively upright posture
Avoid end-range positions
Keep center of gravity of object close to center of gravity of body
Keep center of gravity of object low if possible
Lift symmetrically
Avoid jerking motions

eration. As the water-imbibing capacity of the nucleus is lessened, narrowing of the disc space occurs. This results in increased compressive stresses between the facets (Fig. 4–18). Further narrowing of the disc space results in facet subluxation with the inferior tip of the inferior facet resting against the lamina and the pars interarticularis of the vertebrae below. Extension of the lumbar spine further increases these contact stresses. The joint surfaces respond with patterns of degeneration as the load exceeds joint limits. Rapid impact loading or prolonged, excessive compression have the potential to damage articular cartilage and begin the sequence of joint degeneration.[44, 80]

When structural damage to the surface of the articular cartilage occurs, either by rapid onset injury or by prolonged excessive loads which exceed the physiologic capacity of the joints, the weight-bearing patterns of the joint change. These stresses have the potential to cause further degenerative changes such as denudation of the articular cartilage and eburnation of the subchondral bone.

The weight-bearing limits of the zygapophyseal joint have not been studied *in vivo*. However, it is worthwhile to consider the potential effect of conditions that may keep the joint excessively loaded. For example, a weak abdominal wall most often alters the way in which forces reach the zygapophyseal joints. This weakness results in an increased rotary motion of the pelvis, which increases the extension of the lumbar spine (Fig. 4–19). This extension increases the compressive load on the zygapophyseal joints. A structurally shorter leg on one side, or relative tightness of the anterior hip structures can also alter weight-bearing function of the lumbar facets in the frontal and sagittal planes, respectively (Fig. 4–20).

Each of these examples is used to illustrate the weight-bearing function of the zygapophyseal joints. The manner in which the weight line moves through the lumbar spine determines the amount of compressive loading required by these joints. If ground or trunk forces exceed the physiologic capacity of the joints, degeneration patterns of the hyaline cartilage

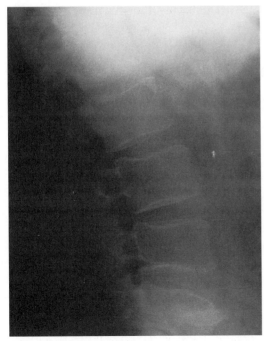

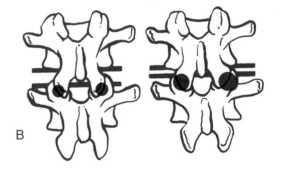

Figure 4–18. *A* and *B*, A lateral radiograph *(A)* revealing a degenerated L5–S1 segment. Note the adaptations of the vertebral body, specifically the created convex–concave weight-bearing surface of the posterior third. This loss of disk height results in narrowing of the neural foramen and increased compression to the facet joint *(B)*.

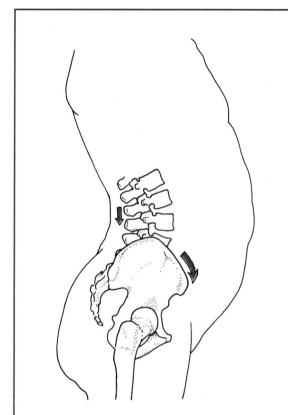

Figure 4–19. Weakness of the abdominal wall results in an increase in the anterior rotary motion of the pelvis. This motion increases extension and compression loading to the lumbar facets.

and subchondral bone of the apophyseal joint may result.

Degenerative Patterns of the Lumbar Facets

The two different planes of the facet surfaces reveal different patterns of degeneration. With advancing age, the cartilage of the anterior (frontal plane) aspect of joint becomes fibrillated and parts of the facet are denuded of their cartilaginous surface, with sclerotic changes occurring in the underlying subchondral bone. The cartilage of the posterior (sagittal plane) aspect of the facet surface shows cartilaginous "splits" that are oriented parallel to the facet cartilage–bone inter-

face. These cartilage splits are like "bacon strips" fitting like templates in the cartilage surface, and are attached to the inner wall of the zygapophyseal joint capsule.[84]

The degenerative changes in the articular cartilage seen in the specific regions of the facet provide some insight as to the loads that are applied to the facet surfaces. The anterior (frontal plane) aspect is primarily loaded in compression. Compression of the two facet surfaces occurs as a result of the anterior shear of the lumbar segment with the normal lordosis, and the anterior shear that occurs during lumbar flexion and lumbar extension.

The posterior (sagittal plane) aspect of the joint is subjected to shear stresses between the cartilaginous surfaces as a result of sagittal plane motion between the facets (flexion and extension), and the anterior shear between the two joint surfaces due to the lumbar lordosis. Shear stresses over the facet surfaces "peel" the strips of cartilage from the joint surface while these strips remain attached at the periphery to the capsule. It is perhaps these template strips of cartilage that are responsible for the "locked back" syndrome, which is occasionally relieved by manipulation techniques that place a distraction force between the facet surfaces, possibly displacing the cartilaginous strip temporarily.

The degenerative changes seen in the articular cartilage of the facets can be compared to cartilaginous degeneration in the knee. The frontal plane aspect of the facet is loaded in compression in a manner similar to the tibiofemoral articulation. Those compressive stresses can lead to a degenerative pattern featuring chondrocyte changes, fibrillation and crevices of the cartilaginous surface, denudation of the cartilage cover, and sclerosis of the subchondral bone resulting in degenerative joint disease of the tibiofemoral articulation. The sagittal plane aspect of the zygapophyseal joint is loaded with shear stresses in a manner similar to the patellofemoral articulation. The degenerative changes seen with shear loading of the patellofemoral joint are cartilage softening and peeling away of the cartilage surface in strips, closely resembling the degeneration pattern seen in the sagittal plane aspect of the lumbar facet.

Despite this understanding of the degenerative process, the relationship between pathoanatomical changes of the zygapophyseal joints and pain is still unclear. Joints that appear markedly degenerated with imaging studies can be asymptomatic, while normal

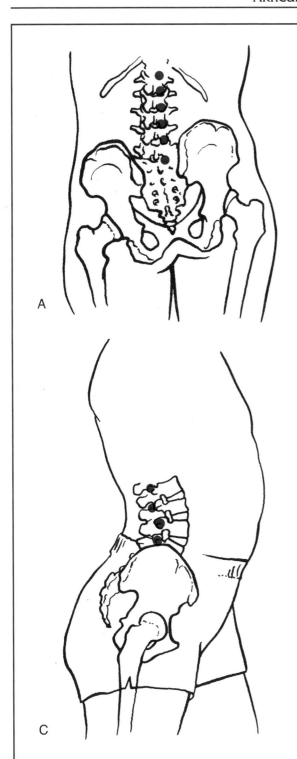

A

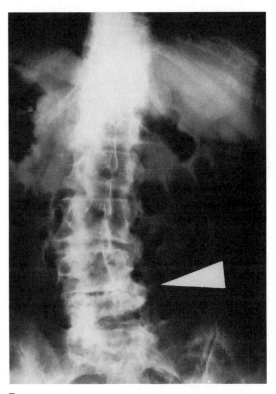

B

C

Figure 4–20. *A,* With an asymmetric frontal plane positioning of the pelvis, there is increased compressive loading to the facets on the long leg side. *B,* Radiograph of patient with leg length discrepancy (asymmetrical frontal plane) showing accelerated degeneration on long leg side. *C,* Tightness of the anterior hip structures results in increased compressive loading to the facets during pushoff phase of gait since the femur cannot be brought back to hyperextension. Therefore the lower extremity is placed behind the body by extending the pelvis under the lumbar spine.

appearing joints may be the source of pain.[70] As discussed below, it is perhaps not simply pathoanatomical changes that are responsible for the pain syndrome but biochemical changes as well.

INTERVERTEBRAL DISC

The intervertebral disc transmits loads through the spine and its position between two vertebrae provides for the flexibility of the functional spinal unit. This flexibility allows the spine to flex and extend, laterally bend, twist axially, and also allows for small excursion in translation. The disc acts as a shock absorber, distributing applied loads throughout the complete disc. It is influenced not only by forces directly applied to it but by forces applied to the zygapophyseal joints as well.[42] The intervertebral disc is always under load as a result of muscle contraction, body weight, and ligamentous tension. Ultimately, the mechanical properties of the intervertebral disc depend on the molecular makeup of the disc matrix.

The intervertebral disc can be considered to have three components, the annulus fibrosus, nucleus pulposus, and cartilaginous endplates (Fig. 4–21). Because the cartilaginous end-plates are intimately related to the intervertebral disc both anatomically and mechanically, they are considered an essential component. Although they do not cover the complete surfaces of the superior and inferior aspects of the intervertebral disc, they are in relation to a significant portion of it. The first structure to be damaged with excessive compression applied to the vertebral body intervertebral disc unit is the cartilaginous end-plates.[33]

The major macromolecular constituents of the disc are proteoglycans, collagen, and water. In addition to these constituents, a relatively small (2–5 percent) proportion of the disc matrix consists of cells. The relative proportions of these components vary depending on such diverse factors as the region of the disc being analyzed (annulus fibrosus, nucleus pulposus, or cartilaginous endplate), spine position, spinal level, age of the disc, and state of degeneration.[78, 87, 107] The proportions of the major disc constituents vary in different regions of the disc. The outer aspect of the annulus has a high collagen but low water content, while the inner annulus is very similar to the nucleus in that it features high water and proteoglycan

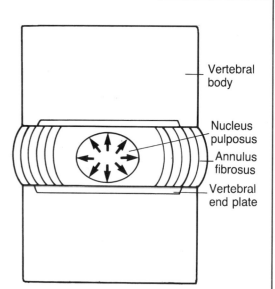

Figure 4–21. The three components of the intervertebral disc—the vertebral body, nucleus pulposus, annulus fibrosus, and vertebral endplate.

content. Thus there is a gradient of the molecular constituents throughout the annulus and one moves centrally toward the nucleus. The cartilaginous endplate has a higher collagen and lower proteoglycan content.[100]

The composition of the disc changes with age. The greatest changes are seen in the nucleus, which demonstrates fewer proteoglycans, different proportions of specific proteoglycans, and less water. More than 85 percent of the nucleus consists of water in the young discs. This decreases to approximately 70 percent in the adult, and decreases even further with advancing age.[78, 91, 92]

The adult human disc is the largest avascular structure in the body, and therefore nutrients are supplied to the cells of the disc from the blood vessels in close proximity. The primary routes for nutrition are through the cartilaginous end-plate and the peripheral parts of the annulus fibrosus. The cartilaginous end-plate begins to calcify with age and this may accelerate disc degeneration by decreasing fluid movement through the endplate. The transport of nutrients to the cells in the discs is largely a diffusion mechanism. Animal models of the disc *in vitro* suggest that immobilization or exercise has a significant opposite effect on disc cell oxygen consumption and lactate production.[51] Exercise increases the rate of solute transport while fusion of the spine decreases oxygen consumption and increases lactate production.

The outermost aspect of the annulus fibrosus appears to be the only part of the disc that is innervated (Fig. 4–22).[12, 141] The posterior aspect of the annulus is innervated by the sinu vertebral nerve, the posterolateral aspect by the branches of the gray ramus communicantes, and the lateral aspect by direct branches from the ventral rami. The function of the nerve supply is thought to be nociceptive as well as proprioceptive because encapsulated and nonencapsulated receptors have been traced in the annulus.[73] Some suggestion of nociceptive potential for the annulus also comes from discography studies. In discography, injections of contrast medium or saline into the nucleus of symptomatic discs have been noted to reproduce familiar back pain in some patients, especially with annular tears that extend to the periphery.[2] However, the mechanism of pain production and the tissues responsible for pain with discography have not been fully elucidated.[130]

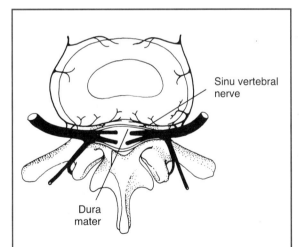

Figure 4–22. Innervation of the intervertebral disc. The posterior aspect is supplied by the sinuvertebral nerve, and the lateral and anterior aspects by the gray ramus communicante and direct branches from the ventral rami.

Nucleus Pulposus

The nucleus pulposus occupies the posterior-central aspect of the intervertebral disc. It consists of mucoid material, cells that resemble chondrocytes, and a loose array of collagen and reticular fibrils. The proteoglycan component of the matrix gives the nucleus pulposus its water-imbibing capacity. As the intervertebral disc ages, there is a decrease in water and proteoglycan components, a change in the types of proteoglycans, and an increase in collagen. Additionally, fibrillation of the nucleus pulposus occurs.

Water is the primary component of the nucleus but the water content fluctuates as a result of several factors. Water is expressed from the nucleus with sustained loads, and is imbibed with removal of the load.[120] Load to the disc occurs as a result of muscle contraction, ligamentous prestress, body weight, and ground reaction forces. Muscle contraction results in the largest compressive force to the intervertebral disc, and consequently postures in which a strong spinal extensor muscle contraction ensues result in increased pressure within the nucleus. Intradiscal pressure is thus strongly influenced by postures and movements of the spine.

As a result of the broad spectrum of motions and postures one assumes with work and activities of daily living, the fluid content does not remain constant because the nucleus pulposus is subjected to cycles of loading and unloading. Such cyclic compression is essential for optimal disc nutrition. Degenerative changes that occur in the nucleus are not only caused by the aging process, but may also be a consequence of interrupted nutrition to the disc. If the loading–unloading cycle is disturbed, the health of the nucleus pulposus may be jeopardized.[86]

With only a limited blood supply, especially at the inner aspects of the disc, the continual changeover of fluid in the nucleus—that is, its ability to be hydrated and dehydrated in a cyclical manner—is important. The health of the nucleus relies on this changeover of fluid, which in turn is facilitated by movement of the spine. The passage of this fluid both into and out of the nucleus pulposus is through the surrounding annulus and especially through the cartilaginous end plates. The cartilaginous end-plates provide an indirect communication link between the rich vascular supply of the cancellous bone of the vertebrae and the central regions of the disc.

Annulus Fibrosus

The orientation and organization of the collagen framework of the annulus fibrosus is striking enough to be seen with the naked eye (Fig. 4–23). The annulus is organized as a series of concentric lamellae that completely encircle the nucleus pulposus. If the layers are peeled back from the periphery, the fibers of the lamellae can be seen to have an oblique orientation which are anchored to the adjacent vertebral bodies and cartilaginous end-plates. The collagenous fibers in individual lamellae are oriented at approximately a 65-degree angle relative to the axis of the spine.[53] This orients the fibers of the lamellae at approximately 25 degrees with the plateau of the vertebrae. The fiber orientation of each successive lamellae alternates, so that fibers of two successive layers are oriented 90 degrees to each other. This creates a crosswoven appearance of the annulus (Fig. 4–23B). The collagen fibers of the annulus fibrosus in each layer are organized in a manner similar to fibers in tendons and are well-suited to resist tension in the direction of the fibers. There is a higher tensile stiffness in the outer annulus than the inner annulus.[30] The annulus is particularly well-suited to resist torsional loads owing to the oblique fiber orientation, but a crosswoven framework provides resistance to all motions of the spine including translations. Thus the annulus fibrosus might be considered as one of the key ligamentous restraints to spinal motion.

The type of collagen in different areas of the annulus is also region-specific. Brickley-Parsons and Glimcher[18] have shown that type I and type II collagen occupy specific regions of the intervertebral disc. There is a remodeling process that occurs from adolescence to early adulthood and results in a different collagenous makeup on the posterior aspect of the lumbar discs— a region subjected to more compression due to the lumbar lordosis as compared with the anterior aspect of the disc, which may have increased tensile stresses. This remodeling process is a type of redistribution of collagen based on imposed demand.

The collagen framework of the annulus provides the functional spinal unit its flexibility. Even though collagen is relatively inextensible, the annulus has the capacity for deformation, especially because the adjacent lamellae can move in relation to each other. The oblique angle of the collagen fibers also changes during spinal motion. As the disc becomes compressed, for example, the orientation of the fibers is altered so that the fibers become more horizontal. This means that the collagen fibers become closer to parallel with the vertebral body as axial compression forces are placed on the disc. Likewise, bending and torsional movements cause a reorientation of the collagen fibers.[63]

In forward bending the posterior annulus is stretched, the anterior annulus is compressed, and the collagen fibers coursing anteriorly and superiorly on the lateral aspect of the disc are subject to increased tension. In a like manner, torsion causes a strain on

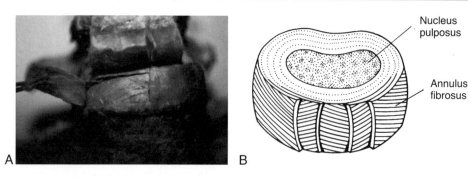

Figure 4–23. *A*, Section from the cadaver illustrating the orientation of the collagen framework of the annulus. *B*, Orientation of the collagen framework at approximately 65 degrees to the long axis of the spine. Crosswoven appearance of successive lamellae of the annulus is due to alternating fiber directions at each layer.

the collagen fibers that are oriented in one particular direction, but slackens the fibers that are oriented in an opposite direction (Fig. 4–24).

The thickness of the collagen bundles varies depending on the region of the annulus being examined. The annulus is thicker in the anterior and lateral regions and thinner posteriorly. This may be due to the eccentric position of the nucleus, which requires the posterior layers to occupy less surface area than the anterior or lateral layers or less binding substances between adjacent lamellae.[75] The posterior aspect of the annular rings is thinner and not as firmly held together, which may make them more vulnerable to degeneration. One of the earliest signs of disc failure resulting from aging, injury, or degeneration is a delamination of adjacent lamellae. Shear stresses are one of the most significant stresses resulting in lamellar separation.[119] Excessive shear stress therefore adversely affects both the intervertebral disc and the zygapophyseal joints.

Cartilaginous End-Plates

Because the intervertebral disc is predominantly an avascular structure, it is largely dependent on the passive diffusion of nutrients through the cartilaginous end-plates. In addition to this contribution, however, the cartilaginous end-plate provides a barrier that minimizes the possibility for loss of proteoglycans from the intervertebral disc.[17]

In addition to this nutritive function, the cartilaginous end-plates contribute to the mechanical function of the spine. They provide a physical barrier for the nucleus pulposus into the vertebral body, and the end-plate distributes part of the hydrostatic pressure exerted on it by the nucleus pulposus. The collagen fibers of the end-plate are oriented horizontally, and the pressure of the nucleus has a "bowing" effect on the cartilaginous end plate. This "bowing" produces a tensile force to the collagen framework of the end-plate, in much the same manner as the tensile forces are imparted to young bone in greenstick fractures. By orienting the collagen fibers horizontally, the tensile forces are resisted, and the end-plate supports the hydrostatic pressure.[100]

Anatomically, the cartilaginous end plate is continuous with the intervertebral disc. The collagen fibers of the disc continue into the end-plate by turning approximately 120 degrees from the lamellae of the outer annulus and 90 degrees from the nucleus.[100] The chemical components of the end-plate are also similar to those of the intervertebral disc: proteoglycans, collagen, and water. These three key chemical components are present in the end-plate, annulus fibrosus, and nucleus pulposus, but in different proportions. The different proportions ultimately contribute to the physical and functional differences of the intervertebral disc and the cartilaginous end-plate.

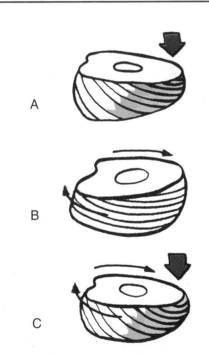

Figure 4–24. *A,* During forward bending, there is a compressive load to the anterior aspect of the annulus and a tensile load to the posterior annulus. *B,* Due to the oblique orientation of the annular fibers, torsion increases the tensile load of the annular fibers. *C,* Flexion with torsion places a significant tensile stress through the posterior aspect of the annulus.

Intervertebral Disc Mechanics

The intervertebral disc is well designed to attenuate shock and transmit the wide array of forces and

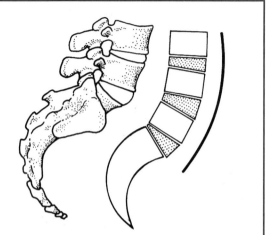

Figure 4–25. The lumbosacral and L4–L5 intervertebral discs are wedge shaped with the anterior height of the lumbosacral disc often twice the height of the posterior height.

moments imposed upon it. Along with the zygapophyseal joints, it receives the total compressive load of the spine. The intervertebral discs between the L4–L5 and L5–S1 vertebrae are wedge-shaped with the anterior height of the L5–S1 disc often being twice the height of the posterior aspect (Fig. 4–25). This wedging is one of the major structural reasons for the lumbar lordosis.[33] In the upper lumbar spine, the discs have a more evenly distributed anterior and posterior height rela-

tion. The wedged-shape of the last two discs makes it difficult to compress the anterior height to such an extent that the posterior height becomes much greater than the anterior height.[93]

When compressive load is transferred to adjacent vertebral bodies, it traverses the cartilaginous endplate, annulus, and nucleus. The nucleus can be distorted but being primarily a liquid, it cannot be compressed. As a result, the primary function of the nucleus is to receive the vertical forces (trunk and ground forces) and redistribute them radially in the horizontal plane, this plane being perpendicular to the long axis of the spine (Fig. 4–26). The internal pressure of the nucleus increases ring tension in the annular lamellae, which increases the stability of the functional spinal unit. The unique "synergy" between the nucleus and the annulus is one in which the nucleus converts a vertical load into radial pressure that is resisted by the tensile properties of the annulus.

The nucleus must have a sufficient fluid volume to develop the necessary pressure to push against the annular rings. The younger intervertebral disc has a greater volume of water and therefore exerts more pressure. With a less hydrous, desiccated nucleus, the load transference to the annulus is altered because nucleus fluid pressure is decreased. As a result, there is less tension in the outer layers of the annulus and increased compressive stress to the annulus lamellae with the degenerated nucleus.

Two factors contributing to increasing the compressive load to the nucleus are muscle contraction

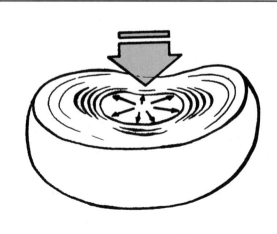

Figure 4–26. The unique synergy between the nucleus and annulus is such that axial compressive force through the nucleus is redistributed in a radial direction to the inner walls of the annulus. This results in increased tension within the annulus, increasing stability of the spinal segment.

and ligamentous prestress. Because the powerful spinal extensor and psoas major muscles cross the functional spinal unit relatively close to the axis of motion, they exert a compressive load to the intervertebral disc upon contraction (Fig. 4–27). However, even in the resting state, there is compressive load to the functional spinal unit as a result of ligamentous "preload."[54] The ligamentous prestress to the functional spinal unit increases the stability of the flexible spine just as muscle contraction also affords the spine greater stability.

Nachemson and Morris[85] measured the pressure developed in the disc under various compressive forces, and because the needle was inserted into the nucleus pulposus region, intradiscal pressure has come to be synonymous with the pressure within the nucleus pulposus. These experiments shed great light on force transmission through the intervertebral disc. They demonstrated that forces were transferred into the disc as body positions were changed, which recruited different trunk muscles. Total intradiscal pressure is a summation of the pressures generated as a result of spine positioning, muscle contraction, and ligamentous prestress. There is a fundamental difference between describing the nucleus pulposus as the component of the intervertebral disc that "absorbs compressive loads" versus "redistributes compressive loads." The annulus fibrosus, working in concert with the nucleus is actually the structure more adept at accepting compressive forces. Markolf and Morris[75] demonstrated that enucleated discs respond very nearly the same as discs with the nucleus pulposus intact when compressive forces are applied, but only for short periods of time. Compression stresses placed over the segments for prolonged periods need nuclear pressure to maintain annular wall tension.

Pure compression of the disc does not cause extrusion of the normal nucleus even in experiments in which the annulus is intentionally damaged and compression forces are applied.[121] Bending and torsional loads rather than compression are considered to be the most damaging to the intervertebral disc.[32] Since rotation and lateral bending are coupled motions, the tension and shear stresses are increased in the disc with these motions.

For the nucleus pulposus to escape the confines of the annulus fibrosus, several conditions are essential:

1. The nucleus must be desiccated, much like a tuft of wet wool becoming fragmented.
2. The nucleus must still have a large fluid volume to exert pressure.
3. The wall of the annulus must weaken. This can be due to injury or degeneration that results in decreased stiffness of the annular rings (altered hysteresis). The posterior aspect of the annulus is particularly susceptible to this, since it has less mass.
4. The annular walls cannot exert an equal and opposite force against the radial pressure of the nucleus.

When the proteoglycan content of the nucleus pulposus is no longer able to hold the nuclear matrix together, the nucleus pulposus becomes partially desiccated. This may occur with mechanical stresses, but it is most likely to occur as a result of biochemical changes within the nucleus itself. Evidence exists for the protein of the nucleus pulposus to serve as an antigenic agent.[77] An autoimmune reaction, with its attendant inflammatory response, may contribute to breakdown of the nucleus pulposus. This antibody–antigen reaction perhaps occurs as a result of defects in the

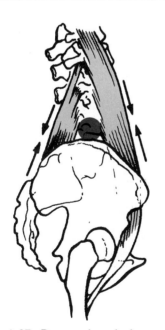

Figure 4–27. Because the spinal extensors and the psoas major cross the spinal segment relatively close to the axis of motion, they increase the intradiscal pressure as a result of the compressive force between the adjacent segments.

cartilaginous end-plate from various mechanical insults. With the barrier between the nucleus pulposus and the rich circulation of the vertebral body disrupted, the protein of the nucleus pulposus is exposed to the circulating antibodies and may possibly trigger such a response.

Intradiscal pressure also contributes to "unloading" of the facets of the zygapophyseal joints. Nucleus pressure exerts superiorly and inferiorly directed forces that essentially attempt to "push the vertebrae apart" which potentially unloads, or more accurately, lessens facet compressive force (Fig. 4–28). Although the zygapophyseal joints are weight-bearing structures, they are responsible for only a small proportion of weight-bearing. Dunlop and co-workers[29] have shown experimentally that peak pressure between the zygapophyseal joints increases significantly with loss of disc height and with increasing extension. These higher contact pressures could possibly damage the facet articular surfaces and result in degenerative disease of the lumbar joints. Therefore, another role of the nucleus may be mechanical in nature by helping to "unload" the zygapophyseal joints. To this end, a cause-and-effect relation between disc space narrowing and zygapophyseal joint degeneration has been suggested.[42]

Another role of the intervertebral disc may be proprioceptive. By having a structure that causes a distraction force between the vertebral bodies, a certain tension develops within the supporting connective tissue structures. The capsular tissue has been shown to be rich with various types of mechanoreceptors and nociceptors, and the disc itself is supplied with nerve fibers in its outermost layers.[73, 138] Gracovetsky and Farfan[43] have suggested that the disc receptors may be more completely viewed as stress receptors, since they are biologic transducers recording the various stresses placed on these connective tissue structures.

The distraction force exerted by the nucleus pulposus between vertebral bodies helps place the capsular tissues at a certain preset tension. This tension stimulates the stress receptors, which in turn starts a centripetal flow of afferent information to the central nervous system. By the nucleus pulposus exerting this pressure and helping to maintain this slight preset tension on the surrounding tissues, small movements in any of these innervated tissues further stimulate the receptors because of their distortion. This increases the barrage of signals into the central nervous system, which in turn can result in a variety of reflex motor responses.

The wide range of postures and movement patterns used in lifting, for example, points out that each person's efferent motor output is subject to variations. These variations in turn are probably caused by the unique and individualized afferent input into the central nervous system. The nucleus pulposus potentially contributes to this afferent neurologic input by affecting tension in the surrounding connective tissues, thus influencing the mechanoreceptor system.

Intervertebral Disc Injury and Disc Disease

The difficulty in clearly defining the difference between age-related changes of the intervertebral disc and frank disc disease lend to the dilemma of establishing evaluation and treatment approaches that have universal agreement. Degenerative changes are not typically viewed as pathological until the structural and biochemical sequelae of disc degradation result in symptoms or signs such as pain, discomfort, and neurological signs. The earliest signs of degenerative changes in the disc include the loss of water content in the nucleus pulposus and evidence of tears in the annulus fibrosus.[52, 89] As a result of such changes, the disc space begins to narrow and the stability of the motion segment becomes compromised, increasing aberrational loading patterns and accelerating the

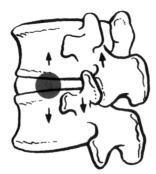

Figure 4–28. Pressure within the nucleus results in a slight "distraction" force between the adjacent segments, potentially decreasing the compressive load between the facets.

degenerative changes in other structures. Abnormal motion as a result of disc degeneration may also sensitize the dorsal root ganglion leading to increased nociception (see Chapter 2).[130]

The annulus fibrosus must withstand the multiple stresses that arise from compression, torsion, bending, and shear. From a structural standpoint, it appears that the posterior aspect of the annulus is most vulnerable to damage.[19] The posterior region is narrower and the lamellae are thinner and are subject to large tensile loads with forward bending and torsion. Consequently, damage can readily occur in this region.

Annular injury is an important aspect of disc pathology. Once the annular rings lose their stiffness from being overstretched, overcompressed or are damaged as a result of their inherent viscoelasticity being exceeded, they are no longer as effective in stabilizing or limiting the motion of the vertebral bodies and in containing the pressure of the nucleus. The pressure by the nucleus pulposus is now exerted against an area of less resistance. As a result, buckling of the annulus occurs, resulting in the well-known disc bulge (Fig. 4–29).

Which stresses cause this breach or weakening of the annulus that precipitates nuclear herniation? There are many potential insults. The annular lesion may be the result of an accumulation of microtrauma or abnormal stresses to the annulus. It may also weaken because of isolated trauma, such as excessive torsion to the spine, prolonged periods of vibration, and excessive and prolonged loading. Prolonged extension stresses—for example, in excessive lordotic posturing—might place greater than normal compressive forces

on the inherently weaker posterior annulus. This in turn may result in structural fatigue of the collagen, and ultimately may weaken the fibers, making them more susceptible to injury.

Torsional forces can damage the collagen fibers of the annulus. Flexion of the lumbar spine combined with torsion submits the oblique collagen fibers to forces that would tend to increase their length. When these forces are applied the fibers of the disc are subject to large tensile stresses. From this point the analogy with any ligamentous tissue in the body can be made. If the viscoelasticity of the fiber under tensile stress is exceeded, permanent elongation or collagen fiber tearing occurs. The stiffness, normally imparted by the connective tissue of annulus, is now lessened by the injury.

Fatigue loading of the collagen of the annulus might also occur as a result of prolonged, static forward-bending forces, which place tensile stresses (tissue "creep") on the posterior annular wall. Repeated forward bending might result in structural fatigue of the collagen located in the posterior aspect of the annulus fibrosus. A sudden, high-velocity force that exceeds the elastic component of the collagen might also damage the posterior aspect of the annulus. In either case, the lamellae of the annulus are sufficiently distorted to render it structurally weaker.[79]

The annular injury that might occur as a result of forward bending, or forward bending with combined torsion of the trunk, is difficult to distinguish clinically from other soft-tissue sprains and strains. During a forward-bending motion, the axis of rotation is in the region of the nucleus. As the motion proceeds, the instantaneous center of rotation gradually moves anteriorly. Regardless of the exact position of this axis, all structures that are posterior to the axis of rotation are subject to tensile stresses. Positioning the patient who has incurred this forward-bending injury in a posture that extends the lumbar spine has the effect of removing the tensile forces on all structures posterior to the axis of rotation. This is an effective way to rest or immobilize tissue. As a result, the referral pain pattern may diminish because injured tissue is not held in an elongated position. To attribute pain relief only to altered disc mechanics ignores all of the other tissues of the spine.

The various terms utilized for herniations of the intervertebral disc are often confusing (Fig. 4–30). A *protruded* disc is one in which the central mass of the disc intrudes into the ruptured inner fibers of the annulus.

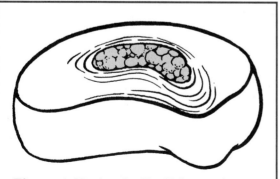

Figure 4–29. Annular "buckle" occurring as a result of loss of ring stiffness of the annulus and nuclear pressure.

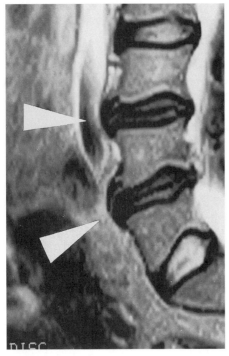

A

Figure 4–30. Lateral view of a magnetic resonance imaging (MRI) scan *(A)* revealing two level anterior protruded discs. Note the degeneration or darkness of these two intervertebral discs as compared to the discs above, L2, L3, and below, L5–S1. *B, C (transverse views),* and *D (sagittal view)* are MRI scans depicting extruded nucleus pulposus. *E* and *F* are lateral views (MRI) of sequestered nucleus pulposus; note how one example shows the migration of disc material superior *(E)* and the other inferior *(F).*

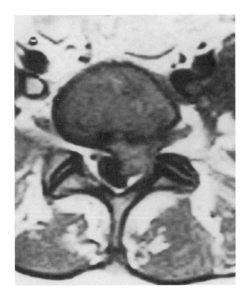

B

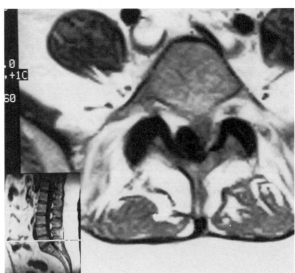

C

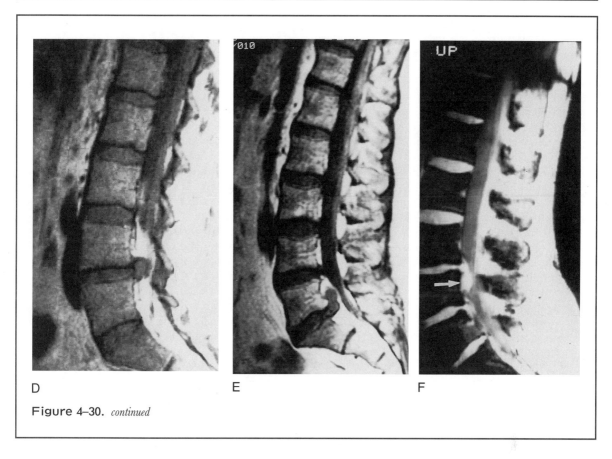

D   E   F

Figure 4–30. *continued*

The peripheral fibers of the annulus remain intact but a general bulging of the disc ensues. An *extruded* disc is one in which the nuclear material has penetrated the outer walls of the annulus but the protruding tissue is still connected to the central part of the disc. The *sequestered* disc is one in which the posterior longitudinal ligament is ruptured and one or more fragments of the herniated material present in the spinal canal. These free fragments have the potential to migrate in different directions, and may lodge in the region of the intervertebral foramen. In the lumbopelvic region, 90 percent of disc herniations are at the L4–L5 or L5–S1 vertebral levels. Usually the protruded distal material affects the next most caudal nerve root. Because of the location of the cauda equina in the spinal canal, a very large midline herniation may compromise several nerve roots. Disc herniations can consist of nucleus pulposus, annulus fibrosus, cartilaginous end-plate, or combinations of these elements.[140]

If we now combine postural positions that have a high intradiscal pressure with spine motion, then movement of desiccated nuclear material is enhanced because it is under high pressure. The younger, gel-like nucleus pulposus is more effective in exerting a higher pressure against the annular walls when compared with the older nucleus, which is more fibrous and has more collagen. These age-related changes of the nucleus pulposus help to explain why disc pathology is more common in young adults (20–45 years old) than in the elderly.

But structural and biomechanical aspects of disc pathology are only part of the etiological spectrum concerning the disc's role in back pain. Since large disc herniations that appear to compress neural elements are known to be asymptomatic, and small disc herniations noted on imaging studies may be more painful than larger ones, there is clearly more to disc pathology and degeneration and their relationship to pain than simply pathoanatomical changes.[117, 134] In fact, there is strong evidence that the signs and symptoms of patients with disc pathology may be more fully explained by inflammation as a result of biochemical factors alone or combined with mechanical factors rather than only mechanical factors.[101] Two broad mechanisms contributing to the inflammatory sequelae to disc pathology have been suggested, and most likely both mechanisms operate simultaneously. One is centered upon immunologic responses; that is, the degenerating disc initiates an antibody–antigen reaction that leads to the cascade of biochemical events promoting inflammation.[11, 38, 76] Herniated discs appear to induce a proliferation of monocytes and macrophages that express inflammatory mediators, further propagating inflammation and inducing a cellular and vascular reaction along the margins of the herniated disc.[25] Another mechanism of inflammation might be directly from various enzymes associated with the discal material itself, independent of an immune response.[20, 102, 103, 114] Extruded nuclear material appears to be a noxious agent causing axonal degeneration and damage to the myelin-forming Schwann cells of the axons through complex biochemical reactions.[88] In both instances, the biochemical milieu lowers the threshold for mechanical stimulation, especially in pain-sensitive tissues within proximity of the herniated discal material, such as the posterior longitudinal ligament, outer aspect of the annulus, dural sheath of the nerve root, and epidural vasculature. Disc degeneration obviously involves a disruption of the biochemical balance within the spinal canal.

An inflammatory state associated with disc pathology may also help explain the relief of symptoms with nonsteroidal anti-inflammatory medication and epidural injections.[24] The fluid stasis associated with inflammation may also explain the relief of symptoms with passive joint mobilization, active range of motion, and exercise.

Thus, a complete understanding of disc injury and disc disease, and their relationship to low back pain, must recognize the structural and biomechanical aspects of the disc while also considering the immunologic and biochemical mechanisms essential to the development of signs and symptoms of associated discal and spinal canal pathology. Inflammation is not only a key but is perhaps the essential component of low back pain. As a result of this understanding, the rationale for treatment strategies is better explained along an inflammation and fluid stasis paradigm than a structural one.

FUNCTIONAL INTERPLAY OF ZYGAPOPHYSEAL JOINTS AND DISC

Now that the zygapophyseal joints and disc have been reviewed in some detail, the previously introduced concept of an interplay between these articulations and the various tissues of the spine should be revisited. Mention has been made of sagittal and horizontal plane motions to give the reader the opportunity to visualize joint activity during movement. However, it is important to continually return to this concept of tissue interplay to better appreciate the mechanics of movement.

To further demonstrate these mechanics, the forward-bending motion will be briefly discussed. This gives us the opportunity to describe the functional interplay between the zygapophyseal joints, intervertebral disc, and posterior spinal ligaments. Using this example also underscores the fact that lumbar tissues work synergistically during movement patterns to provide for the contradictory demands of mobility and stability.

The example of forward bending is chosen because of the extent to which this motion is carried out throughout the activities of daily living. As the trunk begins to bend forward and the motion arrives at the L4 segment, the weight line moves anteriorly causing anterior shear, and intradiscal pressure is increased. A compressive force is generated at the anterior aspect of the L4–L5 disc between the L4 and the L5 vertebral bodies. The anterior compressive force generated into the relatively incompressible nucleus acts now as a fulcrum around which the remainder of the motion can take place (Fig. 4–31). This is a type of "bump and lift" action of one vertebrae upon the subjacent vertebrae.

As the forward motion continues, a tensile stress is imparted to the zygapophyseal joint capsules, and the anterior shear stress of the superior vertebrae on the inferior vertebrae increases. This anterior shear is counteracted by the oblique annular rings on the lateral aspect of the intervertebral disc that travel in a posterior and inferior direction and by the frontal plane orientation of the zygapophyseal joint.[115]

As the fibers of the annular rings become taut, and the articular cartilage of the inferior articulating process of the L4 vertebra engages into the articular cartilage of the superior articulating process of the L5 vertebra, the upward sliding movement at the articu-

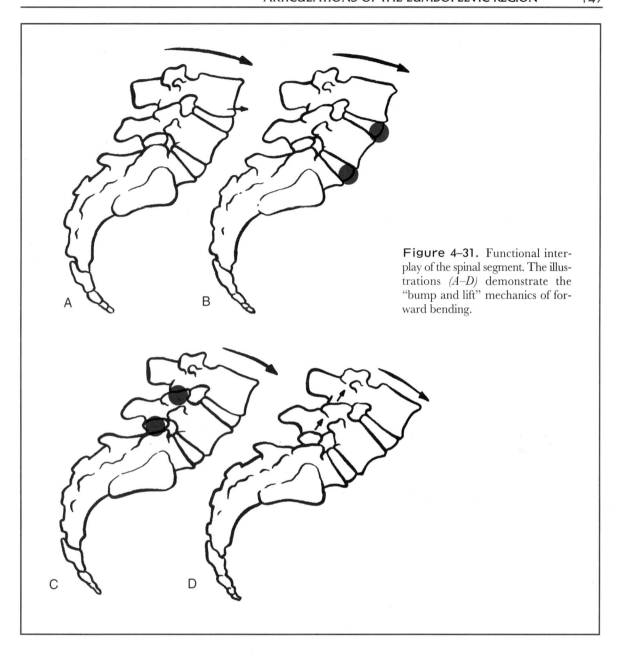

Figure 4–31. Functional interplay of the spinal segment. The illustrations *(A–D)* demonstrate the "bump and lift" mechanics of forward bending.

lar cartilage interface continues. The upward motion of the inferior articulating process is checked by the joint capsule and the posterior ligamentous system.

As the forward bending motion continues, the posterior shear stress is countered by the annular fibers that course interior and anterior, and the interspinous ligament fibers that course superior and posterior. A

dynamic posterior shear force also occurs due to the contraction of the deep erector spinae that are attached to the lumbar transverse processes. These deep erector spinae muscles travel from the iliac crest to the transverse processes of the lumbar vertebrae. They act as lateral guy wires and represent muscle vectors that would be capable of contracting in synchrony to assist in controlling the anterior movement inherent in normal forward bending. This posterior shear exerted actively by contraction of these muscles may theoretically decrease the compressive load that occurs at the frontal plane aspect of the facet cartilage during forward bending. This represents end range motion of that segment.

As the motion is then transferred down to the next lower segment, the same scenario begins. However, at the L5–S1 segment, the forward shear has another significant check in the form of the iliolumbar ligament. This ligament, with its attachment to the transverse processes of the L5 vertebra, comes into play very quickly to stabilize the segment. As the L5 vertebral body compresses the anterior aspect of the intervertebral disc, the posterior bony elements of the vertebra, which include the transverse processes, are "lifted" upward and anteriorly, away from the iliac crest. This movement results in a tightening of the iliolumbar ligament, thus creating a check to these forces of forward bending.

The mechanics of the L4–L5 segment and the L5–S1 segment are subtly different because of the presence of the iliolumbar ligament at the lumbosacral junction. In the absence of this major passive restraint at the L4–L5 level, there exists the potential for increased anterior shear forces, resulting in increased joint compression (frontal plane). Although this particular example deals specifically with the example of forward bending, note also that the iliolumbar ligament helps stabilize the L5–S1 segment in rotation, although this restraint is not afforded the L4–L5 segment. This explanation of the function of these two segments may offer an explanation as to the reason for the increased incidence of injury and slightly greater evidence of pathologic changes at the L4–L5 segment.

It should now be better understood how the zygapophyseal joints work in conjunction with many tissues of the lumbar spine during motion. It is also easy to appreciate how altered function of any of these tissues may result in altered mechanics of forward bending (or any other motion) at the zygapophyseal joints.

THE SACROILIAC JOINTS

The two paired sacroiliac joints have been the source of considerable controversy for many decades as well as the subject of many studies. The reader is referred to studies published more than 50 years ago to gain an appreciation of the historical perspective.[1, 21, 94, 104] The sacroiliac joint has long been used by anthropologists as a skeletal target to determine the age of the specimen. It is well accepted that the joint is an extremely stable structure because of its bony configuration and ligamentous support. There are recorded cases in which severe trauma caused fractures of the ilium and sacrum, but failed to disrupt the sacroiliac joints.[22] The ligaments of this joint are among the strongest in the human body.[137]

Anatomy—Bony Elements

The innominate bone is composed of three segments: the ilium, ischium, and pubis. The paired innominates provide four surface projections—the anterior superior iliac spine, the iliac crest, the posterior superior iliac spine, and the pubic tubercle—that can serve as landmarks for palpation (Fig. 4–32). The ilium is the portion of the innominate that articulates with the sacrum to form the sacroiliac joint, and thus the terms iliosacral and sacroiliac are appropriate anatomical references when referring to this articulation.

The sacrum is a mass of irregularly shaped bone formed by the fusion of five sacral vertebrae and perforated by four pairs of neuroforamina. Over 80 percent of the articular surface of the sacroiliac joint is formed by the first, second, and third sacral segments.[112] The sacrum is wider superiorly than inferiorly, and broader anteriorly than posteriorly (Fig. 4–33). Its overall shape roughly resembles a truncated pyramid with the base located superiorly and anteriorly.

The body of the S1 vertebra articulates with the body of the L5 vertebra by way of the lumbosacral intervertebral disc. Compression and shear loading also occur at the lumbosacral zygapophyseal joints. The plane of the zygapophyseal joints between L5 and S1 varies between individuals and is often asymmetrical when comparing the right side to the left. The orientation is usually a combination of the frontal and sagittal planes.[115] Both regions—the lumbosacral bone–disc interface and the zygapophyseal joints—transmit weight from the trunk to the lower extremity.

Anatomy—Sacroiliac Joints

The sacroiliac joint is a unique articulation with a highly individualized and unique structure. It is a syn-

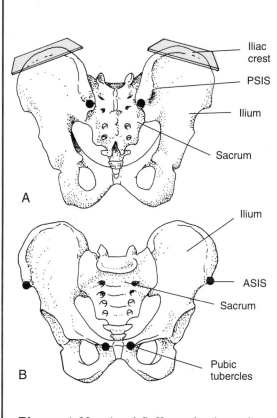

Figure 4–32. *A* and *B,* Key palpation points based upon the bony anatomy of the pelvis: the anterior superior iliac spine, iliac crest, posterior superior iliac spine, and pubic tubercles.

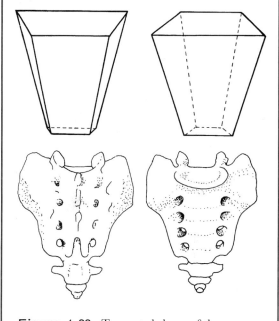

Figure 4–33. Truncated shape of the sacrum. The sacrum is wider superiorly than inferiorly and wider anteriorly than posteriorly.

ovial joint due to the presence of synovial fluid found within the joint cavity, but the interfacing cartilages are of a thicker hyaline variety on the sacral side, and thinner, more fibrous composition on the ilium side. The cartilage on the sacrum is often 3–5 times thicker than the cartilage on the ilium.[9, 16] The adult joint surfaces are marked by a roughened appearance showing several symmetric depressions and raised ridges on the cartilages. The roughened texture results in a joint surface with a higher co-efficient of friction than any other joint.[131] Two vastly different interfacing surfaces, substantially different cartilage thicknesses, and a roughened joint surface make the sacroiliac joint unique, unlike any other joint in the human body, and one apparently structured for stability.

The two sacroiliac joints are "L-" or auricular-shaped when viewed from the side, with the "L" opened posteriorly (Fig. 4–34). Their surfaces are divided into cranial and caudal segments, with the caudal usually being larger.[8, 16] The sacral component of the joint has a more concave profile, while the iliac component is more convex. The orientation of the joint surfaces is not in one of the primary cardinal planes. The sacral surface faces lateral, inferior, and posterior, and, like the iliac surface, is not planar.

This adult bony profile is markedly different from that seen in very young children. At birth, the sacroiliac joint surfaces are smooth and flat, and they parallel the long axis of the spine.[112] In response to changes in growth and the development of upright gait, the joint surfaces change as well as the orientation of their surfaces.[16] Before puberty, the cartilage on the sacral side of the joint is smooth and white, while the iliac cartilage is thin and irregular and appears bluish due to the underlying trabecular bone. During the second and third decades, a ridge develops on the iliac surface with a corresponding depression in the sacral sur-

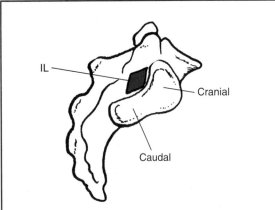

Figure 4–34. Auricular "L" shape of the sacral articular surface. At the junction of the cranial and caudal arms of the sacral facet is the location of the interosseous ligament (IL).

face. The interlocking of this ridge and depression limits the joint motion of the bones to rotation around the X axis (sacral nutation).[10]

A dense ligamentous framework is found both anterior and posterior to the joint cavity (Fig. 4–35). Anteriorly, the anterior sacroiliac ligament traverses the ilium and sacrum and is often blended with the lower aspect of the iliolumbar ligament (Fig. 4–36). Posteriorly, the posterior sacroiliac ligament courses from the posterior iliac ridge to the sacrum. Just anterior to the posterior sacroiliac ligament is the dense interosseous ligament, which is one of the strongest ligament in the human body. It is located at the junction of the cranial and caudal aspects of the "L" (Fig. 4–34). The ligament provides stability to the sacroiliac joint and at the same time permits small, translational movements of the ilium and sacrum on each other as trunk and ground forces converge into the region. Three accessory ligaments also contributing to sacroiliac joint stability are the sacrospinous, sacrotuberous, and long dorsal sacroiliac ligaments (Fig. 4–37). The ligamentous network of the sacroiliac joint and the accessory ligaments helps maintain the positional relationship of the sacrum between the ilia, and minimizes X axis rotation of the bones in response to gravitational and ground forces.

The joint capsule and overlying capsular ligaments of the sacroiliac joint contain unmyelinated and encapsulated nerve endings presumably responsible for pain, thermal sensation, pressure, and position sense.[66] The posterior ligaments and joint capsule are innervated by the lateral branches of the posterior primary rami from L4–S3, while the anterior innervation is from

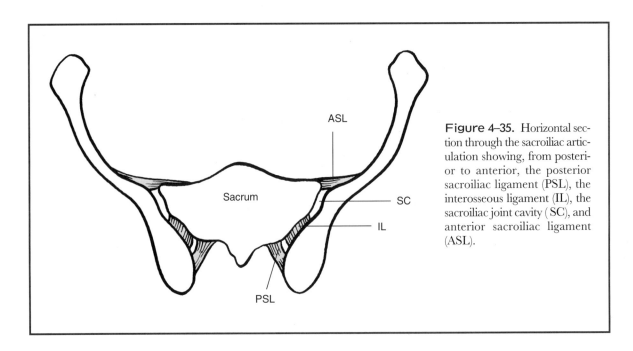

Figure 4–35. Horizontal section through the sacroiliac articulation showing, from posterior to anterior, the posterior sacroiliac ligament (PSL), the interosseous ligament (IL), the sacroiliac joint cavity (SC), and anterior sacroiliac ligament (ASL).

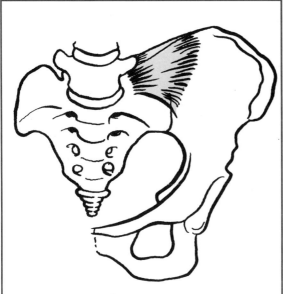

Figure 4–36. Anterior view of lumbosacral and sacroiliac region illustrating how the iliolumbar ligament blends in with the anterior sacroiliac ligament.

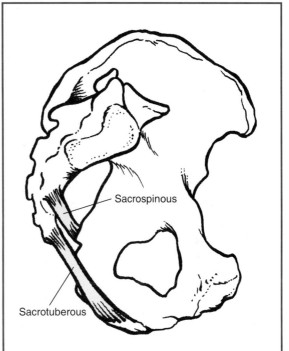

Figure 4–37. Sagittal view of pelvis illustrating the attachments of the sacrotuberous and sacrospinous ligaments.

L2–S2 branches of the anterior rami. The lumbosacral plexus lies directly anterior to the sacroiliac joint as does the psoas major muscle. Because of this broad innervation, sacroiliac joint referral pain patterns mimic those of lumbar pain patterns (Fig. 4–38).[34]

Biomechanics of the Sacroiliac Joint

The sacrum provides the base on which the spine rests. As a result, the sacroiliac joints transmit the loads from the trunk to the lower extremities. The ilium transmits ground reaction forces through the sacroiliac joint to the trunk. In the most simplistic analysis, the sacroiliac joint lies at the intersection of trunk and ground forces.

Numerous motion patterns have been proposed for the sacroiliac joint.[6] The precise model for sacroiliac joint motion, however, and the axes over which these motions occur is largely unknown.[28, 31, 68, 113.] The predominant motion appears to be rotation around the X axis (sacral nutation or iliac torsion), and translation between the sacral and iliac surfaces. Nutation occurs

when there is a forward flexion of the sacrum within the two ilia, while posterior torsion is a rotary force of the ilium on the sacrum (Fig. 4–39). Both result in the same relative positioning of the sacroiliac joint. Counternutation is a backward extension of the sacrum within the paired ilia, while anterior torsion is an anterior rotary moment of the ilium on the sacrum.

Counternutation and anterior torsion also result in the same relative positioning of the sacroiliac joint. Although describing sacroiliac joint motion around the X axis is convenient and allows for systematic analysis of the contributions of surrounding tissues to joint stability, it is a limited model because it is unlikely that motion of the sacroiliac joint occurs around one fixed axis.

In the standing position, the trunk force acts in a direction along the long axis of the spine and converges on the kyphotic and relatively flexed sacrum. The effect of this force through the lumbar vertebral bodies and onto the sacrum is to cause a nutation (flex-

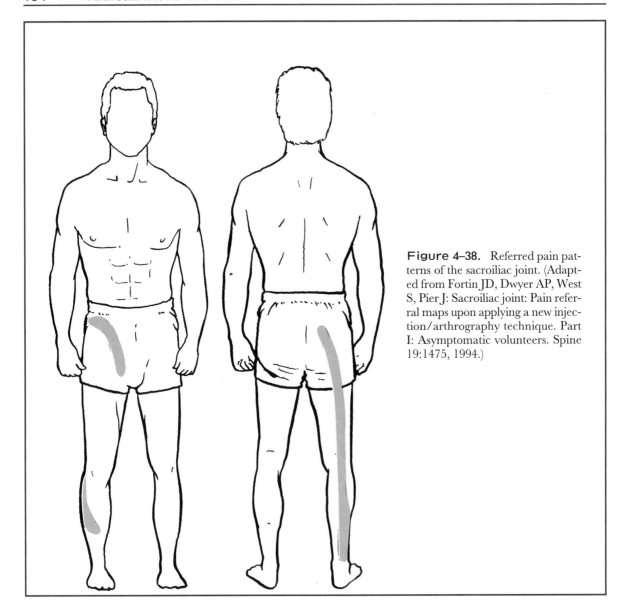

Figure 4–38. Referred pain patterns of the sacroiliac joint. (Adapted from Fortin JD, Dwyer AP, West S, Pier J: Sacroiliac joint: Pain referral maps upon applying a new injection/arthrography technique. Part I: Asymptomatic volunteers. Spine 19:1475, 1994.)

ion) moment of the sacrum within the ilium, and an inferiorly directed shear stress as the weight line converges on the superoanterior aspect of the vertebral body of the first sacral vertebra (Fig. 4–40). Although the plane of the sacroiliac joints is oblique, they are still relatively aligned with the long axis of the spine. Consequently the sacroiliac joints are vulnerable to these two forces—a torque from the nutation moment and a shear from the loading along the long axis of the spine.

In addition to these trunk forces, the sacroiliac joint is simultaneously stressed by the ground force at heel strike, acting through the long axis of the lower extremity and converging into the acetabuium of the pelvis (Fig. 4–41). The result of this force at the sacroiliac joint is also one of torque due to the posterior rotary moment and superior shear of the ilium on the sacrum.

Several factors contribute to sacroiliac joint stability. Vleeming and co-workers have introduced the terms "form closure" and "force closure" to describe mech-

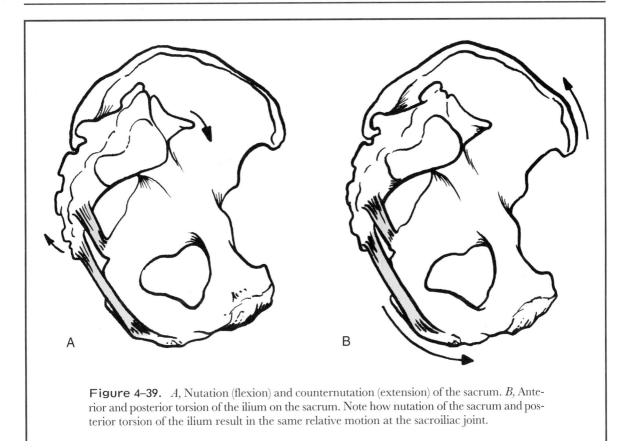

Figure 4–39. *A*, Nutation (flexion) and counternutation (extension) of the sacrum. *B*, Anterior and posterior torsion of the ilium on the sacrum. Note how nutation of the sacrum and posterior torsion of the ilium result in the same relative motion at the sacroiliac joint.

anisms of stability.[110, 111, 124, 126] These terms have clinical utility because they take into account both the structural (osseus, cartilaginous, and ligamentous) and dynamic (musculofascial) contributions to stabilizing the sacroiliac joint. As such, both sets of terms have implications for evaluation and treatment of sacroiliac joint dysfunction.

Form closure is primarily focused on the "fit" of the joint surfaces and those anatomic aspects that relate to "passive stability" of the sacroiliac joint. Stability to the sacroiliac joint in this manner is offered by several means. The wedge-shape of the sacrum being wider superiorly than inferiorly results in the trunk force further seating the sacrum deeper into the ilium as a result of trunk forces. The roughness of the joint surfaces also results in a higher coefficient of friction, which increases joint stability.

Still another mechanism is the trunk force causing a nutation force at the sacrum that increases tension in the sacrotuberous, sacrospinous, and interosseous ligaments (Fig. 4–41). The increased tension results in decreased ability of the sacrum to move within the pelvis, which enhances joint stability.[125, 127] The interosseus ligament is of special interest because the nutation of the sacrum "winds" this ligament tighter, which pulls the sacroiliac joint surfaces together, further increasing the frictional force between the sacrum and ilium.

The various passive mobility tests (see Chapter 5) designed to provoke sacroiliac pain are assessments of the force closure contribution to sacroiliac stability. Tests that purport to assess position or movement by palpation are generally considered to be unreliable.[98] Tests used to create familiar pain by stressing the joint (assessment of form closure) are noted in Table 4–4.[67] It is important to note that the various mobilization and manipulation techniques have little effect on form closure because the instability related to joint dys-

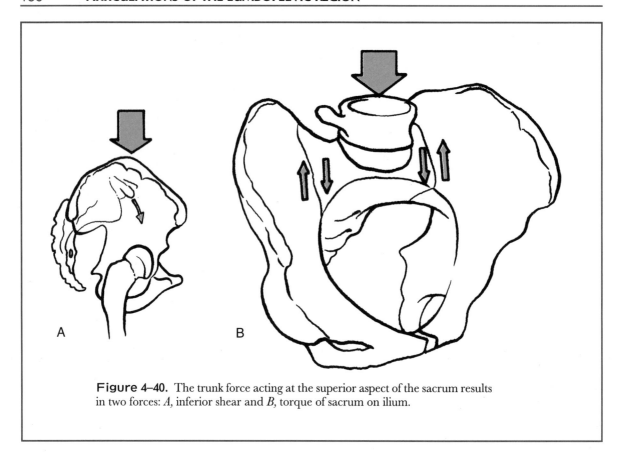

Figure 4–40. The trunk force acting at the superior aspect of the sacrum results in two forces: *A,* inferior shear and *B,* torque of sacrum on ilium.

function is primarily the result of ligamentous laxity. So while manual techniques have practical value in assessment, they have limited utility for treatment. Instead, the coordinated action of the muscles for stabilization becomes of greater importance. Stabilization in this manner is force closure.

Force closure refers to the dynamic stabilization of the sacroiliac joint offered by the musculofascial system. Several of these muscles are reviewed in detail in Chapter 3. Key muscles contributing to force closure of the sacroiliac joint include the latissimus dorsi, gluteus maximus, erector spinae, biceps femoris, and abdominal obliques.

The contralateral latissimus dorsi and the ipsilateral gluteus maximus muscles work in concert through the thoracolumbar fascia.[123] The effect of simultaneous contraction between the two muscles is to create a series of force vectors resulting in increased compression of the sacroiliac joint (Fig. 4–42). This latissimus dorsi–gluteus maximus mechanism allows for

force transference between the arms and the legs through the lumbar spine and sacroiliac regions.

The attachment of the superficial erector spinae to the dorsal aspect of the sacrum through the large erector spinae aponeurosis potentially results in a nutation force vector of the sacrum within the ilium (Fig. 4–43). Nutation is the direction of sacral motion that helps ligamentously lock the sacroiliac articulation due to tightening of the sacrotuberous, sacrospinous, and interosseous ligaments. Furthermore, contraction of the erector spinae (superficial and deep) and the multifidus results in increased tension to the thoracolumbar fascia as the muscles broaden, thereby increasing sacroiliac stability through the same thoracolumbar fascia dynamics implied with the latissimus dorsi–gluteus maximus mechanism.

The hamstring muscles, in particular the biceps femoris, are directly attached to the sacrotuberous ligament (Fig. 4–44). The hamstrings become active just before initial contact in the gait cycle. At initial contact,

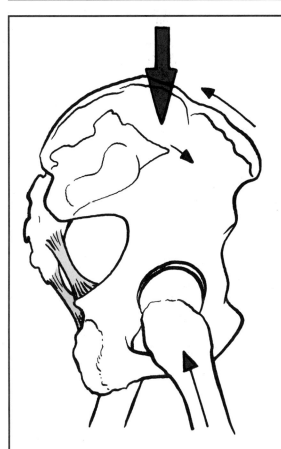

Figure 4–41. At initial contact the ground force results in a posterior rotary moment of the ilium on the sacrum as the force traverses the long axis of the lower extremity and impacts in the acetabulum. This force and the trunk force causing a nutation moment of the sacrum on the ilium result in increased tension to the sacrotuberous, sacrospinous, and interosseous ligaments.

Table 4–4. Provocation Tests: Sacroiliac Joint
Distraction
Compression
Posterior shear of ilium on sacrum
Full ipsilateral hip flexion with contralateral hip extension
Posterior–anterior sacral thrust
Cranial shear
From Laslett M, Williams M: The reliability of selected pain provocation tests for sacroiliac joint pathology. Spine 19:1243, 1994.

ments to the ilium.[14] The action of the abdominal oblique muscles, working over the fulcrum of the interosseous ligament, pull the iliac crests on the right and left side toward the midline, which potentially places the sacroiliac joint in a more close-packed position of joint compression (Fig. 4–45). This joint compression increases frictional force between the sacral and iliac surfaces enhancing joint stability, as well as increasing the compressive force at the pubic symphysis. Compression at the pubic symphysis is also increased via contraction of the hip adductor muscles.

The above discussion lends a scientific rationale for a therapeutic exercise regime for patients with suspected sacroiliac joint dysfunction. An emphasis is placed on the hip extensors, hamstrings, spinal extensors, shoulder extensors, and abdominal muscles. It is interesting to observe that the same emphasis is suggested for lumbar and lumbosacral disorders. The variation between exercise regimes for the different regions of the lumbopelvic area is not that great, which perhaps reaffirms the functional interplay between all components of the lumbopelvic region. Furthermore, it suggests a highly integrated musculofascial system consisting of the upper extremities, spine, pelvis, and lower extremities.

In summary, the forces at the sacroiliac joint are complex and in several planes simultaneously. The rotary forces of the ilium on the sacrum and the torque of the sacrum within the ilium is along a theoretical axis in the frontal plane through the sacroiliac joint and refers to the nutation moment. In contrast, a cranial or caudal shear stress of the ilium on the sacrum would occur around an axis located just posterior to the pubic tubercles.[68] The ligamentous network, bony

the ground force results in a posterior torsional moment of the ilium on the sacrum on the stance leg, and the trunk force is causing a nutation moment at the sacrum. Tension in the sacrotuberous ligament controls the amplitude of these two motions, and this tension through the sacrotuberous ligament is increased with the hamstring contraction.

The internal and external abdominal oblique muscles have a force vector that suggests a contribution to the stability of the sacroiliac joint due to their attach-

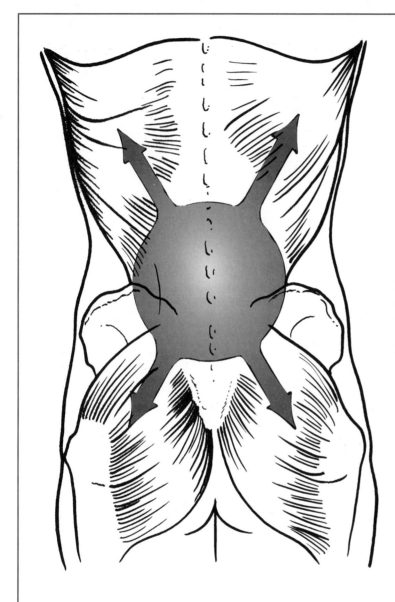

Figure 4–42. The contralateral latissimus dorsi and ipsilateral gluteus maximus are linked through the thoracolumbar fascia system. Contraction of the muscles increases tension to the fascia helping to increase joint compression.

framework, and musculofascial elements all contribute to joint stability.

Sacroiliac Joint Motion

Although appreciable or excessive movement is possible in some people, especially multiparous, post-par-

tum females and individuals with excessive connective tissue laxity, this is not the rule for the general population. Small, accommodating movements occur due to cartilage deformation as the sacroiliac joint surfaces engage and compress together during weight-bearing. Several studies support the concept of limited sacroiliac joint mobility.[62, 113, 128] The range of motion usually in reference to sacral nutation is estimated to be

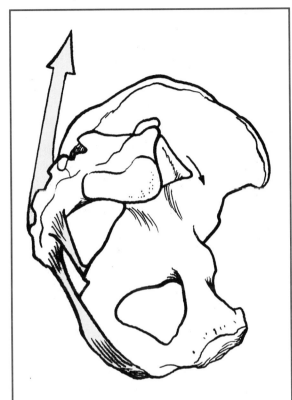

Figure 4–43. Contraction of the superficial erector spinae results in a potential nutation moment of the sacrum. The nutation potentially increases tension to the interosseous, sacrotuberous, and sacrospinous ligaments.

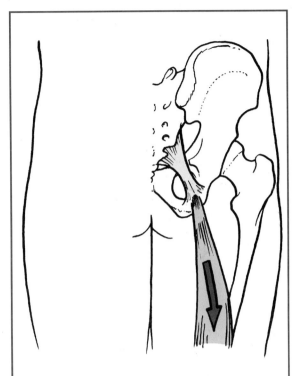

Figure 4–44. The long head of the biceps femoris is continuous with the sacrotuberous ligament. Contraction of the hamstrings increases sacrotuberous ligament tension, potentially increasing sacroiliac joint stability. The hamstrings are active just prior to initial contact in the gait cycle. Initial contact results in posterior rotary moment of the ilium on sacrum and increased sacrotuberous ligament tension via hamstring contraction potentially increases joint stability.

between 0 and 4 degrees with an average of 2 degrees. The shear stress that results in translation between the ilium and sacrum is estimated to be between .5 and 2 mm. Rather than consider actual *movements* occurring at the sacroiliac joint, there is more clinical utility to consider the *moments* that are developed around various axes. These moments are generated by some of the most powerful muscles in the body by virtue of their attachments to the pelvis, as well as by ground and trunk forces. The cartilaginous surfaces compress and seat into each other as the trunk and ground forces are accepted and transferred by the lumbopelvic region during weight-bearing. Therefore, "motion" of the sacroiliac joint is best described as the result of cartilage deformation.

FRONTAL PLANE MECHANICS: ASYMMETRICAL LOADING PATTERNS IN THE SACROILIAC JOINT AND ASSOCIATED LUMBOPELVIC TISSUES

Frontal plane asymmetries are an example of how trunk and ground forces converge into the lumbopelvic region and result in asymmetrical loading patterns of the lumbopelvic tissues. For the purposes of this text,

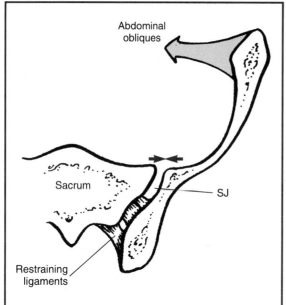

Figure 4–45. Contraction of the abdominal oblique muscles, acting over the fulcrum of the interosseous ligament, increase sacroiliac joint (SJ) and pubic symphysis compression.

frontal plane asymmetries refer to skeletal leg length discrepancies or any structural change resulting in the pelvis being lower on one side. Ground reaction forces reach the lumbopelvic tissues and the resultant forces are attenuated differently than in the symmetrical skeleton.[36, 40, 82, 96] For example, with a structurally short left leg, the pelvis with its sacral base is tilted down to the left side (referred to as a left frontal plane asymmetry for the purposes of this text) (Fig. 4–46). This results in the left sacroiliac joint assuming a more relative horizontal position while the right sacroiliac joint is more vertical. Comparing the forces of the ilium on the sacrum with the symmetrical skeleton, more compressive force is applied to the left sacroiliac joint and more shear stress on the right. Because the sacral base, as it sits within the pelvis, is tilted down to the right, it also results in a side-bending motion at the lumbosacral joint. Consequently, compressive forces are placed on tissues on the concave side of the curve and tensile forces on the convex side of the curve. The longer leg side also has increased compressive forces at the head of the femur. If any of these forces exceed the tolerance of the tissues, there is a potential for tissue injury or accelerated breakdown. Note how the frontal plane asymmetry potentially alters the mechanics at the sacroiliac joint, lumbosacral joint, and the hip. For this

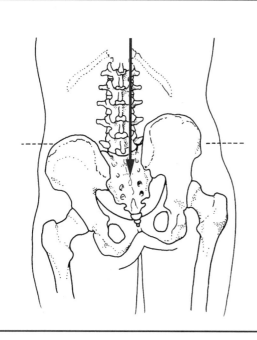

Figure 4–46. With a frontal plane asymmetry the loading patterns of the lumbopelvic tissues is different from one side to the other. On the long leg side, there is increased sacroiliac joint shear, increased compression to the head of the femur, and increased compression of the lumbosacral and lower lumbar zygapophyseal joints.

reason it is extremely difficult to attempt to isolate one tissue at fault, but it is more logical to attempt to improve faulty mechanics that may contribute to the painful condition (see Chapter 5).

SACROILIAC JOINT AND PUBIC SYMPHYSIS: HORMONAL INFLUENCES

The biomechanics of the female pelvis are different from those of the male pelvis. Structurally, the female pelvis is shorter and wider than the male pelvis. The hormonal changes of menses and pregnancy render the female pelvis slightly more mobile, and it has been suggested that this results in an increased vulnerability to sacroiliac joint.[15, 35, 41] Initially, Hishaw[50] and later Weiss et al.[132] described the release of the hormone relaxin during pregnancy. The titer of this hormone, probably in combination with other biochemical changes, appears to alter the stiffness of the connective tissue so that increased motion is available to allow for expansion of the pelvic outlet and to facilitate the passage of the infant through the birth canal. The ischial tuberosities are initially closer together before the infant has moved into the pelvic canal. However, as the infant moves down the pelvic canal, the ischial tuberosities spread, causing an inward motion of the ilia.

Although the biochemical changes may facilitate childbirth, they may potentially render the weight-bearing joints of the pelvis vulnerable to sprain because of excessive motion. This may also include the period during which the infant is breastfed, which also features biochemical changes. Specific sacroiliac joint injury related to pregnancy, therefore, can occur before, during, or for a time after childbirth.

The pubic symphysis has been recognized as a potential cause of anterior pelvis and medial thigh pain since the early 1930s.[1, 21] These authors recognized the vulnerability of this joint, especially with multiparous women, and described osseous changes to its structure.

The pubic symphysis is an amphiarthrodial joint in the anterior aspect of the pelvis that forms a fibrocartilaginous union between the two pubic bones. The pubis is the anterior part of the innominate bone. From its anteromedial body the superior ramus passes up and back to the acetabulum, while an inferior ramus passes back, down, and laterally to join the ischial ramus inferior to the obturator foramen.[137] The superior and inferior rami join anteriorly to form the body of the pubis, which has a symphysial (medial) surface that articulates with the contralateral pubis. The joint surface is lined with a thin layer of cartilage.[37] These joint surfaces are separated by a thick intrapubic fibrocartilaginous disc that is 3–5 mm wider anterior than posterior. The joint also includes a suprapubic ligament that attaches to the pubic tubercles and crests to cover the superior aspect of the joint. The anterior pubic symphysis blends with the aponeurosis of the rectus abdominis muscle, and the posterior aspect is connected by the posterior pubic ligament that joins with the inner abdominal fascia of the transversus abdominis muscle. The thick inferior pubic ligament, or arcuate ligament, forms an arch that spans both inferior rami and stabilizes the joint from compressive, shear, tensile, and rotary forces.[37]

The structure of the symphysis is longer in the vertical direction in males, but the fibrocartilaginous disc is much wider in females and the symphysis pubis undergoes a variety of changes as a result of age, function, and, in females, the special hormonal influences of pregnancy and the mechanical trauma of parturition.[37] This joint connects the two weight-bearing arches of the pelvis that together function to transfer and absorb the ground and trunk forces.

The pubic bone also provides attachment for a number of different muscles. These muscles include the medial thigh muscles: the adductor longus, the adductor brevis, a portion of the adductor magnus, the gracilis, and the pectineus (Fig. 4–47). In addition, the rectus abdominis, the obturator internus and externus through their pubic portion of the obturator membrane, the pyramidalis, and the levator ani are attached. Many of these muscles, especially the medial thigh group, are large and quite capable of exerting significant forces to the pubis and, ultimately, the pelvic joints when the foot is fixed on the ground. These muscles play a major role in controlling the forces that are transferred into this region. The pubic symphysis resembles a bushing that permits tissue deformation and small translatory movements as a result of muscle, ground reaction, and trunk forces.

Several authors have studied the mechanics of this anterior pelvic joint and have concluded that this amphiarthrodial joint has little movement, especially in men and nulliparous women.[37, 65, 122] Walheim and associates looked at mobility *in vivo* by inserting parallel pins on either side of the pubic symphysis at the

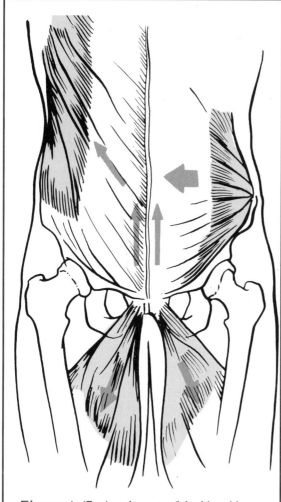

Figure 4–47. Attachments of the hip adductor muscles and abdominal muscles to the pubic rami.

representative of tissue deformation during force acceptance rather than actual joint excursion.

The pubic symphysis can be the site for pathological conditions, such as infectious and inflammatory diseases. The infectious diseases can be characteristic of intravenous drug users, and often involve pyogenic or tuberculous organisms.[108] The most common disease of the pubic symphysis is a self-limiting nonbacterial inflammation of the pubis that can be produced by pelvic surgery, childbirth, or trauma caused by work, play, or sport. The last is often attributed to repeated mechanical sprain or strain to the soft tissues that are attached to this region.[69, 136]

Problems to the symphysis are not commonly seen in the clinic, but they can be recognized by the complaint of anterior pain often exacerbated by mechanical stresses of evaluation, such as posterior-to-anterior compression to the superior ramus of the pubis, resistance to contraction of the previously mentioned medial thigh muscles, and palpation. Tendinitis of the adductor longus or rectus abdominis can be easily mistaken for joint irritation because of the proximity of their attachments to the pubic symphysis. The problems related to treating the region are usually caused by the difficulty in stabilizing the area or controlling the resultant forces that reach it in order to allow healing to occur.

THE HIP JOINT

Because movements of the hip joint ultimately transfer forces to the pelvis and lumbar regions, and the major muscles of the hip joint have attachments to these regions, a brief review of the anatomy and mechanics is warranted. The hip joint is a multiaxial joint with the shape of a ball and socket. Because the complete surfaces of the femoral head and acetabulum are not in total contact with each other, nor are they true hemispheres, it is not a true ball-and-socket arrangement, but certainly approaches one.

The hip joint is very stable because of its design. Its architecture includes the acetabular labrum, which effectively deepens the socket. Because of the depth of the acetabulum, a vacuum effect is created when a distraction force is placed between the head of the femur and the acetabulum. The hip joint has the capability to move actively and passively in all three cardinal planes. There are no accessory movements of the hip except for slight separation effected by strong traction.[137]

pubic tubercles on 15 subjects, all of whom were diagnosed with pelvic instability.[129] The findings revealed that the mean gap at the symphysis was 1 mm, and the forward-to-backward mean motion was 1.1 mm. Rotation was measured to average 0.5 degrees in both planes. The vertical translation varied among the population, but the mean distance was 2.5 mm. These findings support the concept that there is little movement available at the pubic symphysis for the clinician to quantify without sophisticated measuring devices. Like the sacroiliac joint, these small movements are

The hip joint capsule and the reinforcing ligaments provide a measure of joint stability as well as a check for motion. The ligamentous capsule is thicker antero-superiorly, where maximal stress occurs, particularly in standing, while posteroinferiorly it is thin and loosely attached.[137] The capsular ligaments of the hip are divided into iliofemoral, ischiofemoral, and pub-ofemoral. These attachments are named for the areas of the innominate bone to which they are attached (Fig. 4–48). Anteriorly, the iliofemoral and pubofemoral ligaments converge to attach to the intertrochanteric line of the femur, whereas the ischiofemoral ligament originates from the ischium just posteroinferior to the acetabulum and spirals superolaterally behind the femoral neck to attach to the anterior aspect of the femur.

The close-packed position of the hip is full extension, with slight abduction and medial rotation.[137] Therefore, as this position is reached, the capsular ligaments of the hip become taut.[40, 47, 82] This position of the hip corresponds to the hip posture in standing. Although being at this close-packed position minimizes energy expenditure for upright posture, it also contributes to the fact that the hip joint has a higher incidence of degenerative joint disease than do joints that are not close-packed in standing, such as the ankle.[48] As the connective tissue limits of the hip joint capsular ligaments are reached, forces are subsequently transferred to the sacroiliac joints and then to the lumbar joints. Motion of the hip can thus influence pelvic and lumbar mechanics (Fig. 4–20).

The hip is designed as a major weight-bearing joint with an articular cartilage–bony trabecular system that accepts large forces transferred through it.[46, 56, 58] The articular surfaces are reciprocally curved but not completely congruent. The acetabular articular surface is broader and thicker superiorly, where pressure of the body weight falls when in the erect, standing posture. The inferior surfaces of the femoral head do not articulate with the acetabulum during loading and unloading. By contrast, the entire acetabulum is involved in weight-bearing.[23, 45]

Contact and noncontact areas have been studied and both have been found to be involved in the degenerative process, suggesting that contact and a regular pattern of loading and unloading are necessary for normal joint lubrication and nutrition, which contribute to the overall health of the joint.[23, 45, 49] Degeneration patterns range from fibrillation of articular cartilage to osteophyte formation.[57]

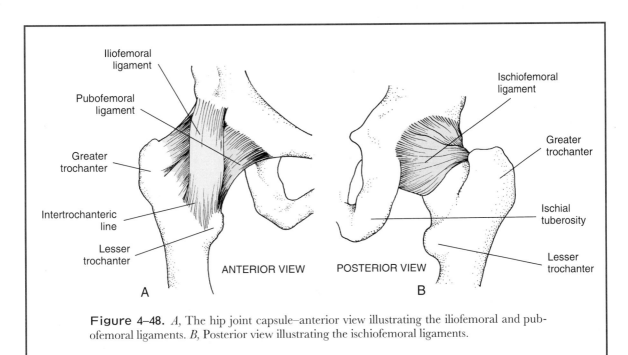

Figure 4–48. *A*, The hip joint capsule–anterior view illustrating the iliofemoral and pub-ofemoral ligaments. *B*, Posterior view illustrating the ischiofemoral ligaments.

The bony trabecular patterns of the femur and the pelvis dramatically illustrate the force transference system of the lumbopelvic region. In the femur two trabecular patterns can be identified. These two trabecular patterns are oriented along compressive and tensile force lines. The acetabulum also reveals a trabecular pattern oriented along lines of stress.

Of perhaps greater interest to the clinician is the trabecular bone growth in response to forces traversing the hip, pelvis, sacrum, and lumbar spine. The trabecular pattern of these tissues reveals that the region is a true weight-bearing hub and works as an integral part of the lumbopelvic functional unit to transfer trunk and ground forces. The articulations of the lumbopelvic region are a linked system, and this linkage is emphasized by the trabecular pattern of the bones making up the linkage.

The femoral head can withstand 12–15 times body weight without destruction. The forces involved in single limb support standing on one leg, owing to the contraction of the hip abductor muscles and body weight, increase the load to 2.5 to 4 times body weight.[58] Running increases the load to approximately 5 times normal body weight.[58] The joint, therefore, is subject to such forces as body weight and muscle contraction.

Inherent in the design of the hip joint is an ability to deform and spread the loads over a larger surface area. This ability decreases the force per unit area and protects the articular cartilage from early degeneration.[44, 81] Although compression is the major force imparted to the hip, it must also attenuate shear, bending, and torsion. The subchondral bone and trabecular pattern of the femur and the pelvis assist the articular cartilage in the transference of these forces.[56]

It is estimated that 10 percent of people under age 30 have a degree of hip arthrosis, and this percentage rises to 89 percent of those over age 65. The ratio of females to males showing degenerative changes is 3:2.[59] As these structural changes proceed, function can be assumed to be altered as well. However, it is not only movement at the hip joint itself that may be altered but also the manner in which the hip joint transfers ground reaction forces to the pelvis and lumbar spine. The hip joint plays a major role in the proper transferral of forces through the axial skeleton. With respect to the lumbopelvic region, the hip plays an integral role and should be closely evaluated.

The clinician should recognize the functional relationships between hips and the low back during the assessment process. For example, tightness of the hip as seen with the figure 4 or FABERS test positions (see Chapter 5, Figure 5–17), results in decreased hip femoral extension during stance phase of gait. As the limits of femoral extension are reached during terminal stance, there is an increased compressive and shear loading between the lower lumbar segments. These relationships are analyzed further in the next chapter.

SUMMARY

We have defined the lumbopelvic unit as the articulations between L4 and L5, L5 and S1, the sacroiliac joint, the pubic symphysis, and hips. Each articulation is unique yet works collaboratively to contribute to mobility, stability, and force attenuation of the lumbopelvic region. There is an important interplay between these articulations, and also the soft tissues, including the muscle–fascial elements, that contributes to movement and weight-bearing by the lumbopelvic region. An understanding of these articulations, the changes associated with pathology, and the effect of the inflammatory process will assist the clinician in the evaluation and treatment of mechanical disorders of this region. These are explored in the next chapters.

REFERENCES

1. Abramson D, Roberts SM, Wilson P: Relaxation of the pelvic joints in pregnancy. Gynecol Obstet (Suppl) 58:595, 1934.
2. Adams M, Dolan P, Hutton WC: The stages of disc degeneration as revealed by discogram. J Bone Joint Surg 68B:36, 1986.
3. Adams MA, Dolan P: A technique for quantifying bending moment acting on the lumbar spine in vivo. J Biomech 24:117, 1991.
4. Adams MA, Hutton WC: The effect of posture on the role of the apophyseal joints in resisting intervertebral compressive forces. J Bone Joint Surg 62B:358, 1980.
5. Adams MA, Hutton WC: The relevance of torsion to the mechanical derangement of the lumbar spine. Spine 6:241, 1981.
6. Aiderink GJ: The sacroiliac joint: Review of anatomy, mechanics and function. J Orthop Sports Phys Ther 13:71, 1991.
7. American Academy of Orthopaedic Surgeons: A glossary on spinal terminology. Chicago, American Academy of Orthopaedic Surgeons, 1985, p.34.
8. Bakiand 0, Hansen JH: The axial sacroiliac joint. Anat Clin 6:29, 1984.

9. Beal MC: The sacroiliac problem: Review of anatomy, mechanics and diagnosis. J Am Osteopath Assoc 81:667, 1982.

10. Bernard TN, Cassidy JD: The Sacroiliac Joint Syndrome. In Frymoyer J (eds): The Adult Spine. New York, Raven Press 1991, p. 2110.

11. Bobechko WP, Hirsch C: Autoimmune response to nucleus pulposus in the rabbit. J Bone Joint Surg (Br) 47:574, 1965.

12. Bogduk N, Twomey LT: Clinical Anatomy of the Lumbar Spine. New York, Churchill Livingstone, 1987.

13. Bogduk N: The innervation of the intervertebral discs. In Ghosh P (ed): The Biology of the Intervertebral Disc. Boca Raton, FL, CRC Press, 1988, p. 135.

14. Bojsen Moller F: Functional anatomy of the sacroiliac joint. (In Danish) Manedsskrift for praktisk laegegerning 4:211, 1988.

15. Borell U: The movements of the sacroiliac joints and their importance to changes in pelvic dimensions during parturition. Acta Gynecol Scand 36:42, 1957.

16. Bowan V, Cassidy JD: Macroscopic and microscopic anatomy of the sacroiliac joint from embryonic life until the eighth decade. Spine 6:620, 1981.

17. Bradford DS, Cooper KM, Oegema TR: Chymopapain, chemonucleolysis, and nucleus pulposus regeneration. J Bone Joint Surg (Am) 65A:1220, 1983.

18. Brickley-Parsons D, Glimcher MJ: Is the chemistry of collagen in intervertebral discs an expression of Wolff's law? Spine 9:148, 1984.

19. Brinckmann P: Injury of the annulus ribrosus and disc protrusions: An in vitro investigation of human lumbar discs. Spine 11: 149, 1986.

20. Brown MD: The source of low back pain and sciatica. Sem Arthritis Rheum 18:67, 1989.

21. Chamberlin WE: X-ray examination of the sacroiliac joints. Del Med J 4:195, 1932.

22. Colachis SD, Worden RE, Bechtol CO: Movement of the sacroiliac joint in the adult male: A preliminary report. Arch Phys Med Rehabil 44:490, 1963.

23. Day WH, Swanson SAV, Freeman MAR: Contact pressures in the loaded human cadaver hip. J Bone Joint Surg (Br) 57B:302, 1975.

24. Dilke TFW, Burry JC, Grahame R: Extradural corticoid injection in management of lumbar nerve root compression. Br Med J 2:635, 1973.

25. Doita M, Kanatani T, Harada T, Mizuno K: Immunohistologic study of ruptured intervertebral disc of the lumbar spine. Spine 21:235, 1996.

26. Dolan P, Earley M, Adams MA: Bending and compressive stresses acting on the lumbar spine during lifting activities. J Biomech 27:1237, 1994.

27. Dolan P, Mannion AF, Adams MA: Passive tissues help the back muscles to generate extensor moments during lifting. J Biomech 27:1077, 1994.

28. Drerup B, Hierholzer E: Movement of the human pelvis and displacement of related anatomical landmarks on the body surface. J Biomech 20:971, 1987.

29. Dunlop RB, Adams MA, Hutton WC: Disc space narrowing and the lumbar facet joints. J Bone Joint Surg (Br) 66B:706, 1984.

30. Ebara S, Iatridis JC, Setton LA, et al: Tensile properties of nondegenerate human lumbar annulus fibrosus. Spine 21:452, 1996.

31. Egund N: Movement in the sacroiliac joints demonstrated with roentgen stereophotogrammetry. Acta Radiol (Diagn) (Stockh) 19:833, 1978.

32. Farfan HF, Cossette JW, Robertson GH, Wells RV: The effects of torsion on the lumbar intervertebral joints: The role of torsion in the production of disc degeneration. J Bone Joint Surg (Am) 52A:468, 1970.

33. Farfan HF: Mechanical Disorders of the Low Back. Philadelphia, Lea & Febiger, 1973.

34. Fortin JD, Dwyer AP, West S, Pier J: Sacroiliac joint: Pain referral maps upon applying a new injection/arthrography technique. Part 1: asymptomatic volunteers. Spine 19:1475, 1994.

35. Fraser DM: Postpartum backache: A preventable condition? Bulletin of Orthopedic Section, APTA 3:14, 1978.

36. Friberg 0: Clinical symptoms and biomechanics of lumbar spine and hip joint in leg length inequality. Spine 8:643, 1983.

37. Gamble JG, Simmons SC, Freedman M: The symphysis pubis. Clin Orthop 203:261, 1986.

38. Gertzbein SD, Tile M, Gross A, Falk R: Degenerative disc disease of the lumbar spine: Immunological implications. Clin Orthop 129:68, 1977.

39. Goel VK, Weinstein JN, (eds): Biomechanics of the Spine—Clinical and Surgical Perspective. Boca Raton, FL, CRC Press, 1990, p. 97.

40. Gofton JP: Osteoarthritis of the hip and leg length discrepancy. Can Med Assoc 104:791, 1971.

41. Golighty R: Pelvic arthropathy in pregnancy and the puerperium. Physiotherapy 68:216, 1982.

42. Gotfried Y, Bradford DS, Oegema TR: Facet joint changes after chemonucleolysis-induced disc space narrowing. Spine 11:944, 1986.

43. Gracovetsky S, Farfan H: The optimum spine. Spine 11:543, 1986

44. Gradisar IA, Porterfield JA: Articular cartilage. Top Geriatr Rehab 4:1, 1989.

45. Greenwald AS, Haynes DW: Weight-bearing areas in the human hip joint. J Bone Joint Surg (Br) 54B: 157, 1972.

46. Greenwald AS, O'Connor JJ: The transmission of load through the human hip joint. J Biomech 4:507, 1971.

47. Grieves GP: The hip. Physiotherapy 69:196, 1983.

48. Gruebel Lee DM: Disorders of the Hip. Philadelphia, JB Lippincott, 1983, p. 1.

49. Harrison MHM, Schajowicz F, Truetta J: Osteoarthritis of the hip: A study of the nature and evolution of the disease. J Bone Joint Surg (Br) 35B:77, 1953.

50. Hishaw TL: Corpus luteum hormone: Experimental relaxation of pelvic ligaments of guinea pig. Physiol Zool 2:59, 1929.

51. Holm S, Nachemson A: Variations in the nutrition of the canine intervertebral disc induced by motion. Spine 8:866, 1983.

52. Holm S: Pathophysiology of disc degeneration. Acta Orthop Scand (Suppl) 251:13, 1993.

53. Horton GW: Further observations on the elastic mechanism of the intervertebral disc. J Bone Joint Surg (Br) 40B:552, 1958.

54. Humzah MD, Soames RW: Human intervertebral disc: Structure and function. Anat Rec 220:103, 1981.

55. Jackson R.P, Jacobs RR, Montesano PX: Facet joint injections in low back pain. A prospective study. Spine 13:966, 1988.

56. Jacob HAV, Huggler AH, Dietschi C, Schreiber A: Mechanical function of subchondral bone as experimentally determined on the acetabulum of the human pelvis. J Biomech 9:625,1976.

57. Jeffery AK: Osteophyte and the osteoarthritic femoral head. J Bone Joint Surg (Br) 57B:314, 1975.

58. Johnston R: Mechanical considerations of the hip joint. Arch Surg 107:411, 1973.

59. Jorring K: Osteoarthritis of the hip. Acta Orthop Scand 51:523, 1980.

60. Kirkaldy-Willis W: Managing Low Back Pain, 2nd ed. New York, Churchill Livingstone, 1988, p. 8.

61. Kirkaldy-Willis WH, Farfan HF: Instability of the lumbar spine. Clin Orthop 165:110, 1982.

62. Kissling R, Brunner C, Jacob HAC: Mobility of the sacroiliac joint in vitro. Z Orthop 128:282,1990.

63. Klein J, Hukins D: Collagen fibre orientation in the annulus fibrosus of intervertebral disc during bending and torsion measured by X-ray diffraction. Biochim Biophys Acta 719:98, 1982.

64. Klein J, Hukins D: X-ray diffraction demonstrates reorientation of collagen fibres in the annulus fibrosus during compression of the intervertebral disc. Biochim Biophys Acta 717:61, 1982.

65. Laban MN, Meerschaert JR, Taylor RS, Tabor HD: Symphyseal and sacroiliac joint pain associated with pubic symphyseal instability. Arch Phys Med Rehab 59:470, 1978.

66. Lamb DW: The neurology of spinal pain. Phys Ther 59:971, 1979.

67. Laslett M, Williams M: The reliability of selected pain provocation tests for sacroiliac joint pathology. Spine 19:1243, 1994.

68. Lavignolle B, Vital JM, Senegas J, et al: An approach to the functional anatomy of the sacroiliac joints in vivo. Anat Clin 5:169, 1983.

69. Le Jenne JJ, Rochcongar P, Vazelle F, et al: Pubic pain syndrome in sportsmen: Comparison of radiographic and scintigraphic findings. Eur J Nucl Med 9:250, 1984.

70. Lewinnek GE, Warrield CA: Facet joint degeneration as a cause of low back pain. Clin Orthop 213:216, 1986.

71. Lorenz M, Patwardhan A, Vanderby R: Load bearing characteristics of the lumbar facets in normal and surgically altered spinal segments. Spine 8:122, 1983.

72. Lumsden RM, Morris JM: An in vivo study of axial rotation and immobilization at the lumbosacral joint. J Bone Joint Surg 50:1591, 1968.

73. Malinsky J: Histochemical demonstration of carbohydrates in human intervertebral discs during postnatal development. Acta Histochem 5:120, 1958.

74. Malinsky J: The ontogenetic development of nerve terminations in the intervertebral discs of man. Acta Anat (Basel) 38:96, 1959.

75. Markolf KL, Morris JM: The structural components of the intervertebral disc. J Bone Joint Surg 56A:675,1974.

76. Marshall LL, Trethewie ER, Curtain CC: Chemical radiculitis: A clinical psychological, and immunological study. Clin Orthop 129:61, 1987.

77. McCarron RF, Wimpee MW, Hudkins PG, Laros GS: The inflammatory effect of the nucleus pulposus: A possible element in the pathogenesis of lowback pain. Spine 12:760, 1987.

78. McDevitt CA: Proteoglycans of the intervertebral disc. In Ghosh P (ed):The Biology of the Intervertebral Disc. Boca Raton, FL, CRC Press, 1988, p. 151.

79. McKenzie RA: Mechanical Diagnosis and Therapy of the Lumbar Spine. Waikanae, New Zealand, Spinal Publications, 1981.

80. Meachim G, Stockwell RA: The matrix. In Freeman MAR (ed): Adult Articular Cartilage. New York, Grune & Stratton, 1972, p. 150.

81. Meachim G: Effect of age on the thickness of adult articular cartilage at the shoulder joint. Ann Rheum Dis 30:43, 1971.

82. Mellin G: Correlations of hip mobility with degree of back pain and lumbar spinal mobility in chronic low-back pain patients. Spine 13:668, 1988.

83. Mooney V, Robertson J: The facet syndrome. Clin Orthop 115:149, 1976.

84. Mooney V: The facet syndrome. In Weinstein JN, Wiesel S (eds): The Lumbar Spine. Philadelphia, W. B. Saunders, 1990 p. 438.

85. Nachemson A, Morris JM: In vivo measurements of intradiscal pressure. J Bone Joint Surg 46:1077, 1964.

86. Nachemson A: Towards a better understanding of lowback pain: A review of the mechanics of the lumbar disc. Rheumatol Rehab 14:129, 1975.

87. Oegema TR: Biochemistry of the intervertebral disc. Clin Sports Med 12:419, 1993.

88. Olmarker K, Nordborg C, Larsson K, Rydevik B: Ultrastructural changes in spinal nerve roots induced by autologous nucleus pulposus. Spine 21:411, 1996.

89. Osti OL, Vernon-Roberts B, Moore R, Fraser RD: Annular tears and disc degeneration in the lumbar spine. J Bone Joint Surg 74B:678-682, 1991.

90. Panjabi MM, Krag MH, Chung TQ: Effects of disc injury on mechanical behavior of the human spine. Spine 9:707, 1984.

91. Pearce RH, Grimmer B, Adams M: Degeneration and chemical composition of the human lumbar intervertebral disc. J Orthop Res 5:198, 1987.

92. Pearce RH, Mathieson JM, Mort JS, Roughley PJ: The effect of age on the abundance and fragmentation of link protein of the human intervertebral disc. J Orthop Res 7:861, 1989.

93. Pearcy MJ, Tibrewal SB: Lumbar intervertebral disc and ligament deformations measured in vivo. Clin Orthop 191:281, 1984.

94. Pitkin HD, Pheasant HC: Sacrarthrogenetic telalgia. J Bone Joint Surg 18:111, 1936.
95. Pope M, Panjabi M: Biomechanical definition of spinal instability. Spine 10:255,1985.
96. Porterfield JA, DeRosa CP: The sacroiliac joint. In Gould JA (ed): Orthopedic and Sports Physical Therapy, 2nd ed. St. Louis, CV Mosby, 1990, p. 553
97. Porterfield JA: Dynamic stabilization of the trunk. J Orthop Sports Phys Ther 6:271, 1985.
98. Potter NA, Rothstein JM: Intertester reliability for selected clinical tests of the sacroiliac joint. Phys Ther 65:1671, 1985.
99. Revel ME, Listrat VM, Chevalier XJ, et al: Facet joint block for low back pain: Identifying predictors of a good response. Arch Phys Med Rehabil 73:824, 1992.
100. Roberts S, Menage J, Urban JPG: Biochemical and structural properties of the cartilage end-plate and its relation to the intervertebral disc. Spine 14:166, 1989.
101. Saal J: The role of inflammation in lumbar pain. Spine 20:1821, 1995.
102. Saal JS, Franson R, Myers, Saal JA: Human disc PLA2 induces neural injury: A histomorphometric study. In: International Society for the Study of the Lumbar Spine. Chicago 1992.
103. Saal JS, Franson RC, Dobrow R, Saal JA, White AH, Goldthwaite N: High levels of inflammatory phospholipase A2 in lumbar disc herniations. Spine 15:674, 1990.
104. Sashin D: A critical analysis of the anatomy and the pathological changes of the SI joints. J Bone Joint Surg 12:891, 1930.
105. Schmorl G, Junghans H: The Human Spine in Health and Disease. New York, Grune & Stratton, 1959.
106. Schwarzer HJA, April CN, Derby R, et al: Clinical features of patients with pain stemming from the lumbar zygapophyseal joints. Spine 19:1132, 1994.
107. Scott JE, Bosworth TR, Cribb AM, Taylor JR: The chemical morphology of age-related changes in human intervertebral disc glycosaminglycans from cervical, thoracic, and lumbar nucleus pulposus and annulus fibrosus. J Anat 184:73, 1994.
108. Sequeria W, Jones E, Seigel ME, et al: Pyogenic infections of the pubic symphysis. Ann Intern Med 96:604, 1982.
109. Snidjers CJ, Slagter A, van Strik R, et al: Why leg crossing? Spine 20:1989, 1995.
110. Snidjers CJ, Vieeming A, Stoeckart R: Transfer of lumbosacral load to the iliac bones and legs. Part I—Biomechanics of self bracing of the sacroiliac joints and its significance for treatment and exercise. Clin Biomech 8:285, 1993.
111. Snidjers CJ, Vieeming A, Stoeckart R: Transfer of lumbosacral load to iliac bones and legs. Part II—Loading of the sacroiliac joints when lifting in a stooped posture. Clin Biomech 8:295, 1993.
112. Solonen KA: The sacroiliac joint in light of anatomical, roentgenological, and clinical studies. Acta Orthop Scand (Suppl) 27:1, 1957.
113. Sturesson B, Selvik G, Uden A: Movement of the sacroiliac joints. A stereophotogrammetric analysis. Spine 14:162, 1989.
114. Takahashi H, Suguro T, Okazima Y, et al: Inflammatory cytokines in the herniated disc of the lumbar spine. Spine 21:218, 1996.
115. Taylor JR, Twomey LT: Age changes in lumbar zygapophyseal joints: Observation on structure and function. Spine 11:739, 1986.
116. Tesh KM, Dunn JS, Evans JH: The abdominal muscles and vertebral stability. Spine 12:501, 1987.
117. Thelander U, Fagerlund M, Friberg S, Larsson F: Straight leg raising vs. radiologic size, shape, and position of lumbar disc herniations. Spine 17:395, 1992.
118. Twomey LT, Taylor JR: Sagittal movements of the human lumbar vertebral column: A quantitative study of the role of the posterior vertebral elements. Arch Phys Med Rehabil 64:322,1983.
119. Urban J: Disc Biochemistry in Relation to Function. In Wiesel S, Weinstein J, Herkowitz H, et al (eds): The Lumbar Spine. Philadelphia, W. B. Saunders 1996, p. 271.
120. Urban JPG, McMullin JF: Swelling pressure of the lumbar intervertebral discs: Influence of age, spinal level, composition, and degeneration. Spine 13:179, 1988.
121. Virgin W: Experimental investigation into the physical properties of the intervertebral disc. J Bone Joint Surg (Br) 33B:607, 1951.
122. Vix VA, Ryu CY: The adult symphysis pubis: Normal and abnormal. Am J Roentgenol 112:517, 1971.
123. Vleeming A, Snidjers CJ, Stoeckart R, Stijnen T: The posterior layer of thoracolumbar fascia, its function in load transfer from spine to legs Spine 20:753, 1995.
124. Vieeming A, Stoeckart R, Volkers ACW, Snidjers CJ: Relation between form and function in the sacroiliac joint. Part I: Clinical anatomical aspects. Spine 15:130, 1990.
125. Vieeming A, Stoeckart R, Snidjers CJ: The sacrotuberous ligament: A conceptual approach to its dynamic role in stabilizing the sacroiliac joint. J Clin Biomech 4:201, 1989.
126. Vieeming A, Volkers ACW, Snidjers CJ, Stoeckart R: Relation between form and function in the sacroiliac joint. Part 2: Biomechanical aspects. Spine 15:133, 1990.
127. Vleeming A, Windgerden JP, Snidjers CJ, Stoeckart R, Stijnen T: Load application to the sacrotuberous ligament: Influences on sacroiliac mechanics. J Clin Biomechanics 4:204, 1989.
128. Vleeming A, Wingerden van JP, Snidjers CJ, Stoeckart R, Dijkstra PF, Stijnen T: Mobility of the SI joints in the elderly: Kinematic and roentgenologic study. Clin Biomech 7:170, 1992.
129. Walheim GG, Olerud S, Ridde T: Mobility of the pubic symphysis. Measurements by an electromechanical method. Acta Orthop Scand 55:203, 1984.
130. Weinstein J: The pain of discography. Spine 13:1341, 1988.
131. Weisl H: Movements of the sacroiliac joint. Acta Anat (Basel) 23:80, 1955.
132. Weiss M, Nageischmidt M, Struck H: Relaxin and collagen metabolism. Horm Metab Res 11:408,1979.

133. White AA, Panjabi MM: Clinical Biomechanics of the Spine. Philadelphia, J. B. Lippincott, 1978.

134. Wiesel SW, Tsourmas N, Feffer HL, Citrin CM, Patronas N: A study of computer assisted tomography: 1. The incidence of positive CAT scans in an asymptomatic group of patients. Spine 9:549, 1984.

135. Wilder DG, Pope MH, Frymoyer JW: The biomechanics of lumbar disc herniations and the effect of overload and instability. J Spinal Disord 1: 16, 1988.

136. Wiley JJ: Traumatic osteitis pubis: The gracilis syndrome. Am J Sports Med 11:360, 1983.

137. Williams PL, Warwick P, Dyson M, Bannister LH: Gray's Anatomy. London, Churchill Livingstone, 1989.

138. Wyke B: Neurological aspects of low back pain. In Jayson M (ed): The Lumbar Spine and Back Pain. Grune & Stratton, New York, 1976, p. 173.

139. Wyke B: The neurology of low back pain. In Jayson M (ed): The Lumbar Spine and Back Pain, 2nd ed. Tunbridge Wells, Pitman Medical, 1980, p. 265.

140. Yasuma T, Makino E, Saito S, Inui M: Histological development of intervertebral disc herniation. J Bone Joint Surg (Am) 68A: 1066, 1986.

141. Yoshizawa H, O'Brien JP, Thomas-Smith W, Trumper M: The neuropathology of intervertebral discs removed for back pain. J Pathol 132:95, 1980.

CHAPTER 5

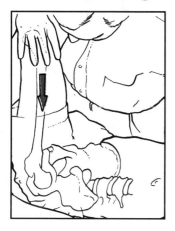

FUNCTIONAL ASSESSMENT OF THE LUMBOPELVIC REGION

GENERAL CONCEPTS

Pathomechanical Versus Pathoanatomical Diagnosis

A point that has been stressed throughout the text thus far is that it is difficult to isolate the exact tissue responsible for a patient's back pain. The potential for pain referral from both the musculoskeletal tissues of the spine and the pelvic and abdominal viscera increases the complexity of the diagnostic process. Therefore, a complete evaluation of the patient with low back pain requires background knowledge of functional anatomy of the spine as well as a comprehensive understanding of pathology, which will enable the clinician to begin distinguishing mechanical from nonmechanical disorders. As it is beyond the scope of this text to present the details of pathology, this chapter will instead focus on an important component of the evaluation process referred to as the *functional assessment*. As the name implies, this evaluation process emphasizes the analysis of function—the use of movement patterns with the application of specific stresses and overpressures to determine if familiar pain is elicited.

This type of evaluation process results in a pathomechanical determination of the problem, rather than a pathoanatomical one. Varying stresses and move-

ments are introduced into the lumbopelvic region and patient's response to these stresses are assessed. With an understanding of the purpose and rationale behind functional assessment, the clinician can then add specific questions or include additional tests that might be indicated to rule out low back pain from nonmechanical causes. The value of such an approach is that it (1) allows the clinician to use the results of the examination as the basis for designing an exercise program around the identified nociceptive mechanics, (2) relates the patient's vulnerable and invulnerable positions and movements to their work and activities of daily living, and (3) provides information about the syndrome to the patient in understandable, practical terms.

In the small percentage of low back pain patients in whom the precise anatomical tissue at fault can be ascribed, there is one group with nerve root signs and symptoms. Classic indicators of nerve root involvement are pain below the knee; increased leg pain on straight leg raising; the presence of conditions in which the leg pain is much more distressing than the spine pain; and reflex, motor, and sensory changes in the lower extremity (Table 5–1). To understand the implications of mechanical and inflammatory conditions of the lumbosacral nerve roots, the neurological screening examination for nerve root involvement was previously discussed in Chapter 2, but elements of the

Table 5–1. Nerve Root Involvement	
Nerve Root Irritation	**Nerve Root Compression**
Leg pain greater than back pain	Myotomal motor weakness
SLR reproduces leg pain	Dermatomal sensory deficit
Gentle spinal movement causes excess irradiation	Muscle atrophy
Extends beyond knee	Reflex changes
Clear demarcation of leg pain/paresthesia	

cxam are repeated in this chapter to keep the neurological examination in the context of the evaluation of the patient with low back pain.

The key to proper functional assessment of the patient with low back injury is determining the position(s) and movements that exacerbate the familiar symptoms, and gaining an understanding of the intensity, frequency, and duration of the pain pattern that motivated the patient to seek professional help. Two of the main goals of the functional assessment are reproducing the pain syndrome with applied stresses, and having the clinician and patient mutually understand the pain pattern. Because of the inherent difficulty in precise isolation of the injured tissue(s) involved in the painful syndrome, this evaluation concept focuses on the forces generated as a result of changes in body position and subsequent muscle contractions that converge in the lumbopelvic region and exacerbate symptoms. It can then be deduced which forces exceed the tissue's tolerance or adaptability, and therefore mechanically and/or chemically stimulate the nociceptive system to give rise to the perception of pain.

Many tests have been devised to evaluate the function and the painful syndrome of the low back region. However, one must always sort through the information gained and decide how it can be used successfully to develop a treatment process that the patient understands. Complex information gained from an evaluation that cannot be reduced to understandable terms or concepts for the patient decreases the chances that the patient will assume an active role in the rehabilitation process. Although neural and discal tissues unique to the spine do lend to its complexity, the clinician should continue to respect basic properties of the primary body tissues, including bone, muscle, and connective tissue and the response of these tissues to injury; the potential for, and estimated healing time of, injured

tissues; and the irreversibility of the aging and degenerative processes.

Not only is the determination of the exact tissue involved in the painful back syndrome difficult but even with current technology, the findings do not always correlate with the clinical symptoms.[15, 20, 25, 33] With the emergence of technologies such as computed tomography and magnetic resonance imaging, structures within and surrounding the spinal canal, including soft tissues, can be better visualized. Although such diagnostic tests are of value, especially in determining differential diagnosis, it is essential that the findings are correlated with and reaffirmed by a clinical impression formed from the history and functional assessment. Low back pain and disability do not increase progressively with age nor do they correlate with the natural degenerative changes of the intervertebral disc.[13, 35] Furthermore, it has become increasingly clear that structural changes are only a small part of the pain picture. Rather, the inflammatory state and biochemical milieu of injured tissues is perhaps more important than structural pathology in the initiation and propagation of the pain syndrome.

In summary, the clinician should remember that (a) as in any region of the body, an isolated lesion is uncommon because it is often associated with an injury process or changes in related tissues; (b) the composition of bone, muscle, and connective tissue and their physiologic properties are consistent in the back—as in any other area; and (c) basing the evaluation system on one specific aspect or tissue of the lumbopelvic region, without considering the mechanism of injury and forces that reproduce familiar symptoms, may hinder the opportunity for achieving long-term results. The goal of a functional assessment is to take the subjective and objective findings and correlate them to the circumstances of the injury or onset to determine the positions of weight-bearing posture of the lumbopelvic region that produce the patient's pain, the pattern of the painful syndrome, the inflammatory status or state of the injured tissue(s), and the appropriate treatment plan to be implemented.

The Concept of Applied Physical Stresses

This assessment system is designed to assist the clinician in determining the applied stresses that increase the patient's pain in antigravity positions. This should initially be established from the standing position and then *substantiated* with tests applying a similar series of stresses in the prone, supine, and sitting positions. In order to be successful with this approach, the clinician must have a three-dimensional understanding of the static and dynamic anatomy of this region, and be able to direct appropriate stresses into and through the spine. This allows the forces generated throughout the tissues of the low back, pelvis, and hips from superior to inferior, inferior to superior, and in all three planes of movement to be visualized as the positional changes of the functional assessment proceed.

The examiner should also gain an appreciation of the irritability of the injured tissue(s) as a result of the magnitude of the applied stresses required to evoke a given painful response from the patient. The intent is to apply these specific stresses in the standing, supine, prone, and sitting test positions to generate movements and forces into the lumbopelvic region and assess matches, or similarities of response, within the functional assessment. If the examiner can effectively use this assessment system to identify the destructive and nondestructive ranges of motion, an appropriate active treatment plan can be developed. It is understood that treatment that involves increased activity promotes muscle and bone growth and minimizes sensitivity to pain.[2, 21, 26, 30] It does not matter what stresses are used to provoke a familiar symptom as long as the clinician can identify the intensity and direction of the force used and the relationship of the applied stress to the pathomechanics of the painful syndrome.

This chapter aims to provide an assessment system for mechanical low back pain. If the clinician is unable to correlate or *match* the findings in the various test positions, then the source of the syndrome may be nonmechanical. The clinician should then be suspicious of the other causes of low back pain such as referred pathology from the abdominal and pelvic viscera, and further diagnostics are indicated.

INFORMATION GAINED FROM THE ASSESSMENT

Several types of information can be gathered from the assessment process. The first is the *syndrome pathomechanics*. The clinician will guide the patient through a systematic series of motions and combinations of motions in order to reproduce familiar pain. The application of overpressure to these motions is used to determine whether the applied overpressure is resulting in increased tensile, compressive, or shear loads, or a combination of these forces. The pathomechanics that reproduce familiar pain, or are recognized by the examiner to be poorly tolerated by the patient due to palpable muscle or motion guarding, are acknowledged by the examiner, and responses to such nociceptive stresses are compared with the patient's responses in the antigravity (standing and sitting) versus gravity-eliminated (supine, prone, or side-lying) positions. Using the same stresses (tensile, compressive, and shear), the examiner is seeking some correlation between the antigravity and the gravity-eliminated positions. The most valuable information regarding the response to stresses placed through the low back is that gained from the standing position. Most patients with mechanical back disorders are symptomatic with weight-bearing positions and pain is eased with lying down. Therefore, it is of most value to gain relevant information from positions that are symptomatic to more clearly visualize the pathomechanics of the problem.

The second aspect gained from the evaluation is a *working assessment*. As clinicians become increasingly responsible for assessing relevant outcomes and gathering data regarding the cost of treatment, it is essential to develop a working classification scheme that allows an easily understood and reproducible diagnostic scheme. Several classification schemes have been proposed.[5, 6, 18] The scheme noted in Table 5–2, which has been previously proposed by the authors, is modeled after the recommendations of the Quebec Task Force.[28] It is recognized that such a scheme is based on symptom description, and requires the examiner to gather most of the information in a well-organized and comprehensive history. However, it's simplicity lends to enhanced clinical utility, and potentially pro-

Table 5–2. Working Assessment: Low Back Pain
Low back pain Back pain with proximal referral Back pain with distal referral Leg pain greater than back pain Leg pain + back pain + neurological signs Post surgery < 6 months Post surgery > 6 months Chronic pain syndrome

Table 5–3. Nonorganic Physical Signs in Low Back Pain: "Waddell Signs"
Tenderness (superficial, nonatomic) Simulation (axial loading, rotation) Distraction (seated straight leg raising) Regional disturbances (weakness, sensory) Overreaction
From Waddell G, McCulloch JA, Kummel E, Venner RM: Nonorganic physical signs in low-back pain. Spine 5:117, 1980.

vides a common understanding of the patient complaint between different clinicians.

The value of a commonly agreed upon starting point (the working assessment or the diagnosis) should not be underestimated. Outcomes, cost effective analysis, and efficacy studies require that a common diagnostic language be used to systematically categorize patients. A meaningful diagnostic classification allows for reliable groupings that can be used for cost-effective comparisons. Furthermore, a common diagnostic language such as that suggested with this working assessment, allows a critical pathway of care or algorithm of treatment to be developed. Algorithms of treatment, which guide the clinician's strategies for intervention along a predetermined set of rules, have been shown to be a cost-effective means of treating patients with low back pain.[41]

The last type of information gained from the assessment is the *syndrome grouping*. In most instances of mechanical low back pain, the syndrome can be categorized into one of the following categories: *acute injury, exacerbation of previous injury,* or *chronic pain syndrome*.[6] The acute injury is fairly self-explanatory and should be viewed similarly to the acute injury process seen in the extremities. The response of the patient to various applied stresses is proportional to the time since the injury and onset of the painful syndrome and the pathomechanics of the injury. Because of the generalizable and predictable healing times of specialized connective tissues, acute injuries are generally those less than 7 weeks old.[28]

Exacerbation of previous injury is perhaps the most common of the three groups. Patients in this category often describe an initial injury or antecedent event,

and then a pattern of pain exacerbations over the course of time with varying pain intensities and varying intervals of pain exacerbations. Even though there is a chronicity to their problem, they are not chronic pain syndrome patients. Instead, their pattern speaks to the limited capacity of previously injured tissue to heal in a way that allows mechanical stresses to be tolerated as effectively as the preinjured state. This syndrome classification also speaks to the age-related, degenerative changes that the specialized connective tissues undergo, and their lowered optimal loading capacity. Patients in this category describe similar recurrent episodes of their own unique low back problem.

The last syndrome grouping, which also serves as one of the categories in the working assessment, is chronic pain syndrome. This syndrome is characterized by the absence of a direct relationship between physical stimulus and pain response. Chronic pain is characterized by persistent pain on a daily basis that persists well beyond an expected healing time, and the syndrome is represented by persistent pain reports despite multiple interventions. Chronic pain syndrome is often characterized by observable pain behaviors such as grimacing, groaning, verbal complaints, and the avoidance of routine daily activities.[29] There may be an overreliance on medications, emotional distress, and a disruption of interpersonal relationships. It is an extremely complex syndrome that, once identified, ultimately requires a comprehensive treatment process consisting of patient education, physical reconditioning, behavioral management, and medication management.[42], The Waddell signs (Table 5–3) are often used as a screen to help identify those patients that may require a more detailed psychological assessment to direct the most appropriate treatment strategies.[39]

PATIENT HISTORY

General Considerations

The first part of any examination is the history. It should be structured so that it allows the clinician and patient to reach agreement and a common understanding of the nature of the problem. This is the first step in getting the patients to recognize that they are an integral part of a successful management program. During the history, the therapeutic relationship between the clinician and the patient is established, and it is also the point in which the educational process for the patient actually begins. For obvious reasons, it should be done in an environment free of distractions or interruptions.

It is important that the clinician ask questions that will elicit information to help discern whether the patient may be having pain of a nonmechanical source, such as abdominal or pelvic visceral pathology. This information also will help determine whether referral for further evaluation is indicated. Descriptions by the patient of fever, night pain, metabolic disease, and bowel or bladder disturbances, factors such as medications currently used, and a medical history of diabetes, vascular disease, and cancer most likely require further diagnostic testing and appropriate referral. Constitutional symptoms and signs such as weight loss or anorexia should be ascertained. If there is a relationship between a female's pain pattern and the menstrual cycle, it should be clarified. One needs to inquire about urinary tract or bowel symptoms, and oftentimes must gather information regarding sexual functions. Lumbar disc disease or spinal stenosis may compromise the cauda equina, resulting in signs of a neurogenic bladder such as overflow incontinence, frequent urination, or acute urinary retention. Prior surgeries—especially abdominal surgeries because of their resultant consequences to the abdominal wall mechanism—should always be described. In addition, the clinician should be familiar with the patient's occupation and have a clear idea of the demands of that job. An intake questionnaire can be used to gain some of the above information, especially that information related to past medical history, but it should not be a substitute for the interview.

Aspects to Consider in Developing the Patient History

The questions that are used in the history (Table 5–4) are designed to provide the examiner with four essential types of information: *pathomechanics history, pain patterns, influencing factors,* and *the effect of the problem on health-related quality of life issues.* Although the intent of specific questions is detailed in the following sections, a summary is provided here so that the examiner will also consider questions that are not listed in Table 5–4; the special needs or circumstances of an individual back pain patient may require that additional questions be asked to further clarify information in any of these four essential categories.

The *pathomechanics history* deals with questions that focus the patient's answers to onset, position of injury, stresses generated during injury, positions and movements that exacerbate symptoms, and the site and extent of the pain. *Pain patterns* refer to the time course and daily pattern of pain, and an assessment of the patient's awareness of their pain pattern. As will be illustrated below, this information is best understood by both the clinician and the patient if it is graphically diagrammed during the interview.

The third aspect to consider is *influencing factors.* Such factors include stressors in one's life such as job stress, family stress, work stress, economic stress, and self-induced stress. It is important that the examiner ascertain how psychosocial factors are influencing the perception of pain or the degree of disability.[3] Failure to relate these factors to the patient's complaint leads to unrealistic treatment goal-setting. Additional influencing factors include how activity affects the pain syndrome, and understanding the pharmacological effects of medications that the patient is taking for either the back problem or other medical conditions.

The last aspect to consider is the affect this problem has on health-related quality-of-life issues. In addition to symptoms, health-related quality-of-life issues refer to elements such as functional status (activities of daily living, recreational activities, social functioning, sense of well being); role function (employment status, disability compensation, work absenteeism, and limitation of work activity); and overall goals, such as the patient's expected treatment outcome and overall expectations. Attention to health-related quality-of-life issues is a relatively new paradigm in cost-effective analysis of treatment outcomes. It is well recognized

Table 5–4. Questions for Patient History
How old are you?
What is your occupation?
Can you describe for me the work you do?
Women: Do you have any children? If yes—
How old are your children?
Have you had any surgeries? Cesarean sections?
Men: Have you had any surgeries?
How long have you had low back pain?
What position were you in when you were initially hurt?
Show me where you have pain. Do you ever have pain or numbness or tingling into your thighs or legs?
Describe previous episodes of back pain and how long these episodes lasted.
What positions or activities increase your pain? What activities are limited by this problem?
How would you rate your level of activity?
How would you rate your level of pain?
How would you rate your level of stress? Is there a relationship between your level of stress and level of pain?
Is your pain worse in the morning upon awakening or is it worse toward the end of the day? Are you more stiff or sore in the morning as compared with the end of the day?
Are you currently taking any medications for your pain?
What do you think is the cause of your back pain?
What would be your goals from treatment?
Special questions related to low back pain:
Have you had any recent weight loss?
Are you experiencing any bowel or bladder disturbances? Do you have numbness in this area?
Does your pain prevent you from sleeping? Is it worse at night?

that it is essential to understand the patient's perception of the problem, and the patient's perceptions are used in many aspects of clinical decision-making and in judging the results of treatment. Gathering such information initially allows a plan to be developed for obtaining meaningful outcome data—that is, data that demonstrate that the treatment process enhanced the patient's quality of life and at what cost.

Specific Questions for the History

Table 5–4 lists a series of questions that allow for a systematic gathering of information related to the patient's low back pain. The questions are designed to provide information regarding the pathomechanics of injury, pain location and pattern, onset and duration of pain, the characteristics of the pain and how it affects activities of daily living and work, external factors that may be contributing to pain propagation, and

the patient's impression of the problem and the goals the patient may have for treatment. How these specific questions relate to these general themes are now discussed.

Pathomechanics of Injury

Answers to questions such as "What position were you in when you got hurt?" "What positions, movements, or activities are limited by this problem?" and "What positions or activities increase your familiar pain?" begin to present a picture of the pathomechanics involved in the pain pattern. Recreating the position of injury, if possible, provides information regarding the biomechanics involved in the painful syndrome. From this information, the clinician can make a judgment as to the compression, tension, and shear stresses involved in the position of injury, and can consider the potential for tissue damage.

If the patient cannot identify a specific position of injury, or if the onset was more insidious, then the questioning should be directed toward determining the type of work and extracurricular activities the patient was involved in prior to the initial onset, as well as determining the motions or positions that now worsen the patient's pain. Following this description of the pathomechanics of injury, it is helpful to get a precise description of pain location.

Establishing Pain Location and Pain Pattern

The location of the pain is a critical piece of information, especially if it is to be used to determine a working assessment. Questions such as *"Where do you have pain?", "Is it all back pain or is it back pain and leg pain?", "Is the back pain more aggravating than the leg pain?",* and (using a body diagram), *"Where on the picture is the area that gives you the most discomfort and any associated pain?"* are all questions that require the patient to describe in detail the areas in which symptoms are most disconcerting, as well as any other regions in which they have complaints. We have found that if the clinician marks the pain drawing according to the patient's direction, rather than having the patient draw, it increases the likelihood that the patient and clinician will expeditiously, and accurately, come to a common understanding of the pain location (Fig. 5–1). Pain drawings arrived at in this manner have provided examiners with valuable information in the diagnostic process.[16]

Since this information is important to the development of the working assessment, it is essential that the clinician and patient come to agreement on where the primary and secondary complaints are located. It is important to determine if the pain is essentially midline, unilateral, unilateral in the back and spread distally, or bilateral with distal referral. It is helpful to have the patient show the examiner the region that is symptomatic rather than simply describe it.

An understanding of the location of pain assists the examiner in planning further questioning and the physical exam. Listening to descriptions of pain location, the examiner begins to consider the tissues in the immediate area as well as tissues that might refer pain to areas described by the patient. A description of leg pain that is greater than back pain, especially when the patient notes that distressing and burning leg pain is along a discrete, fairly well demarcated area, is suggestive of nerve

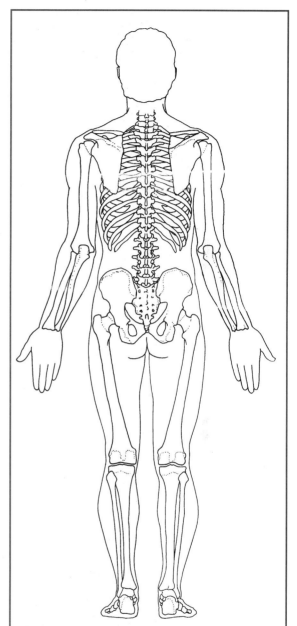

Figure 5-1. Posterior view of the skeleton. This view allows the patient and clinician to indicate the painful site. The drawing can be placed on the same sheet as the graphs (Figs. 5–2 and 5–3), which permits the clinician to complete the history-taking process in a visual manner.

root irritation. Back pain that is clearly more disconcerting than lower extremity pain can be due to any injured tissues of the low back referring pain into the lower extremity. Reaching an agreement with the patient as to pain location is important to the patient's understanding that the centralization of pain (i.e., decreasing referral of pain into the lower extremity) is often a sign of improvement of their condition.[7]

Three types of referred pain patterns into the lower extremity are often described by the patient with low back pain. One is pain in the lower extremity, often the posterior hip and thigh, which tends to be vague and poorly demarcated. Such a pain pattern occurs as a result of the mechanical or inflammatory involvement of any tissue in the spine innervated by branches of the posterior primary rami. This includes joint, capsular, bony, muscular, fascial, tendon, and ligamentous structures. A second referred pain pattern is the radiculopathy pattern along the distribution of a nerve root. This pattern tends to be more discrete and localized and is suggestive of an inflammatory lesion of the nerve root that is now mechanically sensitive. The third referred pain pattern occurs as a result of claudication. This pain is often in both legs and over a very diffuse area. Pain that is exacerbated with walking and relieved with sitting is one of the signs of claudication. Recall that flexion of the lumbar spine increases, while extension decreases, spinal canal dimensions. Because stenosis of the lumbar spine is one of the causes of back pain, activities such as walking uphill (spine is flexed) and sitting, are tolerated, but walking (spine is in extension) increase pain.

Now that the duration and location of the pain and the mechanics of the injury have been determined, the parameters of the pain pattern (onset, intensity, and frequency) should be established.

Onset and Duration of the Problem

Determining the duration of the painful syndrome establishes the length of time the body has had to adapt to the injury, and begins to clarify whether the complaint is an acute injury or an exacerbation of previous injury. Answers to questions such as *"Have you had previous episodes of back pain?", "What were they like?", "How long do the pain episodes last?"*, and *"When did you first have this problem?"* begin to provide a picture of the onset and pain pattern. If the patient has recently experienced the initial injury, then neuromuscular and connective tissue adaptive changes are probably minimal.

Conversely, if the patient experienced the initial injury 7 years ago and has had five exacerbations of the same pain, they are most likely describing similar recurrent episodes and it is probable that adaptive changes have occurred.

Patients with signs and symptoms from disc pathology often describe having had an acute attack of low back pain in their 20s, while engaged in an activity such as lifting or performing heavy work, or after falling or moving abruptly. Approximately 10 years may pass before radicular symptoms appear, and these symptoms are usually preceded by low back pain that lasts for a few weeks.[40]

Graphically representing the history is an excellent way for the clinician and patient to reach agreement regarding the onset and duration or pain. Utilizing a graph that compares the intensity versus time for the entire history, as well as the daily pain pattern, allows the patient and clinician to visualize and agree upon the chronology of the pain pattern (Fig. 5–2). The frequency and intensity can easily be recorded on the graph. Figure 5–3 is a graphic representation of a case study. In this example, the patient states that he sustained a lifting injury 3 years ago. That pain remained for 3 weeks and then gradually and completely resolved. However, the patient reinjured himself at the same level of pain intensity 6 months later. This time the intensity completely diminished but took 4–6 weeks. The clinician should be cognizant of time frames and the mechanisms of healing. Two months ago, the patient reinjured his back at work and the pain intensity has been fluctuating between 7 and 10. The patient has decided to seek professional help and enters the clinician's office with pain at the intensity of 7.

This case presents an example of the exacerbation of previous injury grouping. A graphic representation of the history often allows the examiner to note that patients use self-management strategies to deal with the initial onset of low back pain, but generally seek help when the peaks of pain become too high to be managed, or when the series of pain episodes occurs too frequently without satisfactory pain relief. Thus, the graph demonstrates that many initial bouts of low back pain have a favorable course with resolution over time, but the recurrence is common and increasingly difficult to manage. Recurrence rates following an acute low back pain episode have been estimated to range from 40 percent to as high as 85 percent.[34,36]

A second graph relates intensity and pattern of pain over a 24-hour period. Figure 5–3B illustrates the pat-

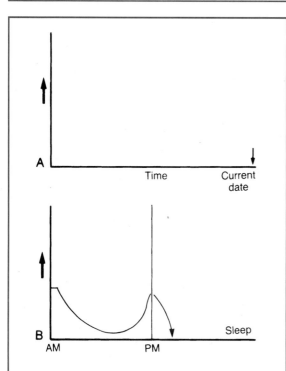

Figure 5–2. *A,* Graph showing the intensity of pain along the vertical and time along the horizontal. This format allows the clinician to take a history with respect to intensity, frequency, and duration of the pain pattern. This simple way of graphically outlining the patient's history is an important tool in that it allows patients to visualize their history, and provides a tangible representation of the history that the patient and clinician can easily discuss. *B,* Graph showing the intensity of pain along the vertical axis, and the morning–evening or 24-hour period on the horizontal, allowing the clinician and patient to agree on the daily pain pattern.

tern of the patient who awakens with stiffness and mild pain; as the day progresses, the pain decreases but begins to intensify toward the end of the day. The patient has no difficulty sleeping. Graphically representing the daily pattern provides the examiner with information regarding the inflammatory state of the tissues. For example, the daily pattern noted in Fig. 5–3B might suggest that the patient awakens with swelling, fluid stasis, and altered biochemical milieu of the injured tissue(s), which chemically stimulates the nociceptive receptor system, giving rise to pain stiffness.[1, 14] As movement begins, the mechanoreceptors are stimulated to help modulate pain, and the forces and pressures generated by muscle contraction help decrease fluid stasis by flushing the fluid environment. These biochemical changes result in decreased nociceptive stimulus and a decreased perception of pain and stiffness. By the end of the day, however, the injured tissue has been subjected to forces that exceed its physical tolerance, and the pain begins to increase (see also Chapter 6, Fig. 6–1).

Conversely, if the patient is most comfortable in the morning and the pain increases after periods of weight-bearing and movement, then that person's antigravity joint and muscle mechanics are unable to keep the tissues in an invulnerable range. The term invulnerable range refers to the range of motion that is within the tissues' tolerance to a given intensity of forces that does not cause further damage. However, as the day progresses and neuromuscular fatigue ensues, the tissues become excessively loaded, increasing discomfort and pain. Quite simply, the injured tissues are "losing the daily battle against gravity." This group of patients responds to rehabilitative activities that strengthen the muscles designed to improve weight-bearing mechanics during the time the patient must counterbalance the gravitational forces, and education that minimizes destructive forces by learning to make the appropriate decisions of activity and rest. Many mechanical low back pain patients describe an increase in pain at the end of the day, which probably represents the inability to maintain the invulnerable range of the injured tissues. The continuous active and passive forces generated to the musculoskeletal tissues during the activities of daily living result in increased pain by the end of the day. On the other hand, rest and unloading these tissues help decrease pain.

After this discussion, the patient reviews the graphs and is asked if they accurately represent his problem. Many patients make subtle changes on the graphs that increase the accuracy of the intensity or the time frames. This is encouraged because the effort of making the graph correct shows that the patient is interested in taking an active role in understanding his problem. The extent of the patient's involvement with the graph may provide the clinician with the first clues about the patient's motivation to recover.

The graphs are important from another perspective as well. The goal of treatment is to minimize the intensity of pain and extend the duration of the pain-free periods. Evidence of reaching this goal can be

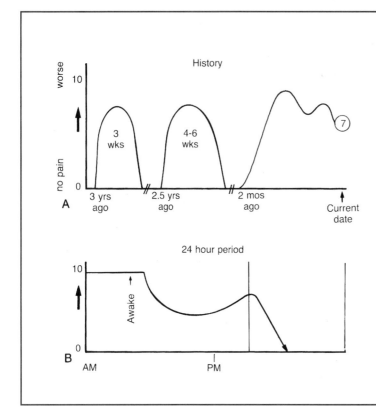

Figure 5–3. *A,* Graph showing an example of a patient who had an injury 3 years ago which lasted for 3 weeks, experienced the same injury 2 1/2 years ago that lasted for 4–6 weeks, and then reinjured himself 2 months ago and has been fluctuating between 7 and 10 for that amount of time. The current rate is 7 on a 10-point scale. *B,* Twenty-four-hour chart showing that the patient awoke with pain and stiffness that gradually declined as the day progressed, but which had increased by the end of the day. The patient did not describe experiencing pain in the evening that altered his sleeping pattern.

read from the graphs, because they represent a tangible record of the patient's pain pattern. Establishing this vehicle for communication provides the clinician and patient with a mechanism to evaluate treatment effectiveness.

The patient must learn to recognize that success in the management of low back pain syndromes is represented by small changes in the intensity, frequency, or duration of pain. If the patient does not experience change after a reasonable number of treatments, then re-evaluation is indicated to redirect the treatment process.

Assessing the Effect of the Problem on Quality-of-Life Issues

Questions such as *"What can't you do because of this problem?", "How would you rate your level of activity?", "How does this problem affect your ability to work?"* and *"How is this problem affecting your ability to work or socialize with others?"* direct the patient's thinking toward his activities of daily living and quality-of-life issues and the effect that the low back pain problem has on them. It is often helpful to ask patients to describe their activity levels on a scale of 10, with 0 referring to no activity and 10 being the normal activity level of the patient. If they respond, for example, that their activity level is "6" as a result of the problem, it is important for the examiner to follow with a question asking if this means that 40 percent of the activities that they were able to do prior to back pain are no longer possible. Asking the questions in this manner allows agreement to be reached between the patient and examiner regarding the interpretation of such subjective values.

Several questionnaires are also available that aid the clinician in assessing the impact of the low back pain problem on a patient's quality of life, and understanding the patient's perception of how the back problem is affecting his activities. Such questionnaires include the Oswestrey Disability Index,[8] the Waddell Disability Score,[38] and the Low Back Outcome Score.[12] These questionnaires have additional clinical utility in that they can potentially serve as measuring tools for assessing outcome as a result of treatment intervention. Other instruments that measure the effect of the problem on quality-of-life measures such as functional status include the Roland-Morris Disability Scale[24] and the SF-36.[17] Use of such reliable and valid questionnaires, as well as directing the questions in the manner described above, help the examiner to better understand patients' perceptions of the impact this problem is having on their lives. Instead of focusing solely on the impairments related to the patient's low back pain, the examiner is now attempting to gain an understanding of the disability associated with the low back pain problem.

Patients who claim their injury is a result of an accident at the work site need to be assessed regarding motivation to return to work. It is often important for the clinician to ask the patient's permission to contact their employer or supervisor to discuss goals and progress of the rehabilitation process. If the patient refuses to grant permission for such a call, then the clinician should expect to run into a conflict in the return-to-work process. For a successful return-to-work process, there must be a communication "triangle" consisting of the employer, employee, and clinician. The clinician should be sure that each member of this communication triangle understand their role in the recovery process to ensure a successful outcome. A lack of communication results in an increased number of treatments and time away from work.

Assessing the Patient's Understanding of the Problem

This category of questions asked during a history deals with directing the patient's attention to the fact that his problem is his responsibility, not the clinician's. Answers to questions such as *"What do you think is the cause of your back pain?"*, and *"What would be your goals as the result of treatment?"* give the examiner a better idea of the patient's perception of the problem. It is also important for the clinician to ascertain the influence of psychosocial stresses on the problem. Asking a patient to "quantify" his stress level, with 0 representing no stress and 10 being extremely high levels of stress, is a simple, yet effective means of communicating this question to the patient. The clinician can define stress to the patient as job stress, family stress, economic stress, or self-inflicted stress. It is often unnecessary to pursue details of the stresses if the patient

replies affirmatively, but it is extremely important to ask the patient if there is a relationship between the stress they are under and the amount of pain they are in. Acknowledging the influence of stress on the perception of pain is critical in setting reachable, realistic treatment goals.

When asked what they think the cause of the problem is, most patients respond with "I don't know." The clinician should encourage some form of answer. This can be done by making a statement such as *"You must have some impression of what is happening in your back. Does it feel like something is grinding, or squeezing, or slipping, or. . . ?"* The clinician should then pause and allow the patient to finish the thought. Although this can be construed as influencing the patient's thoughts, we believe it is important to guide patients toward a verbalization when they cannot describe their perception of the problem. The intent is to gain a clear understanding of how the patient views his problem. If a patient is unable to carry out this thought, the clinician must determine whether the patient is simply unable to express himself or unwilling to divulge the needed information. The clinician, by this time, should be able to judge whether the patient is interested in obtaining a rapid, successful recovery.

In summary, there are many methods of obtaining a good history, and the clinician should develop his or her own method of gathering at least the aforementioned points of information. The questioning should be done in a logical progression, so that the patient can follow the sequencing of the history. If the patient is able to follow the line of questioning and relate one question to another, then he will be better able to assist the clinician in implementing a successful treatment sequence. It is important to stop during the history to begin teaching the patient how the information being presented "fits together." Explaining and illustrating the potential meaning of what has been said are valuable tools of the teaching process. If further questions regarding other medical problems are indicated, they should be addressed. Upon completion of the history, the objective examination begins with the examination from the standing position.

Standing Examination

The standing examination is perhaps one of the most important parts of the physical exam. Information from this aspect of the assessment will ultimately be compared with findings from the supine and prone positions. If the patient is in too much discomfort to tolerate the standing assessment, it may be necessary initially to treat the pain palliatively. However, it is essential that the antigravity nociceptive mechanics be assessed if any long-term benefits of treatment are expected, and if the patient is going to be taught self-management strategies. Table 5–5 lists the essential components of the standing examination, which are detailed below.

Inspection

While the patient stands, the examiner views the patient from the frontal and sagittal plane perspectives (Fig. 5–4). From this position the examiner is looking for any asymmetries or deviations from the expected norm, such as side shifting, listing, or the inability to bear weight on one side compared with the other. The examiner should begin at the occiput and observe the position of the head, shoulders, arms, and scapulae. It is important to note that considerable variations and adaptations occur in the upper portion of the body owing to lumbopelvic disorders. For example, a person who has a frontal plane asymmetry at the pelvis may or may not have uneven shoulders. The upper quarter does not always match the lower quarter in the standing position; this should not be ignored but rather observed and noted.

The inspection continues by following the spine from the upper thoracic region to the sacrum. If scoliosis is suspected, it can be verified by the forward bend test to determine the presence of a rib hump. The contours and the symmetry of the waist angles (i.e., the

angles that the skin fold makes above the iliac crest) should be noted. The waist angles provide one of the best visual cues for frontal plane asymmetries of the lumbopelvic region.

The pelvis is then observed. Attention should be given to the orientation of the pelvis in the three cardinal planes, especially the frontal plane from the posterior view and the sagittal plane from a side view. These can be assessed by observing soft-tissue relationships above the pelvis. If the patient is relatively lean, the examiner can easily observe the antigravity position of the pelvis in the frontal and sagittal positions. The inspection continues down the back of both thighs to the Achilles tendons. These tendons should be vertical. If they are asymmetrical or both bow in, then the calcaneus is likely to be excessively everted and an evaluation of the foot would be indicated.[19] It is important to understand the relationship between foot mechanics and their influence on the normal weight-bearing pattern as the ground forces reach the lumbopelvic tissues.

Structural Examination: Clarifying Frontal and Sagittal Plane Observations

There are numerous ways to carry out a structural examination of the lumbopelvic region. However, the clinician should develop a routine of evaluating every lumbopelvic problem in the same manner. By collecting data in a consistent manner, comparisons can be made among many patients.

The standing weight-bearing examination is one of the most important parts of the overall assessment. Most mechanical low back pain problems are exacerbated by upright positions and movement patterns and relieved by recumbency. The manner in which forces reach tissues is different when the person is standing than when he is supine or prone. It is much easier for a person to place the injured low back structures into nonpainful positions when the forces of weight-bearing are removed.

Four bony landmarks are assessed: the iliac crest, the posterior superior iliac spines (PSIS), the anterior superior iliac spine (ASIS), and the greater trochanters (see Figs. 5–5 to 5–8). The goal with these palpations is to visualize the three-dimensional relationship of the pelvis. The complete extent of the iliac crest is palpated to provide the clinician with information to be used for assessing pelvic position (Fig. 5–5). This

---

Table 5–5. Standing Examination

1. Inspection
   Sagittal and frontal plane
   Structural assessment
2. Gait analysis
3. Gross movement testing
   Combination movements
   Controlled overpressure in all quadrants
4. Neurological screening
   Toe walking
   Heel walking

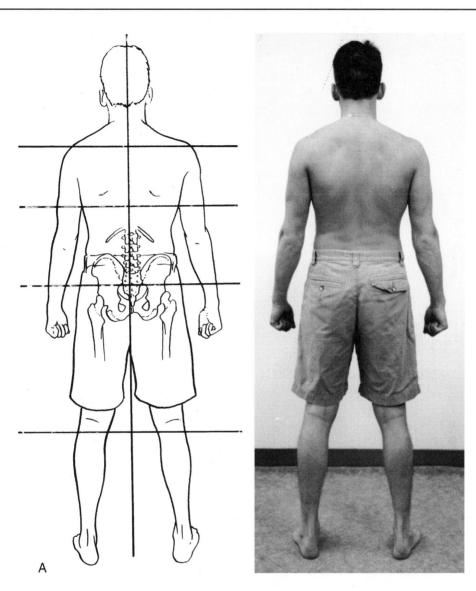

Figure 5–4. *A*, Posterior frontal plane view. *B*, Sagittal plane view. The clinician examines for symmetry and the patient's preferred posture.

assessment is achieved by comparing the bony elements of both sides.

The PSIS's are then palpated by starting caudal to their location and moving the thumbs upward in an attempt to hook under these bony prominences (Fig. 5–6). The "dimples" are surface landmarks that approximate these bony prominences. If the examiner finds these landmarks difficult to locate, he or she can start at the apex of the sacrum and palpate superiorly and laterally along the surface of the sacrum until the edge of the ilium is felt. The large processes palpated in this region are the PSIS. Either technique—

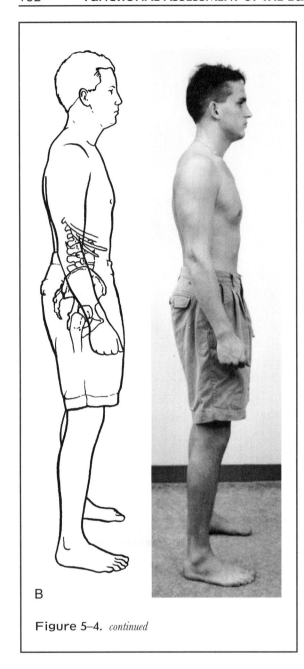

B

Figure 5–4. *continued*

The next palpation point is the ASIS and the iliac crests (Fig. 5–7). The ASIS is a large bony prominence, and it is difficult to palpate a single symmetrical identifying point. Therefore, the complete extent of the iliac crest should again be palpated in conjunction with the ASIS. The frontal plane position and any sagital plane asymmetry should be noted.

The clinician should now pause and assess the findings from these three palpations. These bony landmarks of the pelvis give the clinician a reasonable three-dimensional picture of the pelvis with its accompanying sacral base. The position of the sacral base is important because it helps the examiner visualize the position of the pelvis and lower lumbar spine in the standing posture.

The fourth point, the greater trochanter, is difficult to compare bilaterally because of its size (Fig. 5–8). Therefore, it should be used to help verify frontal plane asymmetries. For example, if the right iliac crest, PSIS, and ASIS are higher when compared with the left, then the greater trochanter should be palpated. If the trochanter is also high on the right and the patient is bearing weight equally on both lower extremities, then the patient has either a skeletally short left lower extremity, an angle difference at the hip, a size variation of one of the ilia, or soft-tissue asymmetries. For the purpose of this text, we prefer to call this type of difference a *frontal plane asymmetry.* Whatever the reason for the asymmetry, the sacral base is now tilted to the left because of the position of the pelvis in the frontal plane. This results in a compensatory lumbar side bending to the right.[9]

Pathomechanic Considerations in Standing: Frontal Plane Asymmetry

In the standing position, a frontal plane asymmetry results in asymmetrical loading patterns through the lumbopelvic tissues (Fig. 5–9).[9, 10, 11, 23, 44] With the left side of the pelvis lower than the right, as assessed from the standing position (referred to as a left frontal plane asymmetry for the purposes of this text), different compressive, tensile, and shear loading patterns are borne by the right and left sides (see also Figure 4–46). On the right side, there is increased compressive load at the hip joint, increased shear stress between the iliac and sacral surfaces, increased compressive stress to the lumbosacral and lower lumbar zygapophyseal joint because they are now in a more close-packed position, and the potential for a decrease in the cranial–caudal diame-

hooking under the PSIS or following the sacrum superiorly and laterally—helps place the two palpating thumbs in relatively the same position on the right and left PSIS. This palpation gives the clinician the perception of the frontal plane position of the pelvis.

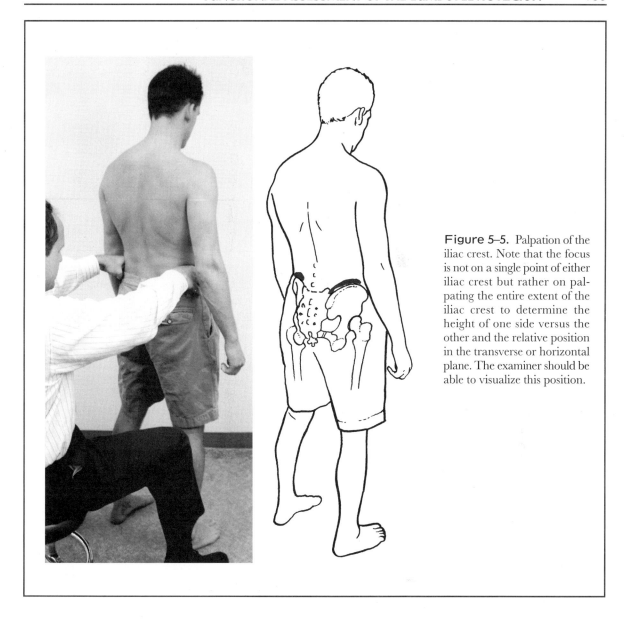

Figure 5–5. Palpation of the iliac crest. Note that the focus is not on a single point of either iliac crest but rather on palpating the entire extent of the iliac crest to determine the height of one side versus the other and the relative position in the transverse or horizontal plane. The examiner should be able to visualize this position.

ter of the neuroforamen on the right. The lumbar changes are a consequence of the compensatory right lateral bending of the lumbar spine that occurs as a result of the convergence of trunk and ground forces to the lowered pelvis on the left.

On the left side, there is increased compression between the iliac and sacral joint surfaces, increased tensile stresses to the soft tissues related to the left side of the lumbar spine including muscular, ligamentous,

and the nerve root complex. Lastly, the right side-bending of the lumbar spine as a result of the left frontal plane asymmetry results in a shear stress to the disc.

Do such asymmetrical loading patterns accelerate the degenerative process of the articular cartilage or render the individual susceptible to injury because of a lowered optimal loading capacity (see Chapter 1)? It has been suggested that the "long-leg side" has an earlier onset of degenerative changes of the hip.[9] Very

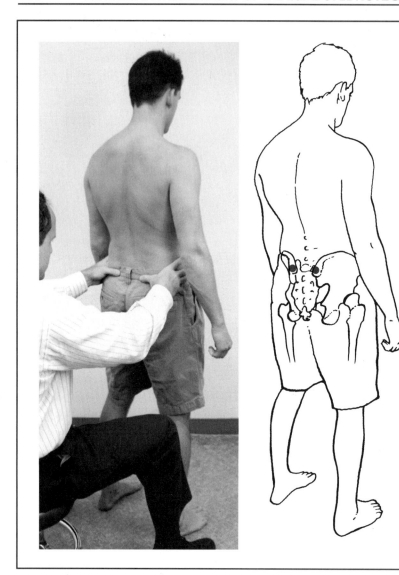

Figure 5–6. The second palpation point is the posterior superior iliac spine (PSIS). The examiner should strive to place the thumb inferior to the PSIS in the "shelf" as the sacrum meets the ilium. This is the most important point in the pelvis because the ledge is the most distinguishable palpation point.

often, individuals with low back pain also have difficulty tolerating extension quadrant stresses to the lumbar spine on the long-leg side from the standing position, which suggests decreased ability of the zygapophyseal joints and their support structures to tolerate compressive loads, perhaps from early facet degenerative changes similar to those seen in the articular cartilage of the hip. As described in Chapter 4, the sacroiliac joint is most susceptible to shear loading. Since increased shear stress is seen on the long-leg side, due to the more vertically oriented right sacroiliac joint, this may result in rendering the sacroiliac joint vulnerable to pain from excessive shear loading.

If a frontal plane asymmetry has been determined, small blocks of known thickness can be placed under the foot on the short side (Fig. 5–9). All points can be palpated again in order to assess symmetry. After placing blocks of the desired thickness under the short side, the patient is asked to equally distribute his weight. The blocks are then removed, and the patient

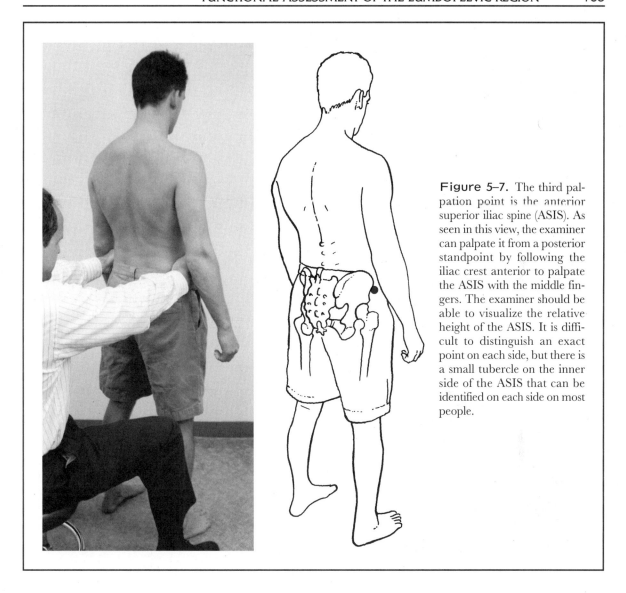

Figure 5–7. The third palpation point is the anterior superior iliac spine (ASIS). As seen in this view, the examiner can palpate it from a posterior standpoint by following the iliac crest anterior to palpate the ASIS with the middle fingers. The examiner should be able to visualize the relative height of the ASIS. It is difficult to distinguish an exact point on each side, but there is a small tubercle on the inner side of the ASIS that can be identified on each side on most people.

is again asked to equalize his weight. This is repeated several times using incremental thicknesses. The patient is then asked about his perception of the height of most comfort. If the patient responds that while he was on the blocks the "pressure" decreased or he was more comfortable, then the patient is conveying to the clinician the height of the correction and the importance of the need to change the loading pattern of his lumbopelvic tissues as an initial step in his treatment regimen. Such a change in the

loading pattern may be initiated by the use of a heel lift.

Other methods of assessing leg length discrepancies have been described but are conducted in the supine, non–weight-bearing position. However, a person's standing, antigravity mechanics are very different from his body mechanics when he is supine. Therefore, the standing assessment using calibrated blocks yields more clinically relevant information because it is in the upright postures that a person usually is symp-

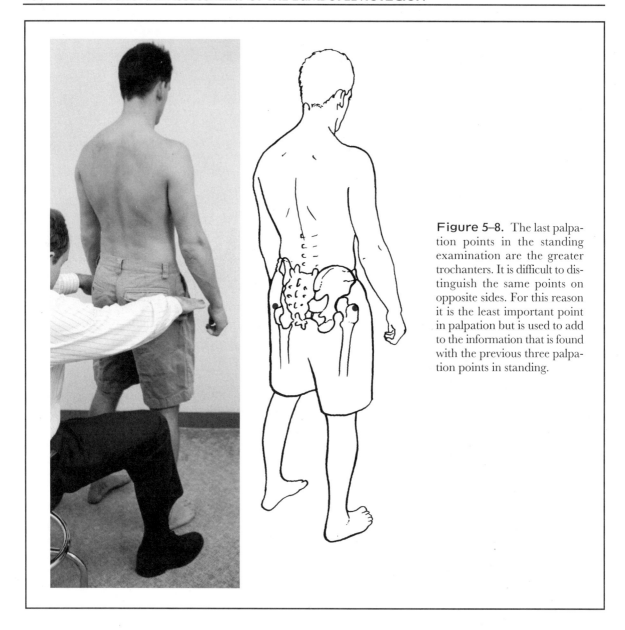

Figure 5–8. The last palpation points in the standing examination are the greater trochanters. It is difficult to distinguish the same points on opposite sides. For this reason it is the least important point in palpation but is used to add to the information that is found with the previous three palpation points in standing.

tomatic. A sit-up maneuver is sometimes used as a measure of "functional" leg length discrepancies, i.e., iliosacral lesions which result in leg-length discrepancies. In this test, the patient is asked to sit up from the supine position to assess which leg assumes a more distal position. If one leg moves further distally than the other, the interpretation is often a functional leg-length discrepancy owing to a pelvic dysfunction. This inter-

pretation, however, ignores the neuromuscular control of the movement pattern that the patient in pain must initiate and complete. In conducting this sit-up test, the clinician assumes that perfectly symmetrical concentric and eccentric contractions occur on the right and left sides of the trunk and lower extremities. This is an unreasonable assumption because a person who is experiencing back pain will guard the injured

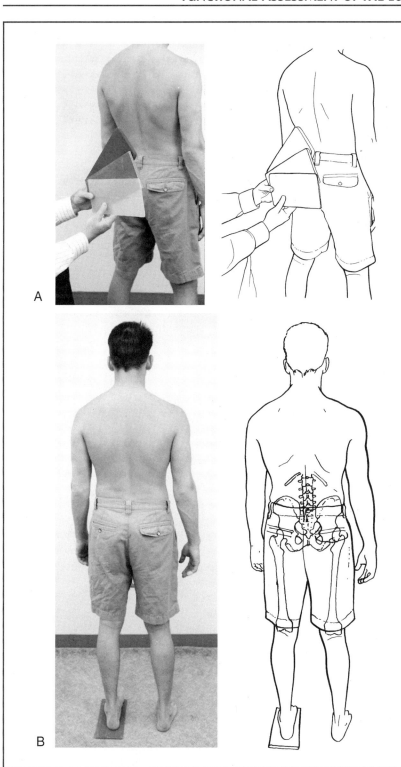

Figure 5–9. *A*, Assessing the frontal plane asymmetry from the standing position using calibrated blocks (4-inch by 14-inch blocks of 1/8", 1/4", and 3/8" thickness). *B*, A 1/4" calibrated block is positioned under the left foot. The patient is placed on and off the block(s) several times, and then asked the question, "At what level do you feel most comfortable?" When a patient replies that one of the blocks is most comfortable, it tells the examiner that a correction is indicated while also determining the height. When a frontal plane asymmetry exists and is correlated to the pain pattern, it often represents a significant part of the overall treatment process.

area and alter muscle activity accordingly. This results in the lumbopelvic segments moving asymmetrically. Therefore, caution must be taken in interpreting the findings of this test as having the same meaning as the antigravity standing evaluation. If we are concerned about the effect of asymmetrical forces reaching tissues, then we need to closely assess the postures and movement patterns that allow this to occur. Drawing conclusions about structural differences from the prone or supine position does not yield functional information because superincumbent and ground forces are removed.

Pathomechanic Considerations in Standing: Sagittal Plane

Chapters 3 and 4 stressed how a weak abdominal wall and tight hip flexors result in increased compressive loads to the lumbar apophyseal support structures. Patients with advanced degeneration of the facets or lumbar stenosis often stand with the buttocks "rolled under the pelvis," a posterior tilt of the pelvis primarily due to hip extensors activity, and they appear to have lost the lumbar lordosis. However, care must be taken in making this assumption because oftentimes this is a posture that is assumed in order to help decrease compressive and shear loads at the lower lumbar spine apophyseal support structures. Likewise, the patients who describe the need to sit after walking a short ways, the rest position of being leaned forward supporting themselves with their hands on their thighs, or the need to lean over a grocery cart when walking in a grocery store, are all describing mechanisms to unload the compression and shear at the lumbar apophyseal joint complex. Rather than assuming that the goal in treatment should be to restore the normal lordosis, it is more reasonable to assume the degenerative processes have resulted in the loss of a certain percentage of back motion, and compression and shear loading tolerance, and the goal will be to optimize function of the remaining invulnerable range of motion. Therefore, when a flattened lumbar spine is seen in this portion of the evaluation, the clinician must determine if this posture is a contributing factor to the nociceptive mechanics, or if the posture is one of protected guarding.

Another finding at the pelvis might be a high iliac crest and ASIS and a low PSIS on one side. Assuming symmetrical weight-bearing, this could be interpreted as a sagittal plane asymmetry when comparing the right side of the pelvis with the left. In this example,

the findings appear to indicate that either the right ilium is fixed in a posteriorly rotated position or the left ilium is fixed in an anterior position. The focus should be on the side where pain is experienced. A broader explanation might be increased muscle activity of the region resulting from afferent nociceptive input. For example, with the right sacroiliac joint positioned in a manner that appears to be posterior torsion of the ilium, it might be concluded that this is a central nervous system strategy to minimize compressive and shear loading at the lumbosacral and lower lumbar zygapophyseal joints on the right side. This might be more likely than concluding that the sacroiliac joint becomes fixed and blocked, especially in males. Such a sagittal plane finding may be more representative of an asymmetrical neuromuscular control mechanism than a fixation of bony elements, especially since the afferent–efferent balance of neurological activity is altered as a result of injury. If backward bending and side bending over the posteriorly rotated side increases the familiar symptoms, the protective guarding is most likely the reason for this sagittal plane finding.

Gait Analysis

An analysis of gait can provide useful information regarding the weight-bearing capabilities of the musculoskeletal system. For example, excessive pronation throughout the stance phase increases valgus at the knee, femoral internal rotation, and increased extension stress to the lumbar spine because of the obligatory downward tilt of the pelvis. Excessive supination of the foot throughout the stance phase potentially results in a decrease in the attenuation of ground forces, which may increase stress to the lumbopelvic region.

More commonly, gait patterns often reveal how the individual is attempting to "unload" the low back. During the push-off phase, there is increased compressive loading at the lower lumbar joints as the pelvis is rotated in a posterior direction on the push-off side. This type of rotary maneuver of the pelvis increases compression and shear loading between the facets. The gait of the patient who cannot tolerate such compressive loads often shows a decreased stride length at the push-off side, and the pelvis is maintained forward on one side as much as possible.

An abnormal gait pattern of patient with nerve root symptoms and signs might also be seen. In addition to the gait pattern being altered because of pain in the back and leg, there is typically weakness of the hip abductors and hip extensors because nerve root pathology may compromise the neural supply to their motor units. The hip abductors are innervated by the superior gluteal nerve carrying primarily the L4, L5, and S1 segments, and the gluteus maximus is supplied by the inferior gluteal nerve carrying primarily the L5, Sl, and S2 segments. Nerve root pathologies affecting the L4 or L5 nerve roots compromise these powerful hip muscles resulting in Trendelenberg and trunk-listing types of gaits.

Gross Movement Testing

Gross movement testing with the patient in the standing position is important in assessing the response of the various tissues to tensile, compressive, torsional, and shear forces. It is important that the clinician be able to visualize how these forces reach the tissues of the lumbopelvic region as movement progresses in the range of motion. Important information is gleaned as the clinician assesses the patient's response to protect the injury. Key questions to ask during the movement testing include whether the movement pattern is making the pain worse and whether it is reproducing the familiar pain that is representative of the chief complaint. The intent is to reproduce the familiar pain in standing through gross movement testing, and then use the supine and prone positions to substantiate the mechanics of the standing examination. Gross movement testing includes active forward bending, backward bending, side bending, and a combination of these motions into the forward- and backward-bending quadrants. Overpressure can be applied to any of these movements in much the same manner as when evaluating the extremities (see Figs. 5–10 to 5–14).

Forward bending is assessed by watching the complete spine and then the pelvis move in a smooth synchronous manner. The examiner is assessing lumbopelvic rhythm as the forces of forward bending proceed from the cervical spine down into the pelvis.[4] The L4–L5 and L5–S1 segments combine for approximately 45 degrees of motion in this plane, and the clinician should be able to detect whether the lumbar and pelvic regions are moving normally. Visualizing the synchronized movements of the spinal segments as the motion reaches the pelvis and continues around the femoral heads is more important than simply assessing whether or not the patient can touch the floor. It is important to note if the patient is not moving in a particular region of the spine. This is most often the result of either true tightness, protective muscle guarding, or both.

The clinician should apply overpressure to the forward- and side-bending motions in varying combinations in an attempt to reproduce the painful response. In order for overpressure to be correctly applied in forward bending, side bending, or a combination of the two motions, it is important that the pelvis be stabilized. Figure 5–10 shows hand placement over the sacrum to stabilize the sacral base while the overpressure force is applied. The overpressure is applied to increase the tensile stresses to the tissues posterior to the axis of motion in the lumbar spine.

The patient is then asked to backward bend. The clinician again observes the preferred movement pattern. Many patients with low back pain backward bend by simply hyperextending at the hips. This is a protective guarding mechanism that decreases the compression and shear forces that accompany extension of the lumbopelvic region. Figure 5–11 shows how the clinician can control the extension motion, directing the force through the lumbopelvic region by applying a compressive force with the hands through the patient's retracted shoulders. This force is applied with an intensity sufficient to create a small, controlled increase in lumbar lordosis or extension. The examiner's hands at the shoulders often detect the guarding by the patient if the forces are poorly tolerated, or the patient recognizes even before the motion is complete that this increases their low back pain.

To assess the movement of backward bending and side bending to the right (Fig. 5–12), the clinician guides the motion with his right hand, by first backward bending the patient and then adding side bending to the right. The left hand maintains the compressive force over the top of the left shoulder. This line of compressive force starts at the left shoulder and travels through the midthoracic spine into the contralateral lower lumbar vertebral segments. The line of force travels into the lumbosacral triangle and then reaches the superior aspect of the sacroiliac joint. The right L5–S1 zygapophyseal joint is now in a closed-pack position, and the force continues through the structures of the sacroiliac joint and into the lower extremity. The examiner's left hand gradually increases the compressive force to this area. Other combinations of forward bending, backward bending, side bending, and rotation can be used in the same manner to identify the pattern that best reproduces the symptom (Figs.

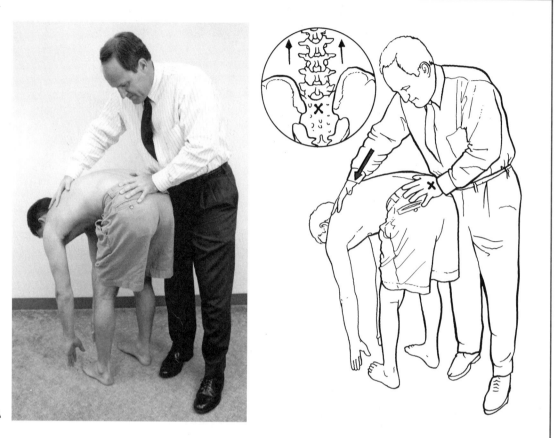

Figure 5–10. *A* and *B*, Overpressure in full-range forward bending *(A)*. Note how the examiner's hands are pushing in opposite directions. The examiner should visualize the compressive forces placed on anterior tissues, and the elongation or stretch loads transferred to the tissues that are posterior to the center of rotation. The spine can be placed in any position, as shown in *B*, where the patient is forward bent and side bent to the left and overpressure is applied. A positive finding is provocation of familiar pain.

5–13 and 5–14). Note how the femoral extension in Fig. 5–14 increases the extension, compression, and shear loading to the left lumbosacral region.

This type of gradual, guided overpressure during gross movement testing from the standing position is probably the most important part of the entire assessment because the subsequent supine and prone assessments are designed to substantiate the pain pattern found with gross movement testing. If the clinician cannot reproduce familiar symptoms in gross move-

ment testing, then determining the correct course of the treatment will be difficult.

A comment is necessary regarding the so-called specific mobility testing of the sacroiliac joint. This test and variations of it were originally designed to evaluate movement of the ilium on the sacrum when the patient flexes the thigh and hip from the standing position. As the hip is flexed, the ipsilateral innominate bone moves through an arc best described as posterior torsion. The clinician palpates the PSIS or the ischial

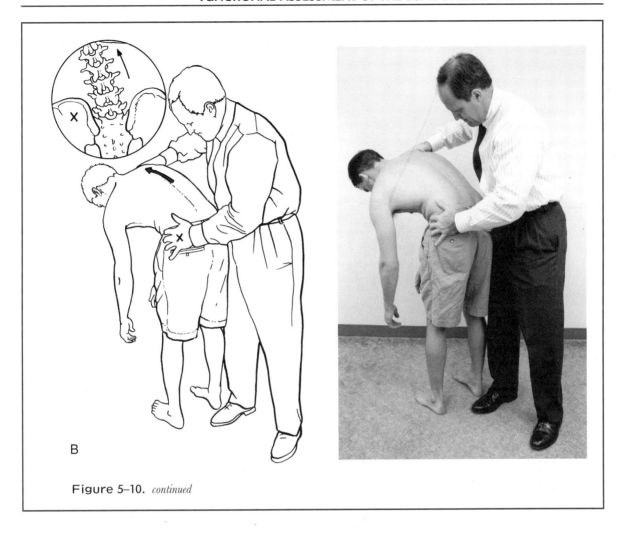

B

Figure 5–10. *continued*

tuberosity and follows these bony landmarks moving in an inferior or a downward direction (Fig. 5–15). This motion can be detected if compared with the relatively stationary position of the opposite PSIS or the second sacral spinous process. If a downward motion occurs, sacroiliac joint movement is considered normal. On the other hand, dysfunction is thought to be present—in particular, a "blocked joint"—if the PSIS or ischial tuberosity moved in an upward direction while the hip was flexing. This interpretation is restrictive, and does not take into account all of the relevant neuromuscular activity that necessarily occurs with the test.

When a person flexes the right hip while standing, the left hip abductors must be strong enough to stabi-

lize the pelvis in the frontal plane. Nevertheless, the pelvis drops on the opposite side as soon as the leg is lifted from the ground, much in the same manner as the frontal plane tilt of the pelvis during gait. This tilt causes the PSIS and ischial tuberosity to assume a more inferior position when compared with the opposite side. This downward motion is not due to sagittal plane posterior torsion but rather to frontal plane tilt.

As the person flexes the hip, and the structures on the posterior aspect of the hip become taut, a posterior torsional force is applied to the sacroiliac joint followed by a flexion force on the lumbar spine. If these forces stimulate the "afferent generator" responsible for pain, the patient reflexively alters the movement to protect the region. Many muscles are involved in

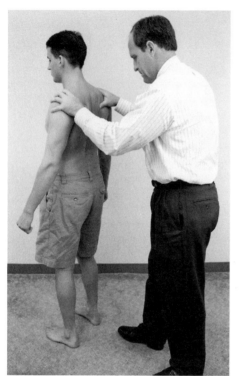
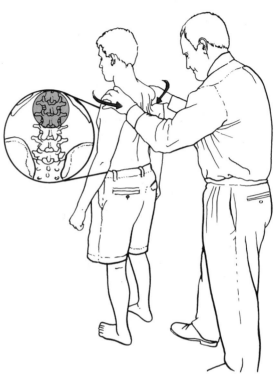

Figure 5–11. *A and B,* Overpressure in backward bending. The examiner manually retracts the scapulae *(A),* which focuses the extension force in the upper part of the lumbar spine, and then a gradual vertical force from above causes extension *(B).* Note that it is most often a very small range of movement.

stabilizing and moving the trunk and lower extremities. For this reason a more accurate interpretation of an atypical movement pattern of the pelvis during the hip flexion test, or any other mobility test, should simply be "altered lumbopelvic mechanics" rather than "a blocked segment."

Neurological Screening from Standing

Two tests can be carried out from the standing position to provide an initial neurological screen. Walking in place on the toes assesses S1 and S2 nerve root function via the gastrocsoleus muscle group. It is helpful to have the patient place their hands lightly on the examiner's hands because the plantar flexor weakness

can be better detected as the patient tries to push down on the examiner's hands to help raise themselves up on the toes while they walk in place. Having the patient rise on both toes simultaneously does not provide information regarding weakness.

Likewise, the patient can be asked to walk in place on his heels to grossly assess the L4 and L5 nerve root function through the anterior tibialis and toe extensor muscle groups.

Supine Testing

With the patient in a supine position the examiner can evaluate hip mobility and place various forces

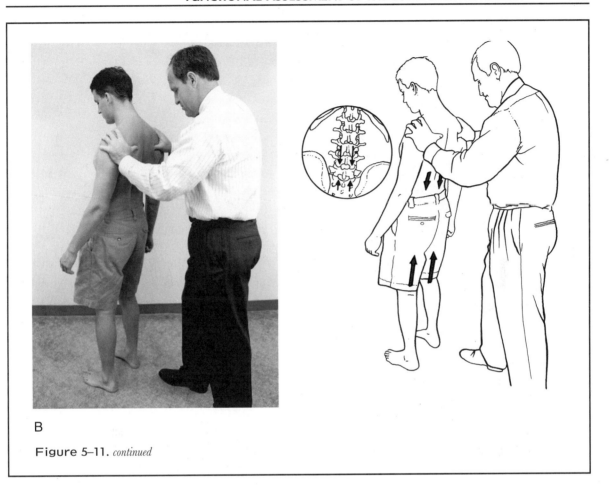

B

Figure 5–11. *continued*

through the sacroiliac and lumbar joints. Much of the neurological evaluation can also be performed in this position. Table 5–6 outlines the sequence of the supine testing position.

Progression of Flexion: Increasing Tensile Stresses

Hip range of motion is an important assessment for low back problems. The examiner must be certain as to when the passive hip motion assessment begins to place forces to the pelvis and then the lumbar spine. When the femur is passively flexed, the hip joint capsule unwinds and the hip joint becomes "open" or "loose-packed." As the hip is moved from the neutral position toward full flexion, tension is increased to the hip extensors and posterior hip cap-

sule, and the femur in essence becomes part of the innominate (Fig. 5–16). As passive hip flexion continues, the motion places a posterior torsional stress of the ilium on the sacrum. There is then a small posterior rotary accommodation of the ilium on the sacrum at the sacroiliac joint.

Once the limits of the sacroiliac joint accommodation are reached and all of the tissue slack is taken up, the ilium and sacrum move as a unit. The continued force of passive hip flexion results in lumbosacral flexion. This inferior migration of the superior articulating process of S1 on the inferior articulating process of the L5 vertebra results in a flexion force at the L5–S1 segment. This motion continues to involve the remainder of the lumbar vertebrae as the tissues tighten in flexion from below upward. The response of the patient to these flexion stresses should be compared

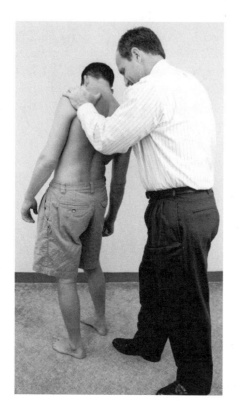
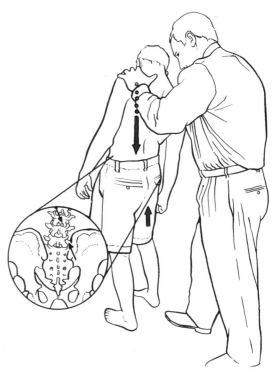

Figure 5–12. Extension quadrant with overpressure in combined motion in backward bending, side bending to the right. The examiner guides with the right hand and applies the compressive force through his left hand. The examiner should be able to visualize the vertical force from the left hand as it passes down through the shoulder, into and through the thoracic spine, down into the right lumbosacral triangle, and through the right lower extremity. This is an excellent test for assessing the response of the right lumbosacral tissues to compressive loads.

with those forward-bending quadrant stresses elicited in the standing examination.

Figure 4 Test

Other hip motions are assessed, and care is taken to determine what is actually hip motion versus pelvic and lumbar motions. The Figure 4 test, or FABER position, is an excellent method to assess the range of motion of the hip joint, joint crepitus, as well as place stress to the sacroiliac and lumbar tissues (Fig. 5–17).

It is essential that the examiner be cognizant of where the stress of the Figure 4 test is focused. Asymmetric differences in the motion between the right and left sides may be revealed with this test. This is especially important to note in patients with unilateral low back pain.

The Figure 4 position moves the intertrochanteric line of the femur away from the ilium and the pubis. This has the effect of placing a tensile force on a significant portion of the hip joint capsule, especially the iliofemoral and pubofemoral portions of the reinforcing capsular ligament (Fig. 5–18). For this reason it is

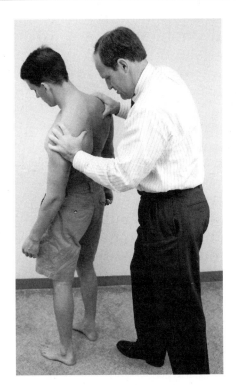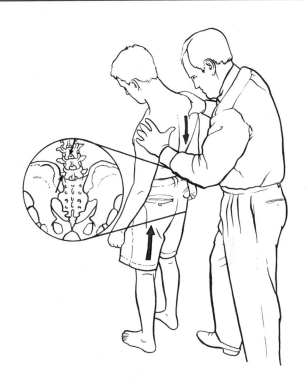

Figure 5–13. Backward bending, side bending to the left, and slight rotation to the right, with a superior-to-inferior overpressure applied through the right shoulder.

an excellent assessment of the extensibility of the hip joint capsule and overall hip joint motion. If the hip adductor muscles are thought to be the cause of the limited range of motion in the Figure 4 position, a contract–relax technique to the adductors can help distinguish between muscle tightness and connective tissue shortening of the capsule.

A tight hip joint capsule can contribute to excessive forces that reach the lumbopelvic joints.[22, 31, 32] Consider the person who walks a great deal at work. Each step the person takes requires creating a hyperextension moment at the hip for effective push-off. If the person has a tight hip joint capsule, the lower extremity is placed behind the body not by femoral extension but rather by anterior torsion and rotation of the pelvis and eventual extension of the lumbar spine. The attempt to extend the hip tightens the anterior hip capsular tissues and increased excessive anterior tor-

sion of the ilium on the sacrum, a forward and downward movement of the sacrum resulting in increased lumbosacral extension and hyperextension of the lumbar spine. Any of these tissues may be symptomatic and, unless the hip range of motion is restored, excessive stresses reach the lumbopelvic tissues contributing to continued damage and prolonged symptoms.

A positive Figure 4 sign may be an indication that femoral extension is limited. If the person with a positive Figure 4 attempts to maintain the same stride length during gait, increased extension stresses to the lumbar spine result. If a limitation in Figure 4 in the supine position is confirmed, and backward bending and side bending on the same side increase familiar symptoms in the standing examination, then this represents a mechanical *match*. In this example, the match represents backward bending and side bending, increasing familiar pain and a positive Figure 4

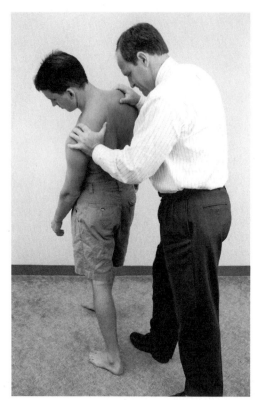
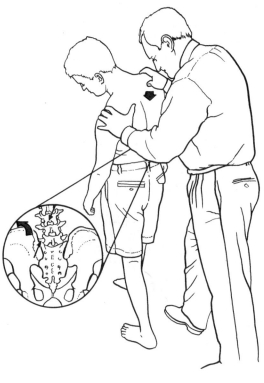

Figure 5–14. Modification of the standing examination that increases the extension, compression, and shear stresses in the left lumbosacral triangle by prepositioning the left lower extremity in extension. By prepositioning in femoral extension (below up) and then backward bending and side bending to the left (above down) with overpressure through the examiner's right hand, the end-range of extension and compression is quickly reached, and the response evaluated. The examiner can vary the leg position, trunk position, and overpressure in any of these examples.

(decreased femoral extension) on the same side. The match refers to the fact that both the lumbar spine and hip maneuvers increase extension, compression, and shear loading in the lumbar spine from above down and below up. It is common to find tightness of the anterior hip on the side of the low back pain.[32]

Straight Leg Raising

The supine lying evaluation continues by performing the straight-leg raise test. The maneuver places a tensile stress to the nerve roots via the sciatic nerve. A positive finding is reproduction of familiar leg pain as the leg is elevated.[27] Maintaining the elevation at the point where pain is initially perceived to assess whether the pain peripheralizes adds significance to the test and represents irritation of the nerve root complex. The straight-leg raise test can be augmented by combining hip flexion with slight femoral adduction and internal rotation. This position increases tensile stress to the sciatic nerve and the L4–S2 nerve roots, owing to the course of the sciatic nerve as it proceeds later-

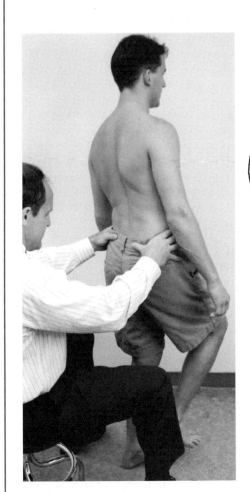

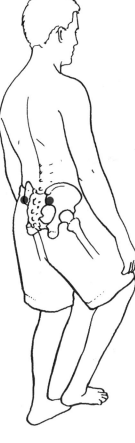

Figure 5–15. The examiner's palpating thumb is at the "shelf" underneath the PSIS, and the patient is asked to actively hip flex. A normal finding would be an inferior motion of the right thumb as the patient actively flexes the right femur.

al to the ischial tuberosity (Fig. 5–19). The examiner should pay close attention to the abdominal wall because it is common to see reflex contraction of the abdominal musculature as the painful point of the straight-leg raise range of motion is approached.

Stresses to the Pelvis via the Femur

From the supine position a variety of stresses can be placed to the sacroiliac joints and support tissues. Figure 5–20 demonstrates the long axis of the femur

Table 5–6. Supine Examination
1. Progression of flexion
Hip $\rightarrow$ Iliosacral $\rightarrow$ Sacral lumbar $\rightarrow$ Lumbar
Assess motion and tissue tension sense
2. Figure 4 Test
Hip $\rightarrow$ Iliosacral $\rightarrow$ Facet compression
3. Straight leg raise
4. Stresses to pelvis via femur
5. Neurological screen

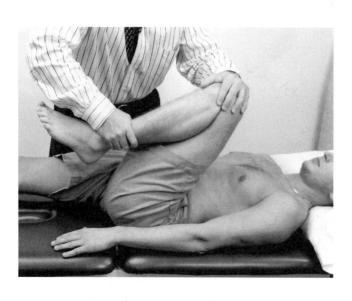

Figure 5–16. Supine lying examination, passive hip flexion. The examiner should visualize the hip joint capsule as it unwinds and comes into an open-pack position at 90 degrees of hip flexion. Continuation of the flexion motion results in a posterior rotary moment on the ilium and ends with spinal flexion. The response to the flexion motion of the lumbar spine should be compared with the responses that were elicited in any of the forward-bending quadrants.

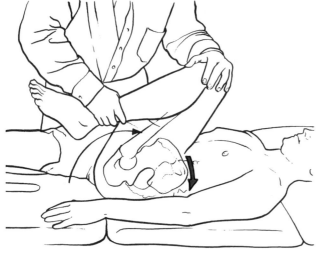

being placed in approximately the same plane as the sacroiliac joint. From this position, a graded force is applied through the long axis of the femur to create a shear force (ilium on sacrum) at the sacroiliac joint. If this maneuver provokes familiar pain, the Figure 4 test also elicited low back pain, the patient has unilateral pain at the sacroiliac region, and the standing extension and side-bending test was painful to the same side,

then a series of mechanical *matches* has been determined.

Using the femur as a lever, a variety of stresses can be directed to the musculoskeletal structures of the lumbopelvic region. Figures 5–21 and 5–22 show some of the stresses to this region. The position of the femur and the amount and direction of the stresses applied help identify the area involved in the painful syndrome.

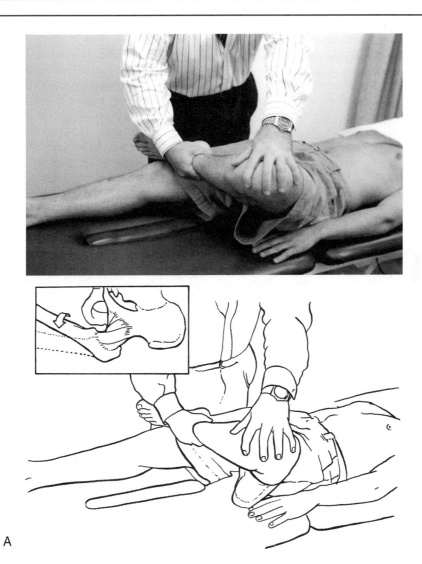

A

Figure 5–17. *A and B,* The Figure 4 test, or FABER position, which shows passive flexion, abduction, and external rotation. The examiner should be able to visualize the passive stretching of the anterior hip muscles and the hip joint capsule as it travels inferior and lateral (see Chapter 4). As the femur is directed toward the table *(A),* the examiner should envision a "gaping" stress to the sacroiliac joint on the left side, and ultimately a small rotary force to the lumbosacral junction. This can be countered and controlled by changing the hand placement to stabilize the opposite ASIS *(B).*

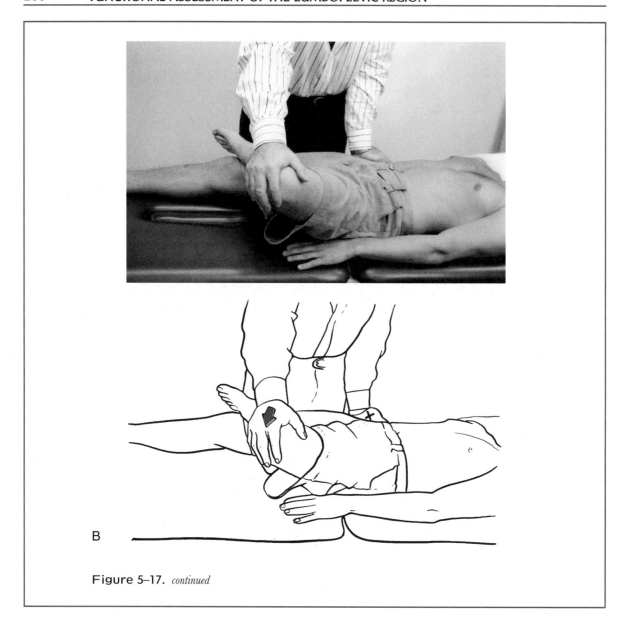

B

Figure 5–17. *continued*

The clinician must be cognizant of how and when the stresses progressively reach the pelvis and are transferred into the lumbar tissues. If the pelvic or lumbar structures are involved in the painful syndrome, the patient should respond with a complaint of familiar pain each time the examiner directs similar stresses to the region, whether from a standing, supine, or prone lying position.

Neurological Screening from Supine

Several neurological tests should be performed in the supine position in addition to the previously described straight-leg raise to rule out nerve root involvement. Specific myotomes can be assessed via muscle testing the quadriceps (L3, L4), tibialis anterior (L4), extensor hallucis longus (L5), and the per-

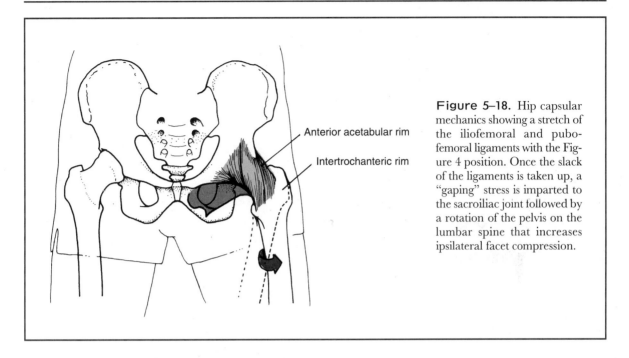

Anterior acetabular rim

Intertrochanteric rim

Figure 5–18. Hip capsular mechanics showing a stretch of the iliofemoral and pubofemoral ligaments with the Figure 4 position. Once the slack of the ligaments is taken up, a "gaping" stress is imparted to the sacroiliac joint followed by a rotation of the pelvis on the lumbar spine that increases ipsilateral facet compression.

oneals (S1, S2). In addition, the supine position provides a relaxed position for the patient for testing the quadriceps, posterior tibialis, or gastrocsoleus reflex. Lastly, sensory screening can be performed from this position to determine if there are localized areas along a dermatome in which sensory perception is absent or significantly altered.

Prone Testing

The patient is asked to lie prone. Table 5–7 outlines the sequence of the prone lying examination. A pillow can be placed under the abdomen to support a neutral position of the lumbar spine. The clinician should consistently use the same method of prone positioning with each patient. This helps to standardize as much of the examination as possible and allows for comparison of findings between patients.

Knee Flexion

Passive flexion of the knee places a tensile stress to the rectus femoris muscle and femoral nerve, as well as other anterior thigh tissues (Fig. 5–23). The rectus femoris muscle attaches to the superior aspect of the

acetabulum and the anterior inferior iliac spine. The examiner pays attention to and palpates any movement of the pelvis as the knee is passively flexed. If there is a decrease in the length or an increase in the stiffness of the rectus femoris muscle, then flexion of the knee can cause an anterior torsional stress to the ilium because of its anterior attachments to the pelvis. The anterior rotary moment at the pelvis is transferred up into the lumbar spine as lumbosacral extension which increases facet compression and shear stress.

With the knee flexed, the examiner can also internally and externally rotate the hip (Fig. 5–24). This repeats a portion of the hip motion assessment from the supine test and provides another piece of information regarding the degenerative state and hip joint mobility. Unlike the supine test, the hip joint is now in 0 degrees flexion, and in a relatively close-packed position. Limited internal rotation from this position is often due to tightness of the hip joint capsule and is one of the first signs of a capsular pattern at the hip. Findings of limited hip motion in this position should be compared with those found in the supine examination, especially if asymmetric hip tightness is seen on the same side as unilateral back pain.

Finally, flexion of the knee, which is maintained while the hip is passively extended, can place a tensile

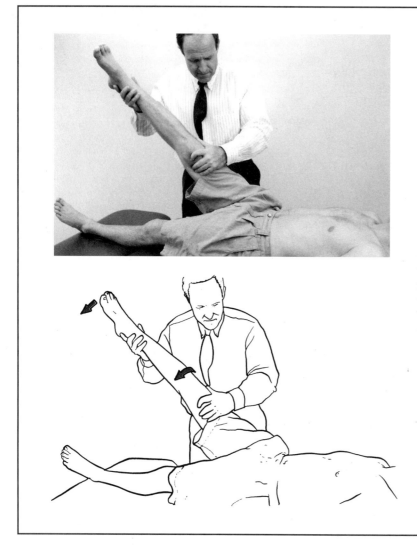

Figure 5–19. Augmented straight-leg raise tests adding adduction and internal rotation to the hip flexion maneuver. This change in mechanics increases the tensile force on the sciatic nerve as a result of the nerve's lateral position relative to the ischial tuberosity.

stress to the upper lumbar nerve roots via the femoral nerve. This position of femoral nerve stretch is an assessment of the response of the L2, L3, and L4 nerve roots to increased tension.

Progression of Extension: Increasing Compression and Shear

After examination of the hip, the clinician begins to assess the pelvis and lumbar spine. The clinician should visualize the approximate plane of the sacroiliac joint, taking into consideration that the sacrum is wider anteriorly and superiorly than posteriorly and inferiorly. If the clinician is unaware of the joint plane and the depth of the tissues related to the sacroiliac joint, then the results from application of forces will be difficult to interpret. Gentle and graded forces are introduced. With the patient's knee flexed, the clinician grasps the anterior distal aspect of the femur with one hand and places the other hand over the ipsilateral posterior ilium. The clinician then passively extends and adducts the femur in a graded manner until he palpates motion at the pelvis (Fig. 5–25).

The analysis of this force is as follows: as the femur is extended and adducted the hip joint becomes close-

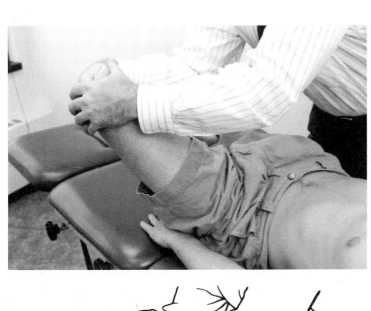

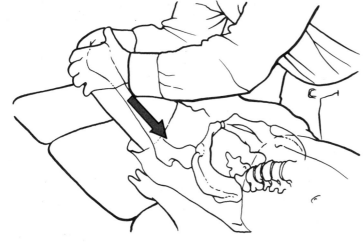

Figure 5–20. Force is directed along the long axis of the patient's left femur during the supine lying examination. The femur is placed in flexion and abduction to align the force with the plane of the left sacroiliac joint. The resultant force is an anterior-to-posterior shear force of the left ilium on sacrum.

packed because the joint capsule, iliopsoas, and other hip flexor muscles become taut. The tightening of these soft tissues results in an anterior rotary stress of the ilium on the sacrum, taking up the 2–4 degrees of motion at the sacroiliac joint. As the passive femoral extension continues, the motion of the pelvis and sacrum creates an extension force at the L5–S1 zygapophyseal joint as the superior articulating process of the sacrum moves on the inferior articulating process of the L5 segment. Coupled with this extension moment is an anterior shear force between the sacrum and the L5 segment. It can also be deduced that this combination of extension and anterior shear results in a tightening of the iliolumbar ligaments bilaterally, an increased compression of the articular surfaces of the L5–S1 zygapophyseal joint, and increased compression to the posterior aspect of the intervertebral disc.

With further lifting of the femur, the extension–anterior shear stress is imparted to the remaining lumbar segments. The protective response of the musculature owing to injury should be recognized. If the forces

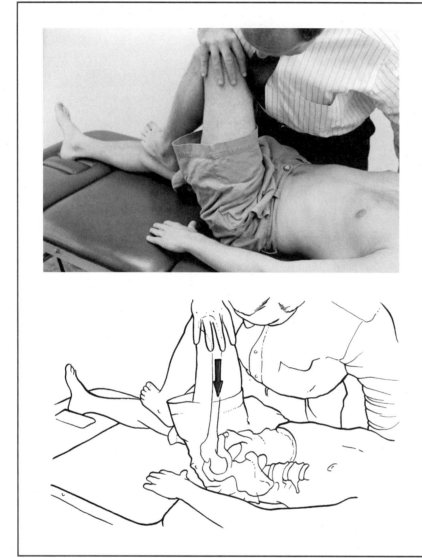

Figure 5–21. Anterior-to-posterior force directed along the long axis of the flexed femur. The resultant force is a compression at the anterior aspect of the sacroiliac joint and a slight gaping stress at the posterior aspect of the sacroiliac joint. It is a direct anterior-to-posterior shear stress at the pelvis.

that accompany the motion generate potentially destructive stimuli to any of the tissues, the clinician may recognize protective guarding of the surrounding muscles, especially in the hip flexors (resistance to the examiner lifting the leg further) as the extension force to the spine is increased. Injury decreases the tissues' threshold to stimuli. A negative finding is painless full range.

The similarity between this motion and that of the backward-bending and side-bending form standing should be appreciated. If compressive loading in the extension quadrant from standing increased familiar pain or was poorly tolerated, the comparable series of stresses in the prone lying examination, this time applied via the femur, should elicit a similar response. This represents another example of a mechanical *match* that is indicative of a mechanical disorder.

The lumbar spine can also be passively prepositioned in extension by having the patient lie prone on elbows. The lifting of the femur into hyperextension by the

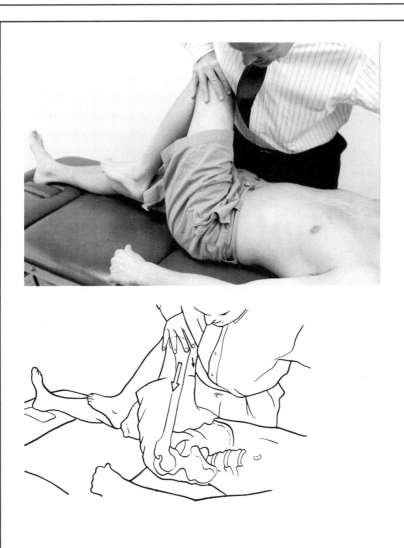

Figure 5–22. Force generated through the femur into the pelvis with the femur in flexion and slight adduction. The examiner applies a stress along the long axis of the femur until all of the tissues have become taut; this imparts a small adduction force to the femur, causing extreme compression at the anterior aspect of the sacroiliac joint and a significant "gaping" stress at the posterior aspect. If the long axis force is not generated through the femur to the pelvis in the initial part of this testing, then a significant compression force to the anterior labrum and iliopectineal bursa results, and the patient experiences groin pain.

examiner loads the lumbar spine in compression and shear more quickly than when the patient is completely prone, and further indicts those structures that are unable to tolerate compression and shear loading in the lumbopelvic tissues. The clinician should be able to visualize the transference of the shear force from the femur and hip joint through the sacroiliac joint, and ultimately through the lumbar spine. The point at which the patient responds to familiar pain in the progression may represent the region of the tissue injury.

Sacroiliac Stresses

The prone examination continues with the examiner placing the hand directly over the patient's midsacrum and applying a posterior–anterior shear force of the sacrum on ilium (Fig. 5–26). This stresses the supporting structures of the sacroiliac joint and compresses the intervening soft tissues under the examiner's hands. The object of this test is not to quantify mobility, but rather to apply a force that may reproduce

Table 5–7. Prone Examination

1. Knee Flexion
2. Progression of extension
   Hip → Iliosacral → Sacral lumbar → Lumbar
3. Sacroiliac stresses
   P–A stresses over sacrum
   Shear stresses of ilium on sacrum
4. P–A stresses over lumbar spine
   Centrally
   Lateral to midline
5. Palpation
6. Neurological screen

the patient's familiar pain. The examiner's hand can then be placed over the PSIS of the ilium and a stress applied along the plane of the sacroiliac joint, resulting in an anterior rotary moment to the ilium, with the intent again being to provoke any familiar pain rather than quantification of motion (Fig. 5–27).

A shear stress to the sacroiliac joint can also be applied by the examiner placing his thumb just medial to the PSIS over the sacrum immediately above the sacroiliac joint line (Fig. 5–28A). The examiner's opposite hand is placed over this thumb and a gradual posterior-to-anterior force is applied by the hand through the thumb and into the tissues (Fig. 5–28B). This pos-

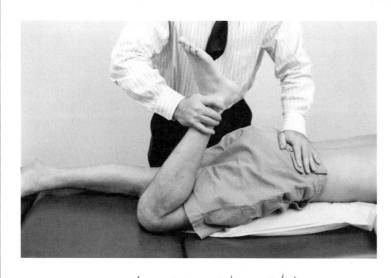

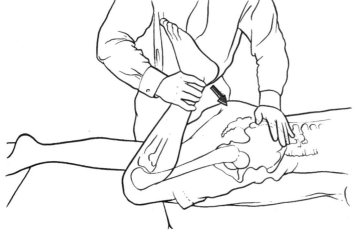

Figure 5–23. Passive knee flexion in a prone lying position that assesses the contractile state of the rectus femoris musculature. A positive sign would be an anterior rotary-type movement of the pelvis before the knee joint reaches 90 degrees of flexion. The opposite side should be assessed for symmetry.

terior-to-anterior force compresses the skin, fat, thoracolumbar fascia, erector spinae aponeurosis, and multifidus muscle. It then reaches the lateral border of the sacrum, with a resulting shear force of the sacrum on the ilium.

Another method of applying shear stress to the sacroiliac joint is via the ilium (Fig. 5–29). The examiner reaches around to the ilium furthest away from him. The opposite hand is placed over the dorsal aspect of the sacrum in order to apply a strong

fixation. The ilium is now pulled posteriorly by the examiner while the sacrum is fixated, creating a shear stress (posterior shear of ilium on sacrum) at the sacroiliac joint.

These tests, like most sacroiliac joint tests, attempt to place controlled forces through the tissues. If symptoms cannot be reproduced and the forces have been specifically directed to the sacroiliac joint structures, the pain is probably not due to mechanical dysfunction of the sacroiliac joint.

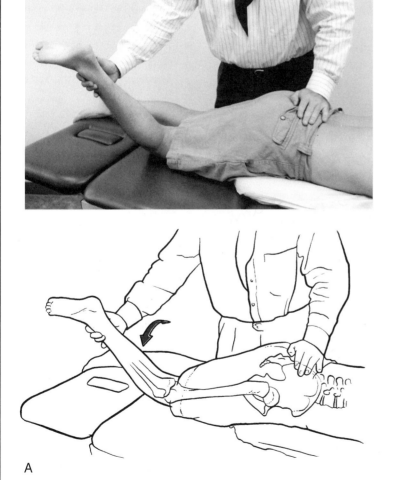

A

Figure 5–24. Prone lying passive internal *(A)* and external *(B)* rotation of the hip joint with the knee at 90 degrees of flexion and the hip at 0 degrees. The examiner should note the change in capsular position with the hip in flexion (supine lying) and in extension (prone lying). In prone lying the hip joint is more close-packed, and one should notice an increased, more rapid onset of resistance if the hip joint capsule is tight. Tightness in internal rotation is one of the main indicators of arthritic changes to the hip joint. The results of this prone lying test should match those found supine.

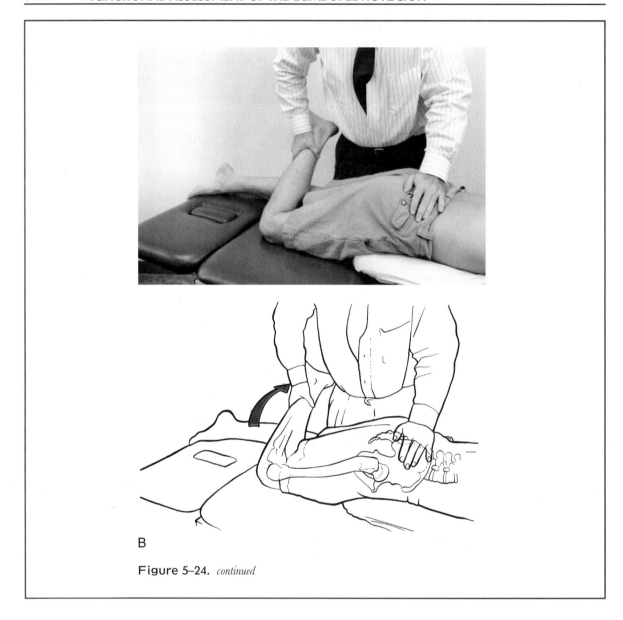

B

Figure 5–24. *continued*

Posterior–Anterior Stresses Over the Lumbar Spine

The prone lying examination continues with the assessment of the lumbar spine. The examiner begins by placing the hypothenar aspect of the hand on the skin of the cranial aspect of the sacrum and applying a posterior-to-anterior force. This results in an extension force on the lumbosacral junction because the force on the sacrum is nutation (flexion). The lumbosacral extension force is created by compression over the cranial aspect of the sacrum, rather than by the previously described long-lever technique using the femur.

The remaining lumbar spine segments are tested in the same manner (Fig. 5–30). The examiner places his hand on the skin and presses downward to impact on the spinous process. A posterior-to-anterior force is applied to each segment (Fig. 5–31). As the force pro-

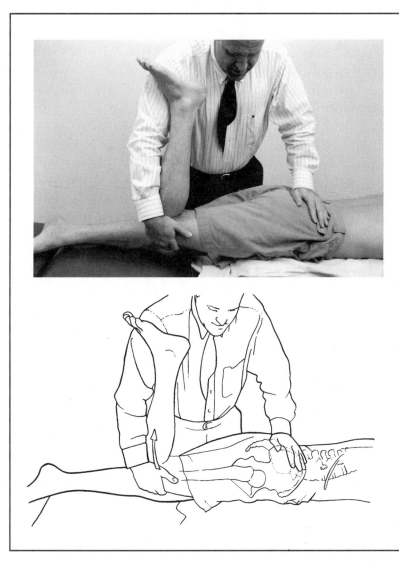

Figure 5–25. Prone lying passive femoral extension. The examiner should visualize the anterior femoral musculature becoming taut, and the hip joint capsule becoming taut, which then imparts an anterior rotary moment to the ilium and eventually an extension force to the lumbosacral junction. Lifting the femur further results in extension up through the remaining lumbar spine segments.

gresses into the spinous process it travels down the bony column into the lamina bilaterally and into the inferior articulating process (IAP) of the vertebra above. As the posterior-to-anterior force gently proceeds, the IAP articular cartilage is engaged into the articular cartilage of the superior articulating process (SAP) of the vertebra immediately caudal. The force causes these two surfaces to compress. Because of the lordotic position of these two vertebrae, an extension moment is generated that increases compression and anterior shear between the lumbar facets.

The force is subsequently transferred to the subchondral bone plate of the articular processes, the bony trabecular system of the vertebral pedicle and body, and finally to the intervertebral disc. This posterior-to-anterior force that began at the spinous process ends with a posterior-to-anterior shear to the vertebral body–intervertebral disc interface of the vertebral segment above the tested level. The goal is not to quantify the amount of motion or diagnose the specific tissue but to assess the capability of the tissues to tolerate these stresses, specifically compression and

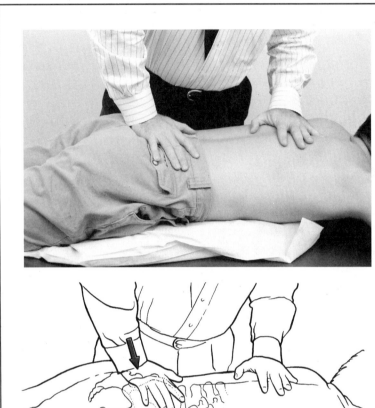

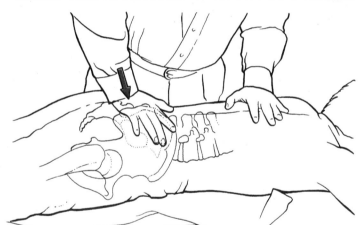

Figure 5–26. Posterior-to-anterior force is imparted through the skin directly over the sacrum, causing a posterior-to-anterior shear stress of the sacrum on the ilium. The examiner should not quantify motion, but rather gradually introduce this force into the sacrum, which stresses those structures that support the sacrum as it is suspended between the ilia.

shear. This test is carried out on the remaining lumbar vertebral segments.

Extension–compression loading stresses can be applied to the lumbar spine other ways as well. For example, while remaining in a prone position, the patient is asked to prop himself up on his elbows. This positions the lumbar spine in end-range extension. The examiner then applies a posterior-to-anterior force (Fig. 5–32). With the lumbar spine passively prepositioned in extension, a posterior to anterior force over the spinous process may elicit pain more quickly if the zygapophyseal joints and related tissues are unable to

tolerate compressive loads due to age related, degenerative changes. On the other hand, often times patients prepositioned in lumbar extension by propping on their elbows have less pain with posterior–anterior compressive loading than they do when the same force is applied in the prone position. We consider this latter finding more representative of instability of the spinal segment. With the patient completely prone, the posterior to anterior stress creates significant shear at the lumbar segments, resulting in increased discomfort and pain. When the patient is prone on elbows, he close-packs the lumbar joints and in-

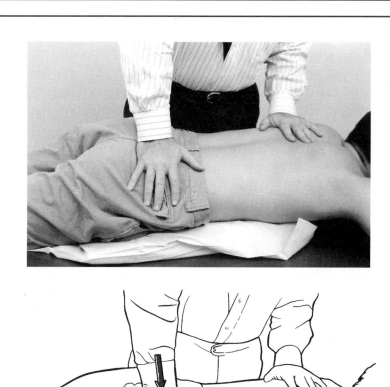

Figure 5–27. Prone lying examination. Posterior-to-anterior rotary force imparted to the posterior superior iliac spine and the right ilium.

creases tension in the anterior tissues, especially the anterior longitudinal ligament. The posterior–anterior force does not result in as much shear motion between the segments, and hence less discomfort.

Rotary Stresses to Lumbar Spine

To complete the assessment of the tolerance of the lumbar spine to passive motion, the examiner can introduce a rotary force to the lumbar spine in much the same manner (see Fig. 5–29B). The examiner places his hand at the midlumbar region, lateral to the spinous processes, and introduces a posterior-to-anterior force to the skin, progressing into the fatty layer, fascia, aponeurosis of the superficial erector spinae muscle, deep erector spinae muscle, and finally over the transverse processes and the lateral aspect of the vertebrae. Once the tissue has been compressed between the examiner's hand and the lateral vertebrae, the force is continued to produce a rotary force of the lumbar spine.

As an example, if a posterior–anterior force was applied over the right paraspinal region, the resultant force would be left lumbar rotation. The motion cre-

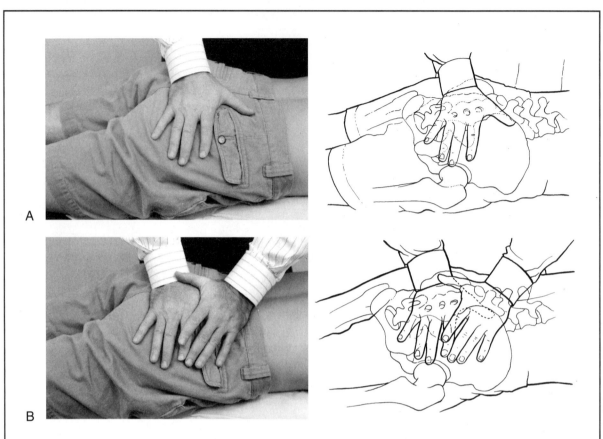

Figure 5–28. *A,* The examiner places the thenar eminence of the thumb at the sacral apex and rotates the thumb to bump into the right PSIS. This places the thumb along the sacrum. The thumb is placed in this position so that the force can be directed through it into the posterior musculature over the dorsal sacrum and then along the sacroiliac joint, creating a posterior-to-anterior shear. *B,* By using the opposite hand over top of the thumb positioned along the sacrum, the examiner can direct the force posterior to anterior until all the slack is taken out of the tissue. Then an angular force downward and outward can be placed, simulating shear force from a posterior-to-anterior aspect of the sacrum on the ilium along the sacroiliac joint. The examiner should visualize the stress being placed at this region, as the sacrum is wider anteriorly than posteriorly. This mainly stresses the strong ligamentous structure of the sacroiliac joint region, both anteriorly and posteriorly.

ates an engagement and compressive load between the inferior articulating process and the superior articulating process on the right side and a rotary and shear stress at the intervertebral disc. This type of passive rotary force can be applied lateral to the spinous processes between the iliac crest and the 12th rib. The rotary stress to the lumbar spine can be enhanced by a counterforce applied through the pelvis (see Fig. 5–29B). The clinician grasps the anterior aspect of the

patient's ilium and generates a rotary force by pulling upward and moving the pelvis on the lumbar spine. This rotary/shear stress can be guided to specific regions of the lumbar spine. The key is to reproduce the symptom and at the same time evaluate the magnitude of the applied force necessary to provoke symptoms.

If the examiner is able to successfully reproduce the symptom in this position, he or she can reposition the

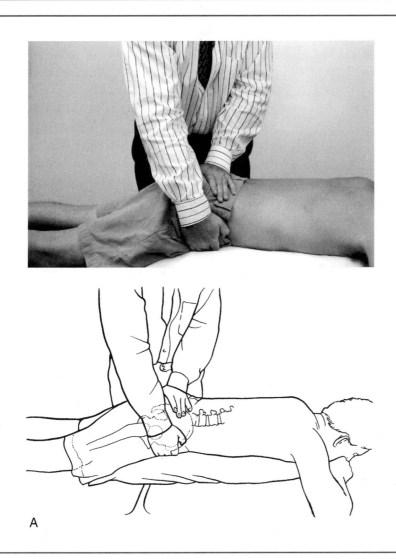

Figure 5–29. *A* and *B*, Imparting passive compressive and shear force to the pelvis and spine. Equal and opposite forces can be directed to converge from above and below to the desired area. The following two examples are *(A)* directed toward the sacrum and *(B)* to the midlumbar spine. The technique is to first push down with the top hand and then gradually pull up from below until the two forces meet, i.e., until all of the available motion is taken up. The clinician should be able to visualize the effect of these movements. A positive finding is reproduction of the familiar symptoms.

patient to further assess the mechanics. For example, if the patient had increased back pain on the right with passive femoral extension, pain with central force directed to the spinous process at the lower lumbar segments, and pain with a left rotary force at the same level, then the examiner can reposition the patient to confirm these painful mechanics. When the patient rises on his elbows, the lumbar spine is placed in extension. Now an applied posterior-to-anterior vertical force will most likely elicit the painful response more quickly. The examiner has thus confirmed the painful force, causing a nociceptive response and created a

mechanical *match,* and can use this important information in biomechanically counseling the patient during the treatment process.

Palpation

The last portion of the prone examination is palpation. As with other aspects of the assessment system, we suggest that the examiner palpate this and any other musculoskeletal area using a consistent sequence. The palpation examination attempts to identify painful areas in the soft tissues, tenderness, muscle

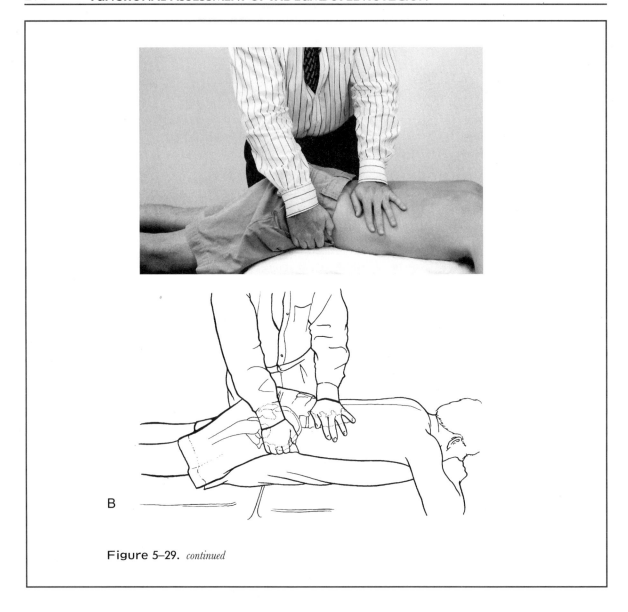

B

Figure 5–29. *continued*

spasm, bony defects, dissimilarities in size, or abnormal tissue textures in the musculature, subcutaneous tissues, and skin. The regions palpated should include the lumbar paraspinal area, central aspect of the lumbosacral spine, along the iliac crest, and the soft tissues inferior to the iliac crest over the posterior hip.

The unaffected region is palpated first. This can be done by first outlining the borders of the last rib, the iliac crest, and the spinous processes. Lateral to the erector spinae muscle is the posterior extent of the external oblique muscle. This area has a softer, spongier consistency than the more medial erector spinae tissues. As the palpating fingers move medial from the external oblique muscle, the lateral border of the erector spinae is reached. The soft tissue can be palpated from the iliac crest to the last rib. The examiner is looking for any painful areas or soft-tissue changes that may signify injury or protective muscle spasm.

The lateral aspect of the erector spinae muscle is the location of the lateral raphe (see Chapter 3). At

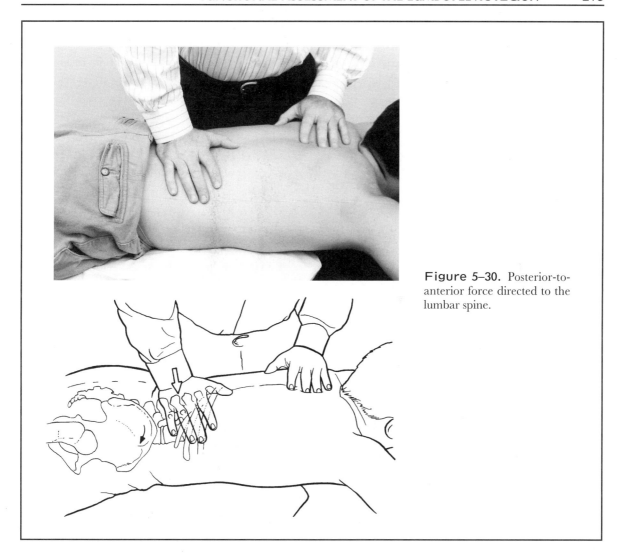

Figure 5–30. Posterior-to-anterior force directed to the lumbar spine.

the inferior aspect of this raphe, at the level of the iliac crest, is an important connective tissue juncture. It is a point where the thoracolumbar fascia, the lateral aspect of the superficial erector spinae tendon, the attachments of the deep erector spinae muscle, the quadratus lumborum muscle, and the lateral one third of the iliolumbar ligament converge to attach to the iliac crest. The cluneal nerves also pass over the iliac crest and near this juncture. This region is frequently tender to palpation, especially in the patient with forward bending and lifting injuries. Consider the forces that this site must withstand with a forward bending, twisting motion. Because the axis for flexion

of the lumbar spine is located in the intervertebral disc, the tissues at this attachment are located a significant distance from this axis.[43] The lumbar tissues must, therefore, tolerate considerable tensile stress due to both stretching and muscle contraction as a person bends forward. The examiner should palpate this region to determine if these tissues might be injured and, more importantly, correlate this with the history and the standing, supine, and prone evaluation.

For example, if a patient with a lifting injury presents with symptoms that can be reproduced with forward bending and side bending to the right in standing, and lumbar flexion created by the end-range hip flexion

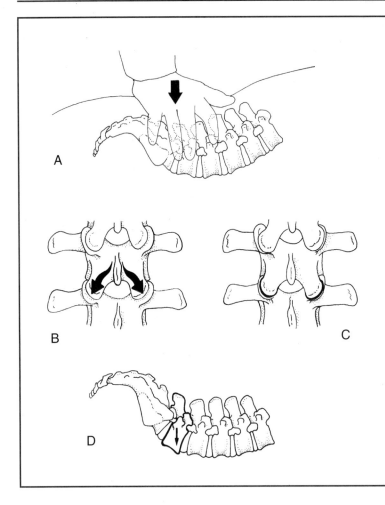

Figure 5–31. Four-step progression showing the force transmitted from the examiner's hand to the spinous process and through the lumbar spine into the abdominal cavity: *A,* Purchasing on the spinous process. *B,* Force transmitted through the spinous process down to the lamina into the inferior articulating process. *C,* Continuing progression down through the spinous process into the lamina, squeezing the apophyseal joints together and causing a small extension force of the inferior articulating process, sliding down the superior articulating process. *D,* The final aspect of the force generated through this system is facet compression and a small posterior-to-anterior shear at the facets and bone–disc–bone interface. If this increases the familiar pain, an analysis of these forces should be carried out to substantiate or match the standing examination.

test in supine is also painful, and if palpation to this region is quite tender, then it is reasonable to conclude that tensile stresses are responsible for the painful syndrome. These findings represent a mechanical *match*.

The region of the supraspinous and interspinous ligaments is then palpated to determine tenderness. This palpation includes the specific regions on each side of the spinous process and the interspinous space. If tenderness elicited by this palpation is the only positive finding, then the examiner has little on which to base a treatment program. However, tenderness from this specific palpation that matches the history and findings from the clinical examination yields useful information, and can be interpreted as indicating injured tissue.

Lastly, the posterior aspect of the pelvis, particularly in the region of the posterior superior iliac spine and

sacrum should be palpated, as well as the superior aspect of the iliac crest and posterior hip muscles. Tenderness on the inferior aspect of the PSIS and just inferior to it may be indicative of long dorsal sacroiliac ligament tenderness indicating involvement of the support tissues of the sacroiliac joint.[37] Tenderness just above and lateral to the posterior superior iliac spine may be representative of deep erector spinae muscle guarding occurring in response to segmental instability of the lumbar spine (see Chapter 3). Posterior superior iliac spine tenderness, increased pain with posterior–anterior stresses to the lumbar spinal segments, decreased pain with posterior–anterior stresses from the prone on elbows position, and pain with extension quadrant testing during the standing portion of the examination might be considered a mechanical match for segmental instability.

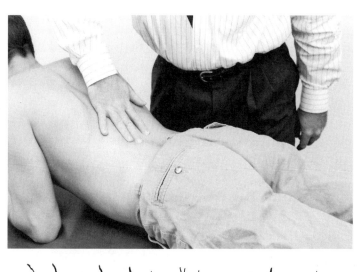

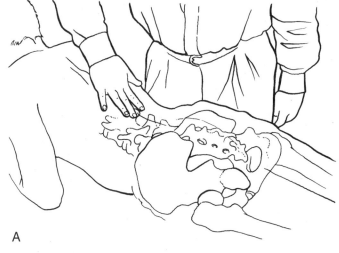

A

Figure 5–32. *A* and *B*, End-range stress to the lumbar spine in extension. The patient is asked to come up on the elbows, and then the index and middle fingers of the examiner's upper hand are placed on either side of the spinous process *(A)*. The examiner's other hand is placed over the index and middle fingers to direct the force to the inferior articulating processes *(B)*. This creates an end-range extension force of the spine when gravity is eliminated. The examiner can gradually move his hands down, indicating testing at different segments. The clinician can also side bend the spine from either above or below and continue the same process, which exacerbates that engagement and extension force on the side toward which the patient is bent.

Neurological Screening

If the neurological screen has not been completed, or if the supine position is not tolerated by the patient, several tests can be performed from the prone position. Myotomes can be assessed via hamstring and quadriceps muscle testing. In cases of suspected weakness of the gluteus maximus muscle, the patient can be asked to "squeeze" their gluteal muscle together, and the examiner may palpate flaccidity in one of the gluteus maximus muscles. The prone position is also an excellent position to assess the gastrocsoleus and tibialis posterior reflexes.

Seated Examination

Table 5–8 lists several tests that can be performed with the patient in the seated position. The Slump test has been described in Chapter 2, and is an excellent way to place specifically graded or maximal tensile stresses to the neural tissues and their dural invest-

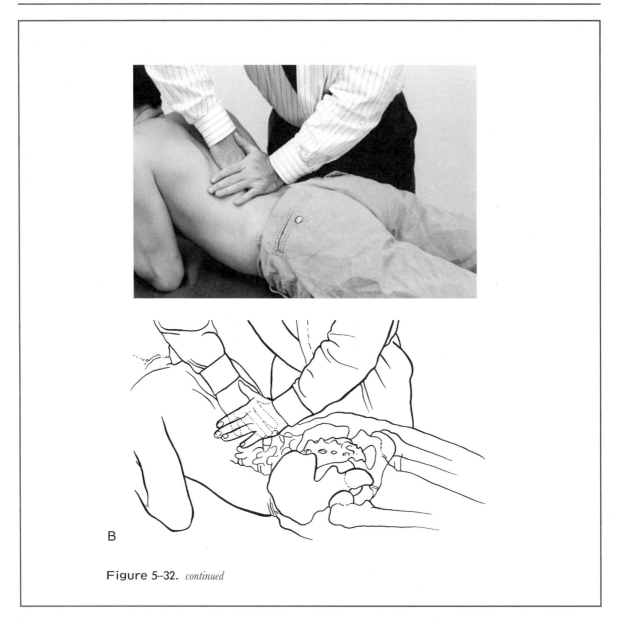

B

Figure 5–32. *continued*

Table 5–8. Seated Examination

1. Slump test
2. Neurological screening
3. Compare pelvis–lumbar relationships to standing
   Structural
   Motion

ments in the spine (Fig. 5–33). Varying degrees of tension to the nerve root complexes and their dural investments are applied by varying the amount of cervical flexion, thoracolumbar flexion, lumbosacral flexion, hip flexion, knee extension, and ankle dorsiflexion. The examiner is looking for reproduction of familiar back pain and peripheralization of pain into the lower extremity.

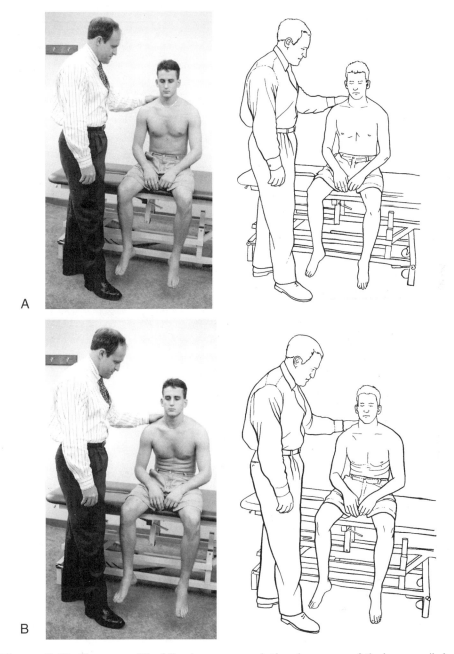

Figure 5–33. Slump test. The following sequence depicts the process of placing a tensile load to the neural complex. The test begins by asking the patient to sit straight *(A)*, followed by the command to slouch *(B)*. The patient is then asked to flex the thoracic and cervical spines *(C)*. After the examiner places an over-pressure to the cervical and thoracic spine, the knee is passively extended (D). This maneuver initially places a superior and anterior force to the dural sheath and nerve root complex followed by an inferior and anterior force that results from passive knee flexion. A positive finding is the reproduction of familiar leg pain.

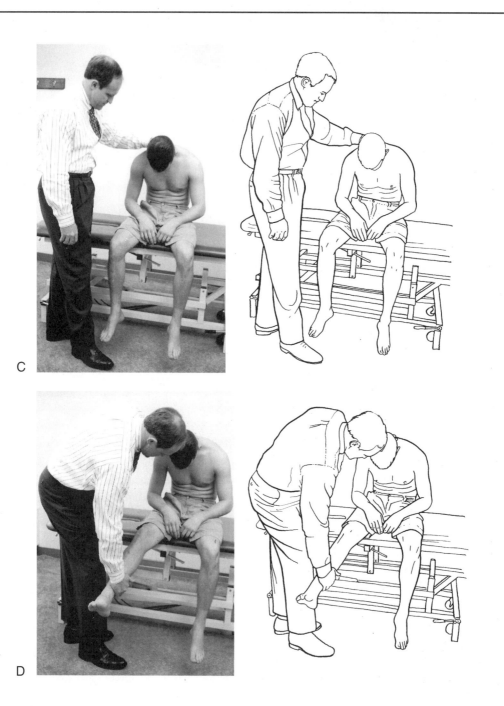

C

D

Figure 5–33. *continued*

Although appearing to be similar, there is not an absolute correlation between the Slump test and the straight leg raise (SLR) test. As the leg is raised in the SLR, sciatic nerve tension eventually causes a caudal and anterior migration of the spinal nerve in the neuroforamen. Irritation of the nerve root or any obstruction in the foramen from a herniated nucleus pulposus or osteophyte is most likely responsible for a positive finding. The mechanics of the Slump test are different. The initial part of the test, a seated "slump," places a tensile stress to the contents of the central canal. The patient is then asked to flex the cervical spine, creating a cranially and anteriorly directed force to the spinal cord and nerve roots. While maintaining this flexed posture, the knee is passively extended. This passive motion places a caudally and anteriorly directed force to the prepositioned nerve root complex. Therefore, the mechanics of the SLR and Slump test are subtly different and do not necessarily correlate. When they do correlate, the low back pain problem is often of greater intensity.

The seated position can also be used to assess specific myotomes: L2, L3 by hip flexor testing, L3, L4 by quadriceps testing, L4 by anterior tibialis testing, L5 by extensor hallucis longus testing, and S1–S2 by peroneal testing. The seated position can also be used to assess the quadriceps, gastrocsoleus, and posterior tibialis muscle reflexes, as well as perform the sensory examination to the lower extremity. Lastly, findings in the seated position can be used to compare with the findings noted in the standing examination, especially when a frontal plane asymmetry has been determined. Bilateral iliac crest heights can be assessed with the patient seated, to help determine if the frontal plane asymmetry is perhaps the result of one innominate bone being smaller than the other, instead of the asymmetry being the result of skeletal differences in the femur, tibia, or foot. When a patient is found to exhibit the same frontal plane asymmetry in standing as in sitting, it is often helpful to counsel them to level their pelvis by placing a small support such as a folded towel under the lower ischial tuberosity to symmetrically load the sacroiliac, lumbosacral, and lower lumbar spine more symmetrically and help redistribute the compressive and shear stresses to the lumbopelvic regions.

SUMMARY

The history should be used to gain pathomechanical information as well as to begin involving the patient in the rehabilitation process. It is important that the history account for psychosocial factors contributing to the pain syndrome, examine the effect the problem is having on the patient's quality of life, and determine the patient's goals for treatment.

The key to the lumbopelvic physical examination is directing controlled forces into lumbar, pelvic, and hip tissues. Each clinical test attempts to apply various degrees of compressive, tensile, and shear stresses from above down and below up. The shear and rotational movements at each specific intersegmental level of the lumbar spine and sacroiliac region are too small to be meaningfully quantified by the examiner. Therefore, the emphasis of the examination should be on the types of force applied and the reproduction of familiar symptoms, rather than on the quantity of movement.

These stresses can be applied in many positions. The goal is to reproduce familiar pain in the standing examination and then substantiate the nociceptive response by the application of similar forces in the supine, prone, or sitting positions to provide the examiner with information regarding mechanical matches. Rather than being concerned with the exact tissue of injury, the examiner is attempting to determine the stresses that are responsible for the injury–reinjury process. Recognition of these destructive stresses is the most important aspect on which to design a treatment program, and teach the patient self-management strategies.

REFERENCES

1. Andriacchi T, Sabiston P, DeHaven K, et al: Ligament: Injury and repair. In Woo SLY, Buckwalter JA (eds): Injury and Repair of the Musculoskeletal Soft Tissues. Park Ridge, IL: American Academy of Orthopedic Surgeons, 1988.
2. Bortz WM: The disuse syndrome. West J Med 141:691, 1984.
3. Burton AK, Tillotson KM, Main CJ, Hollis S: Psychosocial predictors of outcome in acute and subchronic low back trouble. Spine 20:722, 1995.
4. Calliet R: Low Back Pain Syndrome, 2nd ed. Philadelphia: FA Davis, 1981.
5. Delitto A, Erhard RE, Bowling RW: A treatment based classification approach to low back syndrome: Identifying and staging patients for conservative treatment. Phys Ther 75:470, 1995.
6. DeRosa C, Porterfield JA: A physical therapy classification for the treatment of low back pain. Phys Ther 72:261, 1992.

7. Donelson R, Silva G, Murphy K: Centralization phenomenon. Its usefulness in evaluating and treating referred pain. Spine 15:211, 1990.

8. Fairbank JCT, Cooper J, Davies JB, O'Brien JP: The Oswestrey low back pain disability questionnaire. Physiotherapy 66:271, 1980.

9. Friberg O: Clinical symptoms and biomechanics of lumbar spine and hip joint. Spine 6:643, 1983.

10. Giles LG, Taylor JR: Low back pain associated with leg length inequality. Spine 6:510, 1981.

11. Gofton JP: Studies in osteoarthritis of the hip and leg length disparity. Can Med Assoc J 104:791, 1971.

12. Greenough CG, Fraser RD: Assessment of outcome in patients with low back pain. Spine 17:36, 1992.

13. Harris RI, MacNab I: Structural changes in the intervertebral discs. J Bone Joint Surg 36B:304, 1954.

14. Kellett J: Acute soft tissue injuries—A review of the literature. Med Sci Sports Exerc 18:489, 1986.

15. Magora A, Schwartz A: Relation between the low back pain syndrome and X-ray findings. Scand J Rehabil Med 8:115, 1976.

16. Mann NH, Brown MD, Hertz DB, et al: Initial impression diagnosis using low back pain patient pain drawings. Spine 18:41, 1993.

17. McHorney CA, Ware JE, Raczek AE: The MOS-36 short form health survey (SF-36): II. Psychometric and clinical tests of validity in measuring physical and mental health constructs. Med Care 31:247, 1993.

18. McKenzie RA: A physical therapy perspective on acute spinal disorders. In: Mayer TG, Mooney V, Gatchel RJ (eds): Contemporary Conservative Care for Painful Spinal Disorders. Philadelphia: Lea & Febiger, 1991.

19. McPoil TG, Brocato RS: The foot and ankle: Biomechanical evaluation and treatment. In Gould JA (ed): Orthopaedic and Sports Physical Therapy, 2nd ed. St. Louis: CV Mosby, 1990.

20. Moufarrij NA, Hardy RW, Weinstein MA: Computed tomographic, myelographic, and operative findings in patients with suspected herniated lumbar discs. Neurosurgery 12:184, 1983.

21. Nachemson A: Work for all, for those with low back pain as well. Clin Orthop 179:77, 1983.

22. Offierski CM, MacNab I: Hip–spine syndrome. Spine 8:316, 1983.

23. Pope MH, Bevins T, Wilder DG, Frymoyer JW: The relationship between anthropometric, postural, muscular, and mobility characteristics of males ages 18–55. Spine 10:644, 1985.

24. Roland M, Morris R: A study of the natural history of back pain. Part I: Development of a reliable and sensitive measure of disability in low back pain. Spine 8:141, 1983.

25. Rothman RH: A study of computer-assisted tomography. Spine 9:548, 1984.

26. Sandstrom J, Hansson T, Jonson R, et al: The bone mineral content of the lumbar spine in patients with chronic low back pain. Spine 10:158, 1985.

27. Shiging X, Qanzhi Z, Dehao F: Significance of the straight leg raising test in the diagnosis and clinical evaluation of lower lumbar intervertebral disc protrusion. J Bone Joint Surg 69A:518, 1987.

28. Spitzer WO, LeBlanc FE, Dupuis M, et al: Scientific approach to the assessment and management of activity-related spinal disorders: A monograph for clinicians. Report of the Quebec Task Force on Spinal Disorders. Spine 12:S1, 1987.

29. Spratt KF, Lehmann TR, Weinstein JN, Sayre HA: A new approach to the low back physical examination. Spine 15:96, 1990.

30. Stone MH: Implications for connective tissue and bone alterations resulting from resistance exercise training. Med Sci Sports Exerc 20(Suppl):162, 1988.

31. Thurston AJ: Spinal and pelvic kinematics in osteoarthrosis of the hip joint. Spine 10:467, 1985.

32. Thurston AJ, Whittle MW, Stokes IAF: Spinal and pelvic movement during walking: A method of study. Engin Med 10:219, 1981.

33. Torgeson R, Dotler WE: Comparative roentgenographic study of the symptomatic and asymptomatic lumbar spine. J Bone Joint Surg 58A:850, 1976.

34. Troup JDG, Foreman TK, Bazter CE, Brown D: The perception of back pain and the role of psychophysical tests of lifting capacity. Spine 12:645, 1987.

35. Urban J, Maroudas A: The chemistry of the intervertebral disc in relation to its physiological functions and requirements. Clin Rheum Dis 6:51, 1980.

36. Valkenburg HA, Haanen HCM: The epidemiology of low back pain. In White AA III, Gordon SL (eds): American Academy of Orthopaedic Surgeons Symposium on Idiopathic Low Back Pain. St Louis: CV Mosby, 1982, p. 9.

37. Vleeming A, Pool-Goudzwaard AL, Hammudoghlu D, et al: The function of the long dorsal sacroiliac ligament. Spine 21:556, 1996.

38. Waddell G, Main CJ: Assessment of severity of low back disorders. Spine 9:204, 1984.

39. Waddell G, McCulloch JA, Kummel E, Venner RM: Nonorganic physical signs in low-back pain. Spine 5:117, 1980.

40. Weber H: Lumbar disc herniation. Spine 8:131, 1983.

41. Weisel SW, Feffer HL, Rothman RH: Industrial low back pain. A prospective evaluation of a standardized diagnostic and treatment protocol. Spine 9:199, 1984.

42. Werneke MW, Harris DE, Lichter RL: Clinical effectiveness of behavioral signs for screening chronic low back pain patients in a work oriented physical rehabilitation program. Spine 18:2412, 1993.

43. White AA, Panjabi MM: Clinical Biomechanics of the Spine. Philadelphia: JB Lippincott, 1978.

44. Winter RB, Pinto WC: Pelvic obliquity: Its causes and treatment. Spine 11:225, 1986.

CHAPTER 6

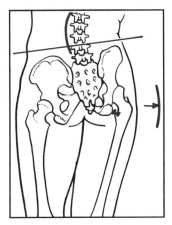

TREATMENT OF LUMBOPELVIC DISORDERS

In the previous chapters, information regarding the natural history of low back disorders and the dilemma of diagnosis for low back pain was combined with a comprehensive analysis of the functional anatomy of the lumbopelvic region. This interrelationship permits the development an evaluation system based on the concept of pathomechanics of activity-related disorders of the low back. In this chapter, the combined information will be linked with the principles of exercise science and the science of soft-tissue healing for the purpose of developing treatment strategies for patients with activity-related mechanical disorders of the low back. Furthermore, it will be suggested that although there appear to be many different therapeutic interventions, more similarities than dissimilarities exist with respect to their effect.

This chapter intimates an active approach toward rehabilitation that appropriately directs the responsibility of recovery to the patient. Rehabilitation is a process in which the focus is on assisting patients in recognizing the parameters of their pain patterns, developing exercise programs to enhance neuromuscular and musculoskeletal capabilities, and gaining information to enhance their self management skills. The exercises that will be discussed and illustrated are based on the relationships that the muscular system has with the fascial systems and articulations of the

lumbopelvic region (see Chapters 3 and 4), and the results of the functional assessment (Chapter 5). Incorporating the findings of the functional assessment into an individualized exercise prescription permits the patient to begin nondestructive exercise early in the rehabilitation process while avoiding reinjury. The sooner the onset of noninjurious activity and the sooner the patient is called upon to make intensity/frequency/duration decisions regarding activity, the sooner and more complete the recovery.

PHILOSOPHY OF TREATMENT

There are four underlying philosophical concepts in formulating the framework for a rehabilitation program:

1. With an understanding of the functional anatomy of the spine, patients with mechanical low back disorders can be treated using the same treatment philosophy as those used in rehabilitation of mechanical disorders of the extremities. At the forefront of this process is early activity at the appropriate point in the healing process; an emphasis on the restoration of function; and the development of neuromuscular

223

strength, power, and endurance to protect the injured or degenerative specialized connective tissues.

2. It is recognized that although the human body has enormous potential for healing, most injured tissue will never be restored to the exact structure, strength, and function as in the preinjured state. Therefore, the role of the clinician is to guide the patient through a healing process that promotes early restoration of function, and effectively prepares the patient for self-management.

3. Injured musculoskeletal and neuromuscular tissues heal with reasonable predictability. If an acute injury is immediately assessed and treated daily for a short period of time (3–4 visits), an accurate prediction of the natural course or time frame of healing and the return to activity can be made. It is also recognized that the late onset of rehabilitation lessens the recovery potential.

4. As previously mentioned, the emphasis should not be directed toward identifying the exact tissue but rather toward identifying the excessive or poorly tolerated physiological stresses that converge into and pass through the injured region, causing the familiar symptoms. Treatment is designed to better prepare the patient to avoid, eliminate, or effectively deal with these physiological stresses.

Treatment of the lumbopelvic region is based on an understanding of the science of soft-tissue healing, the adaptive changes of musculoskeletal and cardiovascular tissues as a result of conditioning and deconditioning, the influence of the central and peripheral nervous systems on motor behavior, and the functional anatomy of the region. These influences form the basis for successful treatment. The rehabilitation process presented in this chapter de-emphasizes a passive approach toward the management of low back disorders, and focuses instead on active restoration of function and improvement of neuromuscular performance.

The progression of a rehabilitation program is influenced in part by the physiology of tissue healing. It should be recognized that vascularized tissues in any area of the body, whether they are contractile or non-contractile, have many similarities in their physiology and response to injury. The biomechanics and physiology of tissues in the low back are similar to those of tissues in other areas of the body and both respond similarly to stimulus. Therefore, the rules of assessment and treatment should be similar in all areas of the

neuromuscular and musculoskeletal systems. To view the low back differently invites treatment that is abstract and unscientific, with the emphasis on "healing the patient" rather than the patient managing his own healing process. More importantly, this type of mismanagement often results in increased tissue dysfunction, frequent reinjury, and chronic symptoms. The patient must understand and assist in the development of the goals of the treatment process.

The emphasis is on *function* rather than pain. Although pain cannot be ignored and certainly needs to be continually and carefully monitored, it should not be the primary focus of treatment. Said more succinctly, a 100 percent pain-free outcome is an unrealistic expectation in most instances.

It should be pointed out, however, that there is one important structure that is unique to the spine and to which no comparison to the extremities can be made. That structure is the intervertebral disc. Mooney [17] suggests that because the healing potential of the intervertebral disc is different from that of other musculoskeletal tissues, perhaps disorders related to the disc should be strongly suspected in that group of patients with chronic and unrelenting pain, e.g., those people who fail to respond in the time period normally allotted for adequate healing of other musculoskeletal tissues.

The essential health of the disc is maintained by a loading and unloading phenomena, and unchanging postures that result in a constant pressure, such as sitting, lying, or standing, lead to an interruption of pressure-dependent transfer of fluid. Thus, even though the intervertebral disc may follow a different set of rules for healing when compared with other connective tissues of the body, passive therapeutic modalities and prolonged rest are also not indicated for the intervertebral disc problem; instead, the encouragement of function remains the primary goal.[17, 20]

INTENT OF TREATMENT

Before discussing the objectives of treatment for lumbopelvic disorders, the intent of treatment can be summarized as follows:

1. To optimize the healing environment.
2. To restore anatomical relations between injured and noninjured tissue.

3. To maintain the normal function of noninjured tissues.

4. To prevent excessive strain from being put on injured tissue.

This summary of the intent of treatment for the healing of collagen structures was first presented by van der Muelen.[27] It can easily be applied to the treatment of lumbopelvic disorders.

Optimization of Healing Environment (First Intent)

The first component of the intent of treatment relates to the clinician's ability to optimize the healing environment to provide for "wound healing." Although "wound" may conjure up thoughts of skin lacerations, torn tissue, and bleeding, this concept should be expanded to include any disruption of the structural makeup of cells or fibers as a result of injury. Thus, there is a potential for the muscles, tendons, ligaments, fascia, intervertebral disc, zygapophyseal joints, or any tissue in the lumbopelvic region to be injured. Low back disorders most likely involve several tissues simultaneously.

The real question that the clinician must answer in this first intent of treatment is how to maximize the potential for the body to, quite literally, heal itself. Therein lies one of the major dilemmas in dealing with low back disorders. It is difficult to create an effective healing environment at the hub of weight bearing that is impacted by a multitude of loads with all antigravity activities.

The low back cannot be immobilized like the extremities; therefore, close attention to the results of the functional assessment is required to determine the forces and loads that reproduce the patient's familiar symptoms. As detailed in Chapter 5, there is an important distinction between performing a low back evaluation to identify a particular tissue at fault and performing an evaluation to assess the stresses that reproduce familiar pain. Biomechanical counseling (discussed below) is teaching patients how these nociceptive biomechanics relate to their activities of daily living. To allow for wound healing and to optimize the healing environment, this aspect is crucial in patients with acute injury as well as in those with an exacerbation of a previous injury.

Restoration of Anatomical Relations Between Injured and Noninjured Tissue (Second Intent)

Injury to tissues results in a cascade of events that proceed sequentially, beginning with the inflammatory process and culminating in a repair that ideally allows for nondestructive movement patterns of the injured region. As soon as possible after injury, controlled nondestructive motions must be properly introduced into the area so that the injured tissues will heal according to appropriate stress lines. Tissues must also be free to glide over, compress onto, and apply tension to surrounding tissues. In short, tissue function is dependent on the surrounding tissues. It is necessary that functional healing involve the activity of the surrounding tissues.

Maintenance of Normal Function of Noninjured Tissue (Third Intent)

Care must be taken to maintain the health and strength of the tissues, with specific attention given to preventing the effects of disuse and altered motor behavior. A phased treatment program allows for early mobilization and recognizes the important balance necessary between activity and wound-healing. The strong argument for early mobilization is in agreement with the data that has accumulated regarding the appropriate length of time for bed rest after the low back injury. There is good evidence to suggest that longer than 48 hours is counterproductive and contributes to catabolic, deconditioning changes.[5] Prolonging the immobilization and bed rest periods for most mechanical soft-tissue injuries invites weakening of the connective tissue structures, loss of muscle and bone strength, neurotrophic functions, and decreased cardiovascular efficiency.[28]

Prevention of Excessive Stress on Injured Tissue (Fourth Intent)

This last major intent of healing requires an understanding of the basic science of tissue healing and the biomechanics of the lumbopelvic region. It necessitates initiating an exercise or activity program that does not continually disrupt the healing process. Therapeutic exercise is important because the lumbopelvic tissues must ultimately accept the various stresses to which they are subjected, yet not at the expense of reinjury, e.g., the introduction of forces and loads in an intensity, frequency, and duration that stimulated growth without exacerbation of the condition. The patient must learn to recognize the relationships that exist between their activities of daily living and the mechanics of their injury and act accordingly.

OBJECTIVES OF TREATMENT

Many approaches and treatment techniques are used in the treatment of low back pain. By considering the objectives of treatment for low back pain, therapeutic interventions can be grouped logically and scientifically and their similarities considered.[6] There are four objectives of treatment, and most interventions relate to one or more of these objectives:[7]

1. Provide biomechanical counseling.
2. Modulate pain or promote analgesia.
3. Generate controlled forces to promote early, nondestructive reactivation of the patient.
4. Enhance neuromuscular performance.

Each will now be discussed with their therapeutic applications.

Biomechanical Counseling

Education of the patient is a critical component of any treatment program, and the educational process often begins during the assessment process. The patient must realize the importance of activity limits. With significant tissue injury of the spine or the onset of age-related degenerative changes in the tissues, the patient and clinician must learn to accept the loss of back function that, most often, cannot be restored. The goal becomes teaching the person how to maximize their activity within new limits. Obviously, the structural changes of degeneration viewed by imaging studies do not improve. The structural changes can stay the same or worsen, but not improve. Once an osteophyte has formed or the disc space has narrowed, the damage is permanent. Tissue that is significantly injured or degenerated cannot attenuate stresses with the same efficiency as normal, uninjured tissue. This is often difficult for the patients to accept, because they have expectations for a permanent "cure." Not only is cure without change an unreasonable expectation, but it leaves the onus of responsibility for care on the clinician rather than the patient. Education in the form of biomechanical counseling becomes one of the most important aspects of a rehabilitation program. In its simplest form, it is teaching the patient to recognize their pain pattern and to minimize the potential for reinjury. Table 6–1 lists several biomechanical counseling considerations for lifting.

Why is biomechanical counseling such an important component of rehabilitation? One of the primary reasons is a recognition of the amount of time a clinician actually interacts with a patient. If, for example, a patient is treated in a clinic three times/week for 45 minutes each session, this represents less than 2 percent of the time the patient is awake and resuming activities of daily living. Therefore, to assume that three 45-minute treatments per week alone will significantly impact the long-range outcome is unrealistic. Certainly there are isolated instances in which mechanical low back disorders with a single causative incident completely respond with one or two treatments and never recur. However, this is not the rule for the typical activity-related low back disorder.

The evaluation and assessment process described in Chapter 5 is the means to determine the information to be used for biomechanically counseling the patient. Each patient has a unique set of limitations that can be determined only through a functional assessment. What might be a vulnerable position or movement for one patient's spine may not be a vulnerable position or movement for another patient's spine.

Patient education also includes teaching patients the importance of recognizing their pain patterns. They must also recognize that tissues of the neuromuscular

---

Table 6–1. Biomechanical Counseling: Guidelines for Lifting

Maintain symmetric, relatively upright posture
Lift object as close to body as possible
Keep center of gravity of object low if possible
Lift symmetrically
Avoid jerking motion
Use moderate lifting speed

and musculoskeletal systems often require up to 12–16 weeks for healing, and that healing is assessed by the small subtle changes to the intensity, frequency, and duration of the pain pattern. For some, this understanding may take weeks to appreciate. The successful clinician is able to teach patients quickly to become aware, understand, and be able to predict these changes—i.e., to take control of their condition.

Modulating Pain or Promoting Analgesia

Interventions helping to modulate pain include the various thermodalities, electromodalities, and medications. However, there is an important difference between symptomatic relief and alteration of the natural progression of the problem. It is ethical to treat pain appropriately, especially with the intent of progressing the patient to the active phase of the rehabilitation process. However, directing treatment with pain as the primary intent is appropriate only for a small, select group of patients who do not show signs of system (segment) degeneration.

The clinician has many therapeutic options available to effectively treat pain. Physical agents, such as thermomodalities and electromodalities, are often used in combination with medications. They promote analgesia, inhibit an exuberant inflammatory process, and decrease the muscle spasm that typically accompanies injury. It is indeed the clinician's responsibility to use these forms of treatment during the acute phase. However, their limits must be recognized. There is no definitive evidence that they greatly accelerate the cellular aspects of the healing process. Rather, they most likely assist in altering the fluid dynamics of the injured area, which replenishes the nutrients required to enhance healing. The result is a temporary desensitization of the injured area, permitting early movement. Early nondestructive active movement is important in functional healing. This concept is further addressed in the next treatment objective.

Generation of Controlled Forces to Promote Reactivation of the Patient

An early return to activity has the most significant impact in the long-term management of low back problems.[2] Therefore, this objective refers to the ability of the clinician to introduce controlled, nondestructive stresses, either passively or actively, through the lumbopelvic region to facilitate and encourage movement by the patient in a fashion that does not exacerbate the condition. The goal of any of these techniques should be to generate a state of improved health and to expedite the patient's return to physical activity. Active, manual, and mechanical treatment techniques that can be included under this objective are noted in Table 6–2.

Previous explanations of the various techniques often focus on their purported effects and their dissimilarities with other techniques. Closer analysis of each treatment technique reveals more similarities than dissimilarities. The authors recognize that each technique has its own mechanics and explanations that represent their dissimilarities. However, the similarities are in their outcome. It is logical to conclude that each technique, either used alone or in conjunction with others, has the same physical effects, as described below:

1. *Influence fluid dynamics.* Fluid stasis,[10] inflammation, and an altered chemical environment of the tissues [31] propagate the nociceptive response and impede the healing process.[27] This is true for all injured tissues in

Table 6–2. Techniques Used to Generate Controlled Forces to Promote Patient Reactivation
PASSIVE MANUAL
Joint mobilization and manipulation
Soft tissue mobilization, massage
Traction
Stretching
Myofascial techniques
Passive range of motion
MECHANICAL
Traction
External supports
Spinal pillows, rolls, wedges
Heel lifts
ACTIVE
Active range of motion
Muscle energy
Strain–counterstrain
Extension–flexion protocols
Contract/relax PNF
From DeRosa C, Porterfield JA: A physical therapy model for the treatment of low back pain. Phys Ther 72:261, 1992.

the low back including nerve root irritation. The manual, mechanical, or active techniques facilitate tissue fluid movement and thus potentially influence the biochemical milieu of the injured region.

Treatment to alter fluid dynamics is essential in the initial stages of the painful condition to maximize functional healing potential. As the treatment is given, blood flow, both arterial and venous, and lymph drainage are stimulated, and temporary relief of pain and stiffness (swollen state) is expected.[10] The rate at which the swollen (static) state reappears is indicative of the extent of the injury. The greater the injury, the quicker the return of symptoms (fluid stasis and biochemical changes). The quicker the return of symptoms, the slower the progression of activity. This finding should direct the emphasis of treatment toward protection, such as crutches, supports, and scheduled periods of rest. The analysis of this rate and extent of return is, in the authors' opinion, the most important piece of information that determines the treatment progression. It is also important to explain this expected outcome to the patient. Figure 6–1 presents a visual that is frequently used for this explanation. This graphic explains the expected short-term outcome of the treatment (i.e., returned symptoms of lesser extent and a longer time between the awareness of symptoms).

This explanation to the patient not only helps him or her understand the physiologic basis for the initial aspect of treatment, but also begins to define the patient's role in improving his or her condition. It is important that a reachable short-term goal is set and met. If the patient and clinician cannot reach this short-term goal, the chances for successful outcomes diminish. Progression toward activities that restore function without exacerbation of symptoms and assisting the patient in quickly succeeding in self-management are the long-range goals.

2. *Generate afferent input into the central nervous system.* Each manual, mechanical, or active technique initiates a barrage of afferent input into the central nervous system. The potential results of such an afferent volley are *modulation of pain* and *altering the state of muscle contraction.* Whenever a change is immediately seen in the active or passive movement pattern or postural positioning of the lumbar spine or pelvis following any technique, it is most likely due to a new and different resting tension of the muscles rather than to bones being "put back in place," or changing the structure of the connective tissue. Altered contractile states of the musculature ultimately effect forces to all tissues, which can result in changes in movement patterns and findings during palpation. This objective of applying controlled forces to promote reactivation of the patient has several implications.

The propagation of pain for most mechanical low back disorders is due to a combination of three important stimuli: *chemoreceptor activation of the nociceptive system, mechanoreceptor activation of the nociceptive system,* and the influence of *emotional/behavioral factors* (Figure 6–2).

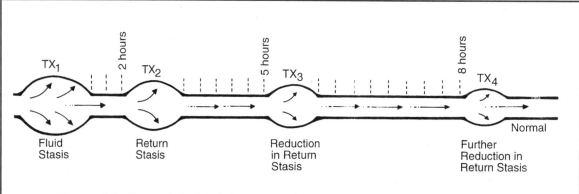

Figure 6–1. Expected physiological outcomes with respect to the state of swelling and fluid congestion of the injured area after four treatments (tx). (From Porterfield JA, DeRosa C: Mechanical Neck Pain: Perspectives in Functional Anatomy. Philadelphia: WB Saunders, 1995.)

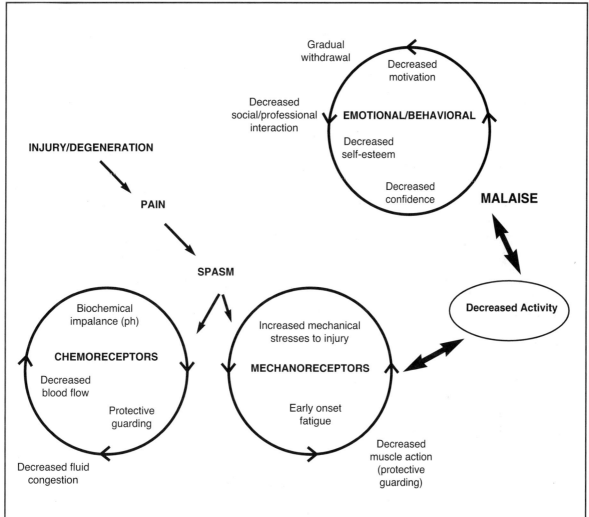

Figure 6–2. The injury/degenerative cycle: Factors affecting the perception of pain. These stimuli can be viewed as three separate "spinning cycles." They include the chemoreceptor, mechanoreceptor, and emotional/behavioral cycles. Pain can be due to each individual cycle or combinations of the three. *Chemoreceptor cycle :* Illustrated here are the nociceptive effects of fluid stasis and altered biochemistry of the injured region, often noted as morning stiffness by the patient. *Mechanoreceptor cycle:* The effects of early onset fatigue and decreasing activity, often noted as pain at the end of the day by the patient, are depicted. *Emotional/behavioral cycle:* Illustration of the influence of psychosocial stressors on the patient. Looked at in terms of "spinning cycles," the clinician is attempting to determine which of the cycles is the most dominant, i.e., which is the one most responsible for the pain perception, which directs the treatment process.

Individually and collectively, these three stimuli influence the perception of pain by enhancing the sensitivity of the neural mechanisms (Figure 6–3).

As previously mentioned in Chapter 5, determining the pain/stiffness status after prolonged periods of rest is one of the keys pieces of information obtained during the history. This information depicts the state of inflammation. For example, fluid stasis and an altered biochemical environment surrounding injured tissue are present in the patient who describes increased pain and stiffness on waking, which subsides or lessens with a gradual increase in movement. Nociception in this case may be the result of the "chemical cycle" noted in Figure 6–2. This is most likely due to the development of fluid stasis during sleep since the forces of muscle contraction are minimal, blood pressure and lymph drainage diminishes, and the patient is not in antigravity and weight-bearing positions. The clinician should consider using the various passive, active assistive, and active motion techniques (Table 6–2) noted under this objective to minimize the "fluid trap." Movement and the forces of muscle contraction poten-

tially "flush" the fluid environment of the injured region.

This is in contrast to the patient with less pain in the morning on waking but with increasing symptoms as the day progresses, suggestive of cumulative mechanical stresses in the upright antigravity posture resulting in activation of the nociceptive system (see Chapter 5). These patients are in essence "losing the battle against gravity." They are more likely candidates for the next objective of treatment (enhancing neuromuscular performance), and less likely to have treatment focused on the various manual and mechanical treatment techniques.

The intensity and frequency of this manual aspect of the treatment process depends on the technique chosen as well as the knowledge and skill of the clinician in recognizing the potential for exacerbation of the injury. Being too aggressive with forces into the "barrier" (painful position) can prolong the inflammatory process of the injured tissues. The clinician is faced with the decision of how aggressive one should be with any of the techniques. Treatment must be pro-

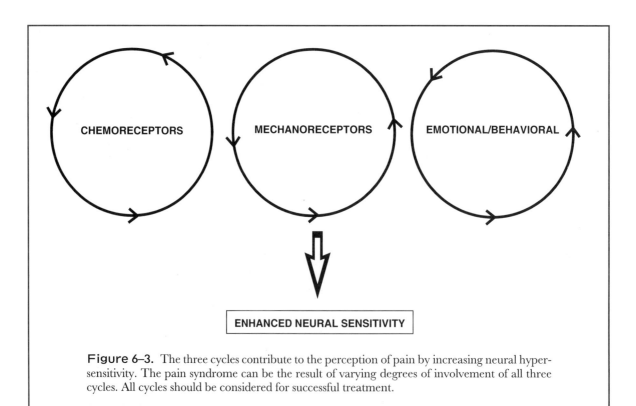

Figure 6–3. The three cycles contribute to the perception of pain by increasing neural hypersensitivity. The pain syndrome can be the result of varying degrees of involvement of all three cycles. All cycles should be considered for successful treatment.

vided carefully to strike a balance between therapeutic recovery and avoidance of reinjury.

The clinician also faces the dilemma of determining when, or if, the techniques should move the injured tissues into the painful movement pattern, i.e., the painful range. During manual treatment especially, the clinician should be sensitive to the "barrier" to movement, i.e., that perception imparted to the clinician's hands when reaching the reinjury limit or what the patients will tolerate in terms of movement or physiologic stress. This begins with the recognition of protective guarding that provides the perception of increased tissue resistance which will eventually reproduce the familiar pain. This is referred to as a firmer end-point or end-feel.

The aggressiveness of manual treatment is often based on such palpatory findings. The treatment process should first be carried out through the invulnerable free-moving ranges of the movement as determined during the weight-bearing or standing portion of the functional assessment. The sooner movement into the painful range occurs without exacerbation of the condition, the greater the potential for enhancing fluid movement, decreasing pain, and restoring painless range. However, with patients in the exacerbation of previous injury grouping (see Chapter 5), return to 100 percent range of motion or being able to tolerate any and all lumbopelvic weight-bearing positions without symptoms is an unrealistic goal. The clinician must quickly realize this fact and begin to assist the patient in understanding the need for and importance of making appropriate changes (position, load, and frequency) to minimize the reinjury process. Making the patient aware of the injury/reinjury cycle is imperative for functional healing, decreased disability, and successful rehabilitation.

There are numerous ways in which the clinician can introduce passive and active assistive nondestructive forces into the tissues. Before incorporating manual techniques, the area should be thoroughly palpated. The goal of the palpation is to identify the boundaries of the injury. Palpation of the injured area is similar to the effect of a pebble tossed into a pond. The epicenter of the injury site is the pebble's entry point, and its gradually diminishing effects on sensitivity are the ripples of the water as they move away from the center. This information, coupled with the recognition of the forces and positions of the injury represent the basis for any technique used. The purpose of the technique is to enhance fluid movement by creating pressure into and through the injured area from many different directions and to passively and/or actively create movement into the injured area to ensure proper alignment of the forming scar (functional healing). This helps decrease pain, but it should be recognized that we "pay a little" in the form of decreased function, for each injury. Figure 6–4 illustrates deep friction/soft tissue mobilization to the superficial tissues of the lumbosacral triangle. This is especially valuable for the acute tensile injuries to the low back tissues represented by pain in the forward bending quadrants and reproduction of pain with tensile stresses to the low back. Two other soft tissue techniques, shown in Figs. 6–5 and 6–6 apply a force to the muscle tissues in a plane perpendicular to the paraspinal muscles and are excellent paraspinal mobilization techniques. Such techniques can eventually result in lumbar joint movement. This type of controlled force to the spine can be modified by simply placing the hips in varying degrees of flexion or extension, increasing lumbar flexion or extension respectively.

Muscle energy techniques (Fig. 6–7) are commonly used to direct controlled forces to specific regions of the lumbopelvic area. By strongly fixing the distal attachments of muscles like the hip flexors, adductors, or extensors, the force of an isometric muscle in contraction generates movement and forces to the lumbar and pelvis. Such techniques, if chosen wisely, appropriately direct loads and forces into and through the injured area. The isometric contraction during the technique helps move fluid and specifically stresses the injured tissues in a controlled manner.

Techniques such as muscle energy, contract–relax, and hold–relax also increase afferent input into the nervous system owing to stimulation of the muscle proprioceptors. Such mechanoreceptor input potentially modulates pain and results in a different neural "setpoint" of the muscle. The muscle facilitates relaxation of the antagonistic muscles, allowing for increased movement over the joints. One could argue that any active, active assistive, active resistive, or isometric contraction has the same result. It is the skill of the clinician to visualize the movement in three dimensions and then relate it to the assessment findings. The proper decisions can then be made regarding the intensity, frequency, and duration of the technique. The process is to create a stimulus via manual, mechanical, and/or active technique, predict the outcome, and then reassess. One of the common mistakes is to subject the patient to too many stimuli during a single treatment session.

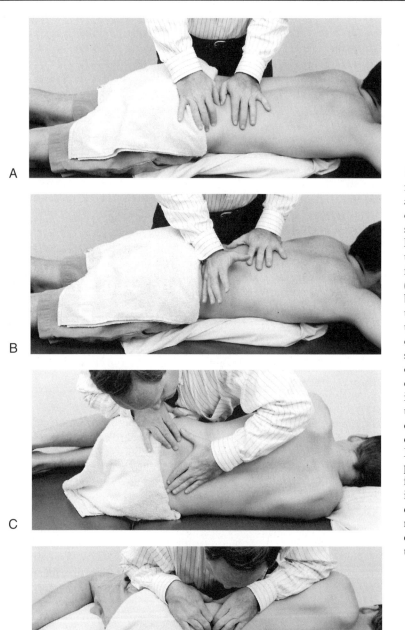

Figure 6–4. *A–D*, Four techniques, two prone lying *(A, B)* and two side lying *(C, D)*, demonstrating deep friction/soft tissue mobilization of the lumbosacral tissues. These techniques are especially useful for acute tensile injuries (pain reproduced with forward-bending quadrants). *A*, Use of the thumbs for deep friction at the inferior lateral attachment of the lateral raphe, a common site for tensile injuries. *B*, Use of the hypothenar eminence to direct forces to the tissues of the iliac crest region. *C*, A superior-to-inferior stroking technique commonly used prior to specific techniques in *A, B,* and *D.* Note the stabilization of the pelvis with the examiner's right forearm and hand. This is important to appropriately control the forces of the treatment. *D*, Specific techniques directed to the left iliac crest tissues.

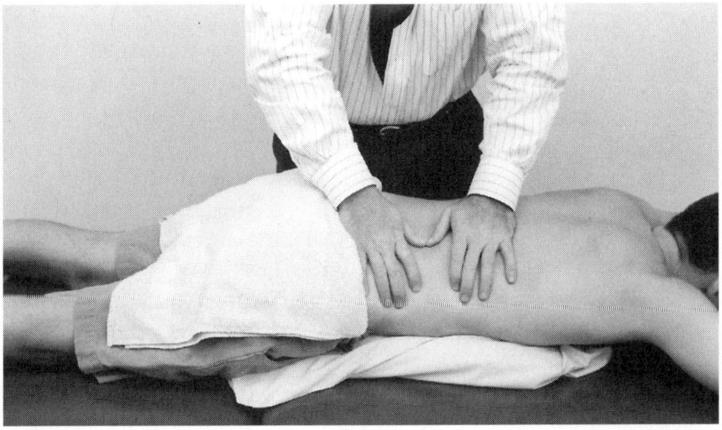

Figure 6–5. With the patient prone, the clinician can apply a force to the muscle tissues perpendicular to the lumbar paraspinals. The thumbs are placed in the space between the lumbar spinous processes and the lumbar paraspinals, and the muscle tissue is mobilized in a transverse direction. The clinician's hands and the patient's skin move as one unit in order to avoid frictional force to the patient's skin.

This makes assessing the effectiveness of each stimulus or technique very difficult.

Another example of techniques in this objective of treatment is stretching. Stretching techniques for the lumbar spine are often integrated into this objective of treatment. For example, the goal of the clinician might be to place stretching or lengthening forces on left lumbosacral musculature that travel superiorly, anteriorly, and medially (i.e., the quadratus lumborum and deep erector spinae). The patient can be positioned in a right side-lying position, over a rolled pillow or bolster (Fig. 6–8). The clinician faces the patient and manually controls, with or without resistance, the contract–relax–stretch maneuver. As the stretch force is released, the patient can be asked to contract against a small resistance. The stretch is then repeated.

This technique of stretching the lumbar musculature can be very effective, but the clinician must, once again, recognize that the position of the lumbopelvic region and the forces related to the stretch potentially make other tissues vulnerable to injury. A compressive force, due to right side bending and a rotary stress, occurs on the right side of the lumbar spine. This position also exerts a tensile force and rotary stress to the tissues on the left side of the lumbar spine. This may or may not be a nondestructive position, depending on the results of the assessment. If, during the gross movement portion of the standing examination, the patient experiences familiar pain on the left side reproduced by backward bending and side bending to the right, then this treatment position would potentially aggravate the condition. The clinician may intend to have the patient move into this potentially painful and vulnerable range, but he needs to be cautious as to the intensity of the contraction and/or the stretch. Only with this understanding, and reassessment, can the clinician determine the effectiveness of the technique. Meaningful reassessment is critical in making decisions regarding future treatment. This is why daily treatment for the acute injury is important. It is very difficult to recognize the subtle changes in the pain pattern at the initial aspect of treatment if 2 or 3 days lapse between treatments. Once the pain pattern is understood and has become predictable to the patient and clinician, then the frequency of treatment should be lengthened. Decisions regarding the number of treatments per week become dependent on the amount of time it takes to recover from training.

The important question is "Should all tight structures be stretched?" The following is offered as a working clinical guideline: *If the forces of the tightness generate unwanted forces and loads into the injured area—stretch the tight structures. If the forces of the tightness generate unwanted loads away from the injured area—avoid stretching of those specific tight structures.* Oftentimes, tightness is a protective guarding mechanism designed to control loads to injured tissues. In these cases, the treatment should be designed to minimize neuromuscular fatigue by positioning for rest, exercise, and enhancing fluid dynamics of injured tissues.

If the clinician finds tightness of the hip when it is placed in the FABER position (see Chapter 5), or a

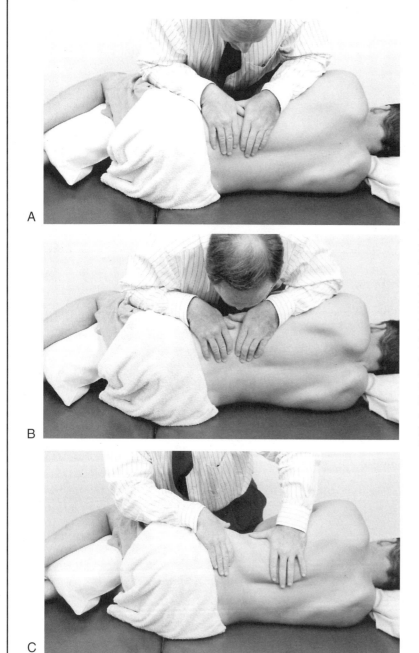

Figure 6–6. *A–E*, Side-lying techniques for frontal plane mobilization of lumbosacral tissues. *A* and *B* demonstrate a technique that utilizes the pelvis and the rib cage to augment mobilization at the hands. Note how the rib and pelvis are separated while the hands push in and lift up. *C* depicts a modification of the same concept. In *D* and *E* note the position of the patient's legs. This position coupled with contract–relax of the left paraspinals permit a greater range of motion.

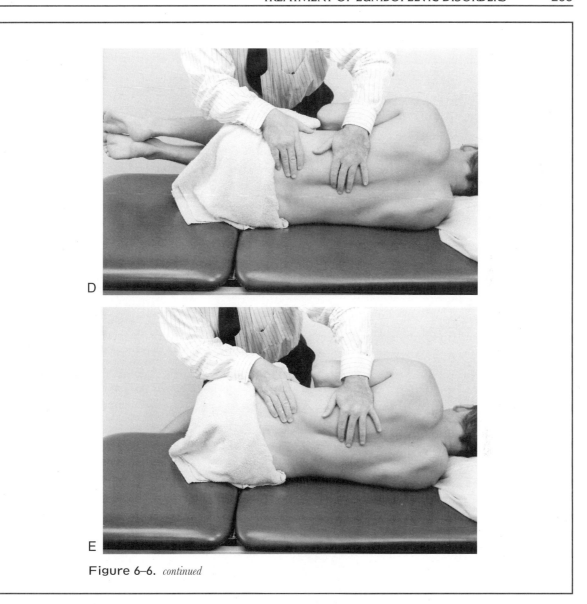

Figure 6–6. *continued*

tightness in hyperextension and internal rotation on the side of lumbopelvic pain, and pain is reproduced with extension quadrant stresses, then stretching techniques for the tight hip are indicated. Tight anterior hip structures have the potential to cause anterior torsional forces of the ilium on the sacrum, and increased extension forces to the lumbar spine when the person is in a standing posture. If the clinician stretches the anterior hip structures and at the same time creates an

extension force to the lumbar spine, reinjury may occur. The lumbar condition continues in this example, only now it is iatrogenic in nature. One of the most common clinical challenges is to stretch the hip joint capsule and anterior thigh musculature without compromising the lumbar spine (Fig. 6–9).

Another means of applying controlled forces into the lumbopelvic region to allow for early activation of the patient is by utilization of a spinal orthosis. The

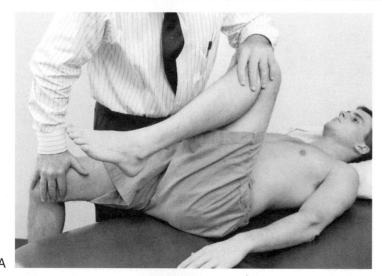

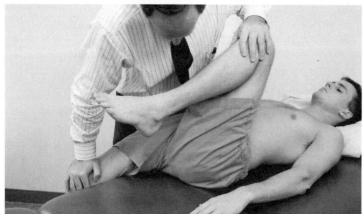

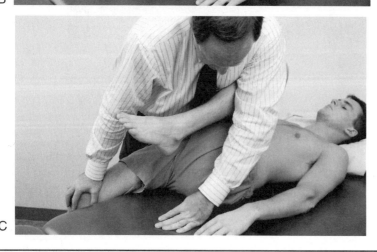

Figure 6–7. *A–C,* Muscle energy techniques, contract–relax techniques, and hold–relax techniques are commonly used to place controlled forces into the lumbopelvic region. *A,* The contraction of the hip flexors, controlled at the distal end of femur, places an anterior torsional stress on the ilium, and an extension stress to the lumbar spine. Following contraction, the hip is passively moved into extension, and then the contraction is repeated. *B,* With the distal femur fixed, the patient is asked to attempt another hip flexion (isometric contraction). This results in an anterior torsional stress to the ilium, compression to the sacroiliac joint and pubic symphysis, and an extension moment to the lumbosacral junction. *C,* A combined technique in which the hip flexors on the right side and the hip extensor on the left are contracted isometrically to place similar forces of greater magnitude to the pelvis and lumbar spine.

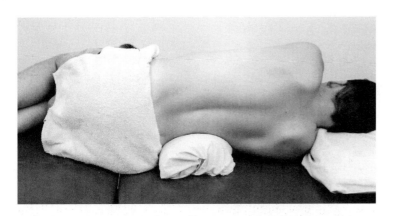

Figure 6–8. The patient is positioned right side lying over a pillow or bolster to create a stretching or lengthening force, or a decreased left side bending force at the left lumbosacral region. If the left arm is placed over the head in complete abduction, the stretching force will be increased. Soft tissue mobilization can also be performed in these various stretch positions, as well as contract–relax techniques.

patient must recognize that the orthosis cannot offer complete immobility of the region, and that use of the orthosis should be accompanied by an exercise program. One of the goals of the rehabilitation program would be to ultimately discontinue use of the orthosis. Nevertheless, it is included under this objective because it often allows for an early return to activity. Figures 6–10 and 6–11 illustrate the use of a lumbar orthosis and a sacroiliac orthosis, respectively. Modifications to accommodate the pregnant population are also shown in Figure 6–11 as laxity of the ligaments of the pelvis in pregnancy may contribute to this type of low back pain.

Enhancing Neuromuscular Performance

The third objective of treatment focuses on exercise, with particular emphasis on physiological and structural changes of the neuromuscular and musculoskeletal systems as a result of resistance training. A basic tenet of musculoskeletal rehabilitation is that optimal neuromuscular function is essential for safe loading of the specialized connective tissues. Improvements in strength, endurance, and coordination are primary goals in rehabilitation and are essential components of neuromuscular performance.[7] Strength, power, and coordination are achieved, in part, by the effect that muscles have on fascia, and how fascia directs loads to the axial skeleton.[3, 24, 29, 30] It is the appropriate increase in tension (pull) to the connective tissue structures, par-

ticularly to supporting ligaments and fascial sheaths, that ensures proper intensity, frequency, and duration of loads that are a result of forces generated by gravity and movement. Another mechanism by which muscle interacts with the fascial elements is by "push." Pushing on fascia is described as the broadening of the muscle within a fascial envelope by either contraction or hypertrophy.[9, 18] Based on the interaction that muscle has with its associated fascial elements, two important goals of exercise are to increase the tension-generating ability of the muscle (affecting the muscle "pull" capacity), and increasing muscle girth or hypertrophy (affecting the muscle "push" capacity). These functions are improved with therapeutic exercise that provides the appropriate training stimulus, i.e., an overload that stimulates the necessary anatomical and biochemical changes required to increase hypertrophy and improve tension-generating ability. The challenge to the clinician is to provide the overload, via appropriate therapeutic exercise, to stimulate growth without exacerbating the painful condition.

The use of the term "training" should not be limited to a description of the activities of the athletic population, but can serve as the global description of applied exercise programs for patients with painful disorders of the spine, particularly the low back. Training the neuromuscular system is essential because the muscles serve as the most important and efficient shock absorbers for the skeleton (see Chapter 3). Training also entails teaching patterns of movement to the patient that minimize stresses to the injured region. The edema control and self-management education-

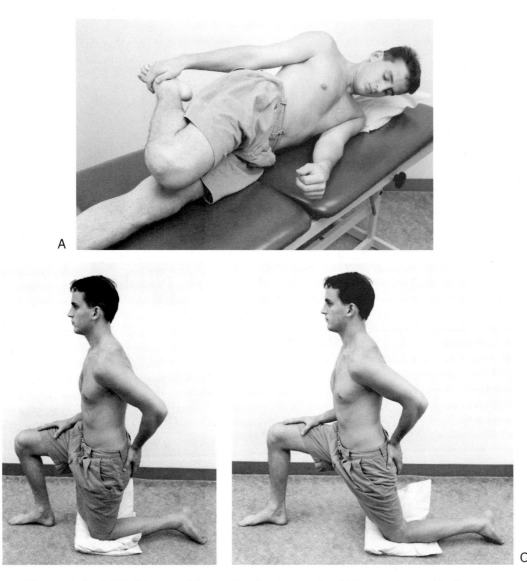

Figure 6–9. *A,* Side-lying stretching position for the anterior thigh musculature, hip flexors, and anterior hip joint capsule. The patient is instructed to maintain the position of his pelvis, via contraction of the abdominal wall, as the force of the stretch reaches it from below. This stabilization of the pelvis minimizes the extension and anterior shear to protect the lumbar spine. *B,* Another example of anterior thigh, hip flexor, and anterior hip capsule stretch in a kneeling position. The patient kneels on a pillow with the leg that is to be stretched. *C,* The patient then moves forward at the hip joint. The left hand augments the stretch by directing an anterior and inferior force to the pelvis. As in example *A,* the patient is instructed to stabilize the pelvis to protect the spine.

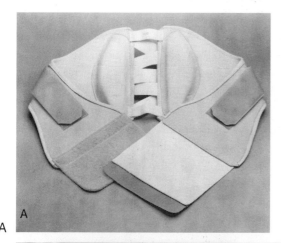

A

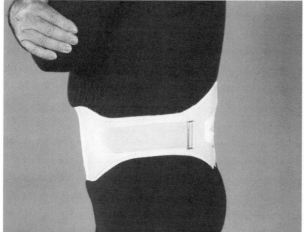

B

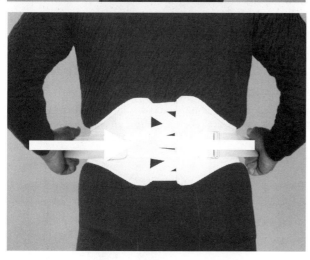

C

Figure 6–10. *A–C*, Lumbar support based on a securing and tightening system designed to create a resultant force of compressing the posterior lumbar tissues into the lamina and spinous process of the vertebral bodies. (IEM Orthopaedics, Ravenna, OH, patents no. 4, 794, 961.)

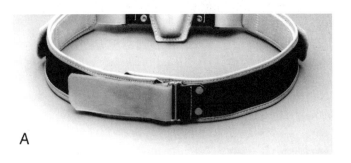

A

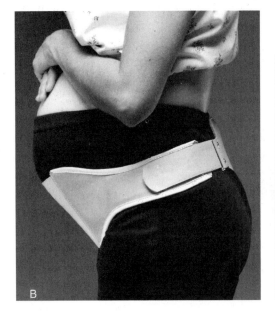

B

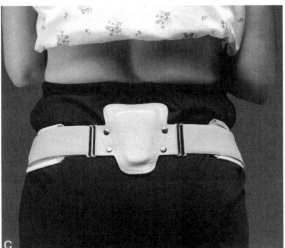

C

Figure 6–11. *A,* Sacral support used to create a posterior-to-anterior force of the sacrum and a posterior rotary movement to the ilium as the belt is tightened (IEM Orthopaedics, Ravenna, OH). *B,* Adaptation of the sacral component for the pregnant population. This uses an anterior window of elastic that allows the belt to conform to the abdomen. Posterior view *C* shows placement of the triangular pad on the sacrum (IEM Orthopaedics, Ravenna, OH).

al approaches of the two previously described objectives are intended to move the patient quickly and rapidly toward focusing on enhancing motor performance.

Although many different techniques are employed to enhance neuromuscular performance—including lumbar stabilization exercises, Feldenkrais techniques, progressive resistance exercises, work hardening, and functional restoration programs—this section of the chapter focuses primarily on resistance exercises designed to induce structural and biochemical changes that increase the strength, power, and endurance of the muscles that pull on fascia and the girth of the muscles that lie within fascia. Training of the muscular system affords patients the opportunity to better control how their weight line passes into and through the injured area (neuromuscular coordination). This helps control the intensity and frequency of the reinjury process. Learning to direct loads to invulnerable ranges (pain-free motions and positions) of spinal movement is the key to successful training. Starting a program in this manner can be valuable because it is the first attempt to train trunk muscles as *stabilizers* or *controllers,* rather than as *prime movers.* This type of stabilization exercise instruction might best be termed proprioceptive and kinesthetic training of the trunk, because the muscles are asked to control spinal position. However, although typical stabilization exercises are an excellent point from which to begin therapeutic exercise, the stimulus most often falls short of providing the overload necessary to increase strength, hypertrophy, and endurance.

When resistance exercises are incorporated into the training program, adaptations occur in the connective tissues and the neuromuscular system.[4, 8, 12, 16, 21, 24] Resistance exercise training results in an increase in connective tissue strength, including the specialized tissues such as bone, ligaments and tendons.[11, 22, 25, 28] The enhancement of connective tissue strength is optimized when exercises are done in weight-bearing positions, and an overload stimulus is provided. Adaptations in the neuromuscular system include muscle hypertrophy, increased resting turgor of the muscle resulting in enhanced muscle stiffness (resistance to deformation), and the development of more efficient patterns of movement indicating not only a muscular change but neural changes as well.

These changes have the potential to occur rather quickly. There can be a 15–20 percent increase in the integrated EMG and force output capability of the neuromuscular system in 4–6 weeks of proper strength training.[15] It should also be recognized that the weaker the patient the greater the strength change. However, the healthier the neuromuscular system, the quicker the recognition of the training effect. Strength changes such as force output, muscle fiber size, and improved efficiency of muscle contraction begin within 6 weeks of initiating a regular resistance exercise program.[15] It is important to make the patient aware that such favorable changes can be expected within this time period as long as they engage in a regular and consistent exercise program.

The training process has four important guidelines:

1. *Begin with submaximal loads and progress to progressive resistance exercise (PRE).*

2. *Take time to develop a safe movement pattern (stroke) for each exercise and continue the resistive exercise until the quality of movement changes (repetitions to substitution).* This ensures that each exercise bout works the tissues to momentary fatigue. As long as the emphasis is on smooth controlled motion, the chances for injury or increased pain are minimal.

3. *Progress to more functional positions.* Weight-bearing (closed kinetic chain) exercise stimulates all aspects of the axial skeleton to control the forces of the resisted movement.

4. *Vary the angles and positions of the exercise loads.* This is prescribed to recruit each aspect of the muscle and related tissues. The patient should be taught to use the first three or four movements to effectively develop the stroke, and then concentrate on the consistency of the resisted movement. This approach de-emphasizes counting repetitions and emphasizes the importance of analyzing movement.

The difficult questions for the clinician designing the exercise prescription relate to establishing the specifics of the exercise program:

- *How much?* This is determined by an estimation of the inflammatory state. This is best monitored by morning stiffness, and how easy it is for the examiner to provoke pain during the physical exam. As previously mentioned throughout this text, the goal of all of the treatment is to decrease the morning stiffness, while increasing the physical activity.
- *How many?* This should not be determined by a "standardized" number of repetitions or number of sets, but by exercising to the point of repetitions to substitution. The clinician must teach the patient that when substitution occurs, the exercise set should be terminated. This is very important because on one day several repetitions of one exercise may be an inadequate stimulus, and on yet another day, due to an increase in their condition, the same number of repetitions may result in further exacerbation or injury.
- *What position?* The optimal postural positions are determined through the functional assessment. Those positions or movement patterns that have been determined to be nociceptive are avoided or loaded minimally during a resistance exercise pro-

gram. Safe exercise can be accomplished by establishing the appropriate load transfer through the injured area by prepositioning or restricting the range of motion. The goal is to permit as much movement and load as possible without exacerbation. There are many variables in the three planes of movement that can be regulated; for example, bearing more weight on one side than the other in standing (frontal plane), externally rotating the femur on the side of the injury to decrease the compressive loads in the lumbosacral junction in standing (transverse plane), tilting the pelvis (sagittal plane) to a safe position, and creating a movement sequence that gently loads the injured tissues.

It should also be mentioned that depending on the extent and age of the injury, full resisted movement or tolerance to full resistance may never be possible. Most people do not recognize that there is decreased load bearing tolerance and changes occur in function as a result of injury. If the patient has a

15-year history of low back pain and has lost approximately 25 percent of normal function, it is unlikely that full return of function is realistic. In this case, the emphasis of treatment should not be on improving the 25 percent lost but on maintaining the remaining 75 percent.

For the exercise to have practical value, it must eventually be carried out in functional positions (specificity of training). Often it is not possible to begin resistance exercises programs from functional positions such as standing, but the exercise program should progress as soon as possible to weight-bearing positions.

The last aspect of the training process entails adequately stressing the muscular system to stimulate anatomic, biochemical, and neural changes by varying the loads and the angles of resistance. This provides varying stimuli that the muscle must respond to. Figure 6–12 illustrates this concept with a standing pull

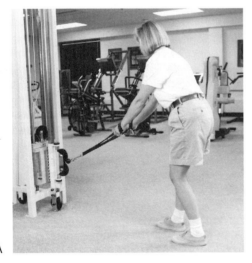 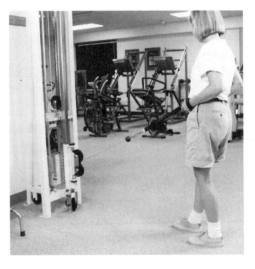

A

Figure 6–12. *A–C,* Varying the angles and positions of resistance. The standing pull exercise is an excellent training stimulus for the extensor mechanism. The technique involves transferring the weight from the front foot to the back foot as the pulling motion proceeds. This protects the spine by keeping it in a neutral position. The exercise can be done as a low pull (sequence A), mid-pull (sequence B), or high pull (sequence C). Note how the standing pull exercise trains the shoulder extensors, scapula retractors, spinal extensors, hip extensors, and quadriceps.

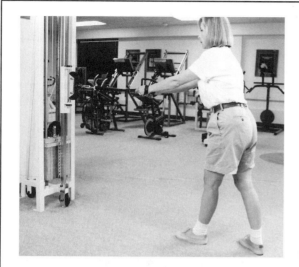
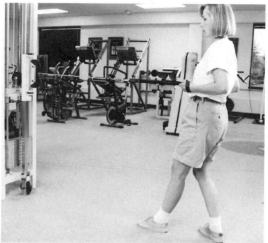
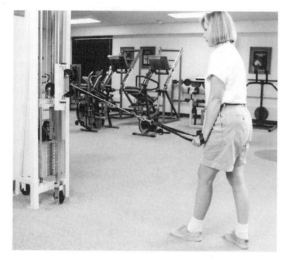
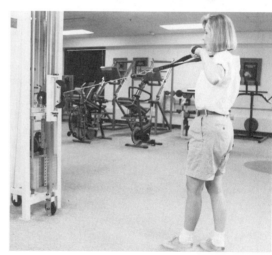

B

Figure 6–12. *continued*

exercise using three different angles of resistance. The patient is pulling low (toward the belt line), then up toward the midchest, and then up toward the eyes. As fatigue sets in with one angle of resistance, the angle can be changed during the pulling stroke to subtly change the demand on the muscles. Standing pull exercises are some of many movements to train the extensor mechanism of the trunk.

Enhancing Neuromuscular Performance: Specific Exercise Considerations

As previously mentioned, the integrated function between muscles and fascia in the lumbopelvic region serves as the basis for exercises designed to stabilize the lumbopelvic region. Therefore, exercises designed to

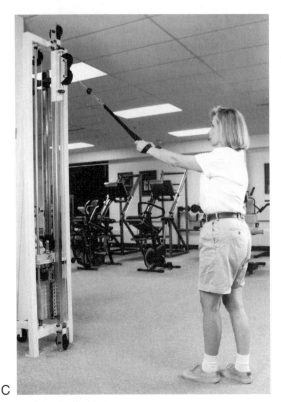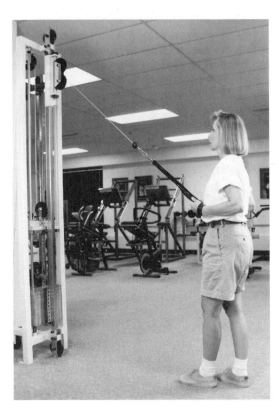

Figure 6–12. *continued*

increase the performance of the musculofascial system of the trunk are indicated for training patients with low back pain. The muscles associated with the lumbopelvic region include the abdominal muscles, posterior spine muscles, and those muscles associated with the pelvis, hip joints, and thighs (see Chapter 3). Within the lumbopelvic region are three important muscle fascial systems: *abdominal mechanism, thoracolumbar,* and *fascia lata.* Exercises designed to enhance neuromuscular performance will be described using these three muscle–fascial networks as the points of reference.

Enhancing Neuromuscular Performance: Abdominal Mechanism

The importance of the abdominal muscles and their various functions has been described in Chapter 3.

Table 6–3 lists a series of exercises designed to improve abdominal muscle strength through either motions of the pelvis on the rib cage, or motions of the rib cage on the pelvis. Figure 6–13 demonstrates movement of the pelvis toward the thorax through multiplanar motion. From this supine position, the thorax position is stabilized, and the pelvis (with the hips and knees fixed in flexion) moves in a diagonal toward the rib cage. If the functional assessment has determined that lumbar extension and rotation are not tolerated, the degree of lumbar rotation can be easily controlled by placing a bolster or pillow on the side of the lower extremity, which helps limit the amount of rotation as the legs and pelvis are returned to the starting position.

Figure 6–14 demonstrates the important supine pullover exercise that takes advantage of the mechanical linkage between the abdominal, pectoralis major, and serratus anterior muscles. In such an exercise it is

Table 6–3. Exercises for Abdominal Muscles

TRAINING FOCUS TO ABDOMINAL MUSCLES: SAGITTAL PLANE MOTION

Supine

  Upward pelvic tilt

  Maintenance of upward pelvic tilt while leg lowering (low back remains fixed against surface at all times)
    One leg lowering
    Two legs lowering with hips and knees remaining bent
    Two leg lowering with knees near fully extended position

  Reverse "crunch"—pelvis rolled posteriorly and slightly elevated off table at end of range via abdominal
    contraction

  Curl-up enhanced by increasing lever arm via position of hands at side, across chest, or lightly touching
    head. Arms should be strongly adducted to bring in pectoral muscles

  Sagittal plane crunch with hips and knees flexed

  Dumbbell pullover. The rib cage moves toward the pelvis while the arms are extended from overhead
    position

Sitting

  Resistance exercise using pulleys

Standing

  Medicine ball catches and throws with partner

  Standing pulleys—arm strongly adducted to side, and rib cage moves toward pelvis

  Pulling abdomen "in" away from beltline

TRAINING FOCUS TO ABDOMINAL MUSCLES: MULTIPLANAR (OBLIQUE) MOTIONS

Supine

  Cross crunch—upper thorax is rotated while maintaining flexed position of hips and knees

  Reverse cross crunch—pelvis is rotated while thorax is fixated and lumbar spine is held firmly against
    surface (hips and knees flexed to 90 degrees and that position maintained during rotary motion)

  Simultaneous cross crunch and reverse crunch

  Alternating bicycle motions with lower extremities

Sitting

  Rotary resistance through use of pulley system

Standing

  Medicine ball rotations with partner (standing)

  Standing pulley exercises with varying angles of resistance

Reprinted from Physical Therapy. DeRosa C, Porterfield JA: A physical therapy model for the treatment of low back
pain. 1992;72:261–264.

important that the motion pattern focus on moving the rib cage toward the pelvis. Exercises for the abdominal muscles that utilize pushing motions should emphasize a strong protraction motion to take advantage of recruiting the pectoralis major and serratus anterior muscles (see Chapter 3). Abdominal exercises from the standing position, utilizing a pulley system to vary the angle of resistance, are shown in Figure 6–15. This is an excellent exercise for the abdominal oblique muscles, and takes advantage of the linkage to the pectoralis major muscles by having the patient "push" the resistance across the body while simultaneously flexing and rotating the trunk over the pelvis. The eccentric capabilities of the abdominal muscle unit are also enhanced as the individual controls the speed at which the trunk returns to the starting position.

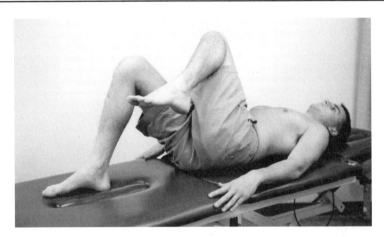

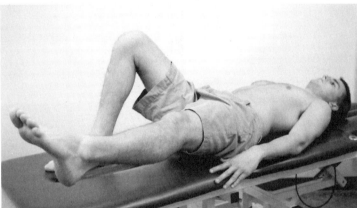

A

Figure 6–13. Supine lying abdominal exercise emphasizing abdominal muscle activity by movement of the pelvis toward the rib cage in a diagonal pattern. *Sequence A* demonstrates one leg only (left). Emphasis should be placed on the movement of the left anterior aspect of the pelvis as it moves diagonally up toward the right shoulder and the return to the neutral position. This exercise can be made more demanding by using both legs with hips and knees flexed *(sequence B)*. Maintaining control of the weight line as it traverses through the lumbosacral region during these movements is critical to minimize the chances for reinjury.

Enhancing Neuromuscular Performance: Thoracolumbar Fascia System

Several key muscles attach to the thoracolumbar fascia in such a way as to have a pulling effect and thereby potentially increase the tension in the thoracolumbar fascia. The latissimus dorsi pull superolaterally, the internal abdominal oblique and transversus abdominus pull transversely, and the gluteus maximus pulls inferolaterally. The superficial erector spinae and multifidus have a portion of their origin from the deep surface of the posterior layer of thoracolumbar fascia, but it is primarily an "enveloping"

relationship that the erector spinae and multifidus muscles have with the thoracolumbar fascia. Hypertrophy of the multifidus may be especially important for the clinician to be cognizant of, because atrophy and degeneration of the multifidus muscle are common histologic findings in patients with chronic low back pain.[13, 19]

Table 6–4 lists exercises for muscles related to the thoracolumbar fascia system. Pulling exercises [pulldowns, rowing-type motion against resistance (Fig. 6–16)] focus the training effect to the latissimus dorsi, while leg presses, squats, lift training, and hip hyperextension focus the training effect to the gluteus maximus (see below). Reciprocal motions are essential for

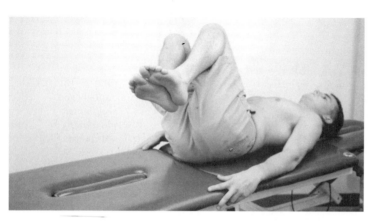

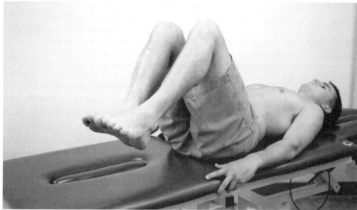

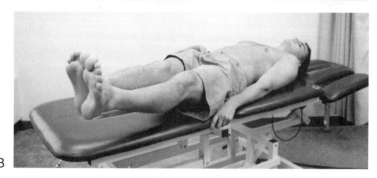

B

Figure 6–13. *continued*

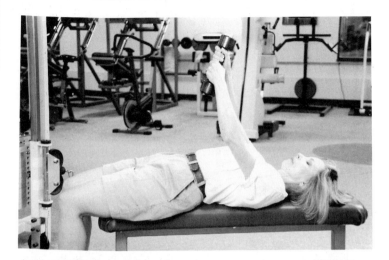
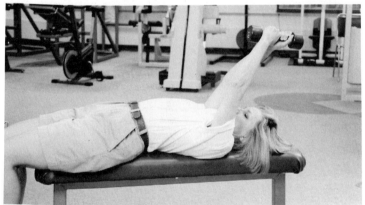
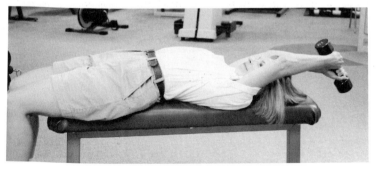

Figure 6–14. *A–C,* Supine pullover exercise with modification. These exercises are safe for most back patients and are excellent for strengthening the muscles of the trunk, i.e., latissimus dorsi, triceps, pectoralis major, serratus anterior, and abdominals. *Sequences A* and *B* show two different leg positions. The rib cage can be fixed or allowed to move depending on the patient's condition. Movement is preferred due to the action (coordination) of the abdominal wall. As in all resistance exercise, the range of motion should start small and progress to the largest possible range while still maintaining complete control. *Sequence C* is recommended after completing set *A* or *B.* This modification of the movement isolates the serratus anterior and abdominal wall. Note the forward and vertical direction of the movement. Stabilization of the pelvis via position of the femur can also be done.

A

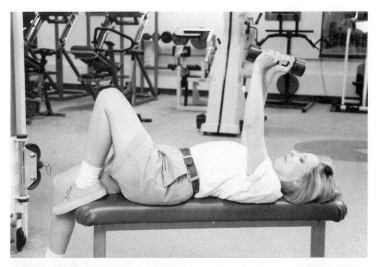

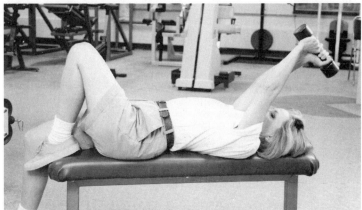

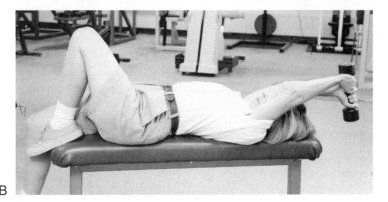

B

Figure 6–14. *continued*

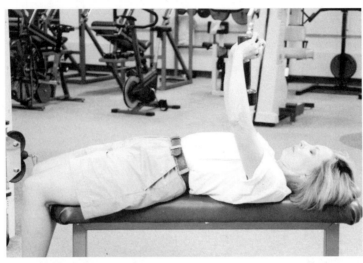

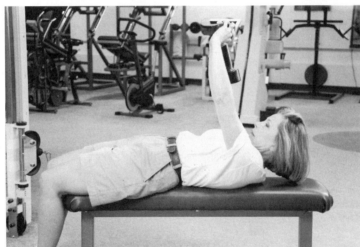

Figure 6–14. *continued*

training the latissimus dorsi and contralateral gluteus maximus.

Resistance exercise training to develop strength and endurance of the extensor muscles of the spine are recognized to have clinical benefit.[1, 14] Training for hypertrophy of the erector spinae and multifidus muscles occurs with resistance exercises emphasizing lumbar extension rather then pelvic motion, such as those done over a hyperextension support or stand-ing lift exercises. Figure 6–17 illustrates prone exten-sion over a high bench. With this type of exercise it is important to note whether the pelvis is fixated or free to move. If the pelvic support (pads or pillows) fixates the pelvis, the hyperextension motion is pri-marily due to action of the spinal extensors. How-ever, if the pelvis is free to move, the hyperextension motion is primarily carried out by the hip extensor muscles.

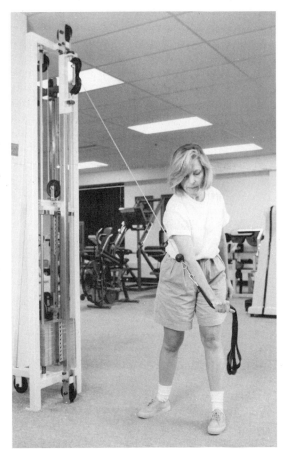 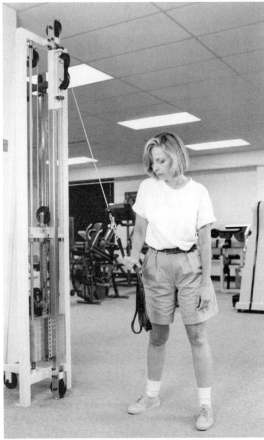

Figure 6–15. *A* and *B*, Standing high pulley exercise for abdominal obliques. In this exercise, the patient is "pushing" via the pectoralis major and serratus anterior while simultaneously flexing and rotating the trunk, and then slowly eccentrically controlling the return to the starting position. This is an excellent way to train the abdominal muscles in the upright antigravity position. Note the small range of motion and the isolation of the motion to the trunk. The emphasis is on bringing the right bottom part of the rib cage down and in toward the pelvis, rather than on the movement of the humerus.

Enhancing Neuromuscular Performance: Fascia Lata System

Tension is increased in the fascia lata system as a result of the strong pull of the gluteus maximus, since its primary attachment is to the fascia. Encased within the compartmentalized fascia lata are the quadriceps, adductor, and hamstring muscles. Of particular importance is the relative hypertrophy of the quadriceps because, like the gluteus maximus, these muscles are essential in the integration of activity between the spine and lower extremity. Contraction of the quadriceps results in a broadening effect within the fascia lata envelope, especially the vastus lateralis, which pushes against the thick lateral wall (iliotibial band) of the fascia lata. The fascia lata system is also extremely important because it is tied to the contralateral tho-

Table 6–4. Training Focus: Muscles of Thoracolumbar Fascia System

LATISSIMUS DORSI
Action: Resisted shoulder extension and/or adduction)
Goal: To increase tension-generating ability

   Pull down exercises (wide and narrow grips)
   One arm dumbbell rowing
   Seated row (from high, mid-, or low pulley)
   Standing pull (from high, mid-, or low pulley)

SPINAL EXTENSORS (ERECTOR SPINAE AND MULTIFIDUS)
Action: Resisted lumbar extension/hyperextension
Goal: To increase muscle hypertrophy

   Back extension/hyperextension over high bench
   Functional lift training (modified "deadlift")
   Seated row: movement from lumbar flexion to
      extension
   Squat exercise
   Dumbbell overhead cleans
   Back extension machines (pelvis fixated)

GLUTEUS MAXIMUS
*Action: Resisted hip extension; returning to upright from
      forward bend*
Goal: To increase tension-generating ability

   Pulley exercises for resisted hip extension
   Leg press
   Squat (weight line anterior to hip)
   Functional lift training (modified "deadlift," gluteus
      maximus/hamstring emphasis)
   Walking lunge (with or without dumbbell resistance)
   Step-ups
   Simulated skating

RECIPROCAL LATISSIMUS DORSI AND CONTRALATERAL GLUTEUS MAXIMUS)
Action: Shoulders/hip extension
*Goal: Utilize mechanical linkage between latissimus dorsi and
      gluteus maximus through thoracolumbar fascia*

   Functional lift training—gluteus maximus emphasis
   Cross-country ski simulators

TRANSVERSUS ABDOMINUS, INTERNAL ABDOMINAL OBLIQUE (SEE TABLE 6–3)

racolumbar fascia system by the powerful gluteus maximum muscle (see Chapter 3). One can begin to appreciate how the muscles of the upper and lower extremities are mechanically linked through the thoracolumbar and fascia lata systems.

Training of the quadriceps for hypertrophy includes exercises such as squats, lunges, and resisted cycling.

Table 6–5 lists several exercises for muscles intimately related to the fascia lata system. The squat exercise is extremely important and can be taught to the patient in several different ways. Note that the squat exercise is essentially teaching patients to raise and lower their body weight against resistance. For many patients, the hip extensors and quadriceps are so weak that their body weight is an overload stimulus.

Whether the squat exercise is performed with or without resistance, the technique taught to the patient should follow the principles listed in Table 6–6. These principles not only assure that the training stimulus is focused on the hip extensors and quadriceps but also increase the safety of the exercise. Of these principles, the most important one for patients with lumbopelvic disorders is learning to "track" the patella over the second toe during the descent. Often patients with weakness of the hip groups and quadriceps, or poor flexibility of the ankles, will track the knees medially by internally rotating their hips and significantly increasing knee valgus. When such a substitution occurs, the hip internal rotation tilts the pelvis anteriorly, resulting in increased anterior shear and compressive load to the lumbosacral region. Tracking the knee over the second toe during the descent phase (lowering the body weight) minimizes this force over the spine, and is an important instruction to give the patient engaging in any squatting or lunge maneuver.

Figure 6–18 demonstrates use of the gymnastic ball to help control the tracking of the patella over the second toe. In this case, the hip adductors are strongly recruited to help with pelvic and hip motion. Figure 6–l9 illustrates lowering the body weight to a bench. This is an excellent way to begin teaching the patient the concept of sitting back, rather than leaning forward. Dumbbells can be used to add resistance to the squat (Fig. 6–20). The exercise shown in Figure 6–21 can only be used if the patient can tolerate vertical loading of the spine. Note that a plumb line dropped from the weight should fall anterior to the hip joint, and posterior to the knee joint to overload both the hip extensors and the quadriceps.

Functional lift training is one of the most effective methods of training the hip extensors and hamstrings from the standing position. Table 6–7 lists instructions for teaching patients the exercise to focus on the hip extensors or the spinal extensors. This exercise should be used with caution when treating patients with forward-bending injuries, and the clinician may need to establish the range of safe forward bending against

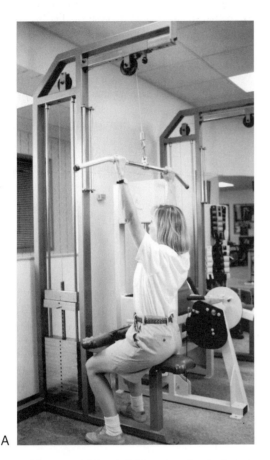
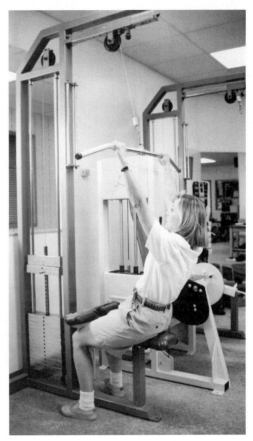

A

Figure 6–16. *A–C,* Exercises for the latissimus dorsi muscles, scapular retractors, and spinal extensors should include the pull down exercise (wide grip—*sequence A*, narrow grip—*sequence B),* and seated rowing exercises *(sequence C).* As in all resistance exercise, as the resistance increases so does the chance for strength gain as well as injury. Therefore, as the resistance increases, the motion should be controlled in an invulnerable midrange. *Sequence A* demonstrates a four-part movement: posteriorly rotate the pelvis, stabilize the spine, lean back, extend the humerus, retract the scapulae, and then slowly isometrically reverse the complete motion. To protect the back, the first and last movement should be at the hip joint and not at the spine. The narrow grip position permits a varied more efficient angle of pull, which will permit the use of greater resistance. *Sequence C,* seated row, is an excellent five-part movement for strengthening the back: forearm supination and spinal extension to neutral, humeral extension, scapular retraction, and slowly reverse to slight tolerable flexion. As with all resistance exercise, the clinician should instruct the patient to limit any aspect of the movement to minimize chances for injury.

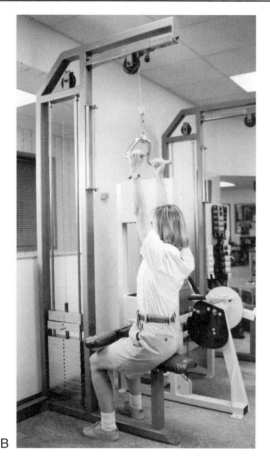
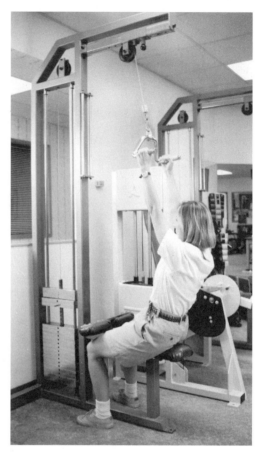

B

Figure 6–16. *B continued*

resistance. We prefer to have the patient keep the knees slightly bent to approximately 20 degrees, as this passively increases fascia lata tension.

The gluteus maximus/hamstring focus (Fig. 6–22) of functional lift training is one of the most effective ways of developing the strength and functional abilities of these two powerful hip extensors. The clinician closely monitors the exercise to be certain the pelvis is moving around the hips during both the descent and ascent of the motion, rather than the lumbar spine moving into flexion and extension. If performed correctly, the patient feels a slight stretch in the hamstrings when bending forward, and the lumbar spine is maintained in extension isometrically during both the descent and ascent phases.

CLINICAL EXAMPLES: PATHWAYS OF CARE CORRELATED TO FINDINGS IN THE FUNCTIONAL ASSESSMENT

Several clinical examples are now provided to discuss how treatment strategies might be incorporated for different clinical findings. The first example, frontal plane asymmetry, might be a finding during the standing assessment, and its potential effect on various lumbopelvic tissues is illustrated. Following the short discussion regarding frontal plane asymmetries, several different pathoanatomic diagnoses will be correlated

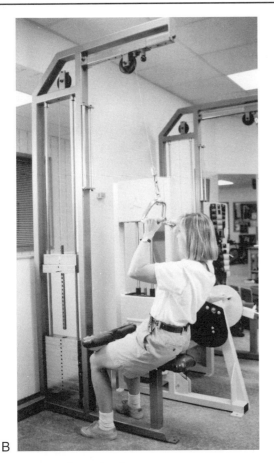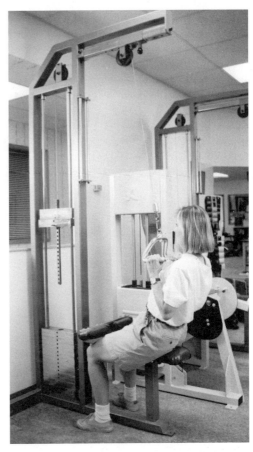

B

Figure 6–16. *continued*

to their pathomechanical counterparts. Treatment strategies based on the pathomechanics noted during the functional assessment will then be matched to the different objectives of treatment.

Clinical Example 1

Frontal Plane Asymmetry

As noted in Chapter 5, a frontal plane asymmetry of the pelvis is referenced by the low side of the pelvis. In a left frontal plane asymmetry, the left side of the pelvis is lower than the right side as seen in standing. This finding might be caused by skeletal differences

and neuromuscular imbalances in the musculature responsible for the frontal plane position of the pelvis. The outcome is an asymmetric loading pattern of tissues in the lumbopelvic region due to the lateral pelvic tilt on the left and the resultant lumbar side bending to the right (Fig. 6–23). Note how this standing posture of the lumbopelvic region results in the weight-bearing line traversing the right posterolateral corner in the lumbar spine.

This frontal plane asymmetry produces a similar convergence of ground and trunk forces to the lumbar spine as would occur with backward bending and side bending to the right. Although the magnitude of the forces is not exactly equal, the convergence of forces in both instances results in a close-packed position

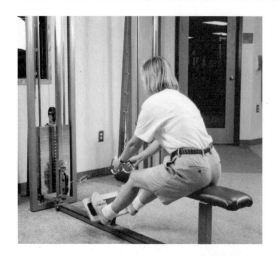

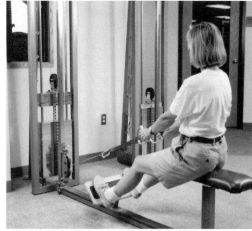

Figure 6–16. *continued*

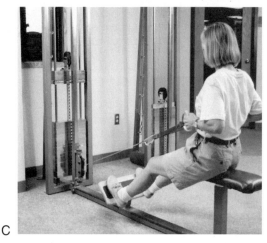

C

of the facets with increased compression and shear stresses. As noted in Chapter 5, there is also increased shear stress to the sacroiliac joint and increased compressive loading at the hip.

The soft tissues surrounding the hip joints are also affected by this frontal plane asymmetry (Fig. 6–23). The right femur (longer leg side) adopts a relatively adducted position with respect to the pelvis, and the left femur is relatively abducted. The lateral musculature of the right hip will be contracting from an elongated position, and the musculature of the left hip will be contracting from a relatively shortened position. Similarly, soft tissues at the hips are subjected to varying compressive and tensile loads. This

increases the potential for tissue irritation. Soft tissue diagnoses often seen with such frontal plane mechanics include piriformis syndrome due to increased tensile stresses to the deep rotators of the thigh, and trochanteric bursitis due to compression bursa by the gluteus maximus, both on the longer leg (relatively adducted hip) side or iliotibial band friction (Fig. 6–23). Heel strike on the short side, in the presence of weakness, can create increased frontal plane motion of the pelvis (down on the left in this example) and a varus force to the long-leg side.

This varus moment creates asymmetric loads that can result in an overload or tissue breakdown in any of the sites listed in Table 6–8. It should be recognized

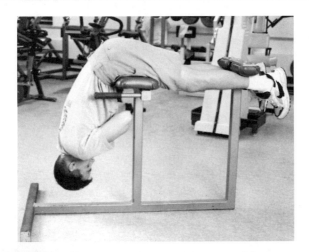

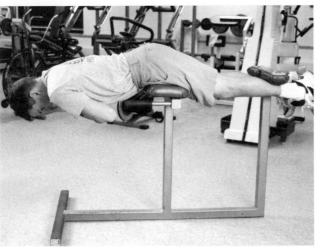

A

Figure 6–17. *A–C,* Prone extension exercises (two positions) over a high bench. The exercise can be modified based on the position of the pelvis on the pad. *Sequence A* demonstrates the best position for strengthening the back extensors. The pelvis is maximally placed or stabilized on the pad. *Sequence B* shows a forward pelvic position. This position permits movement of the pelvis, which effectively adds the hamstrings and gluteus muscles. *Sequence C* demonstrates the stabilized pelvis and the introduction of resistance, a barbell plate grasped across chest. The instructions to the patient for any of these exercises should be to tuck your chin, squeeze your buttocks together, pull your elbows into your side, and then come up.

that the anatomic regions closest to the convergence of ground and trunk forces, such as the L4–L5 and L5–S1 segments, sacroiliac and hip regions, are the most vulnerable to breakdown. When a patient has complaint of peripheral conditions (see Table 6–8) in the absence of direct trauma, the clinician should be searching for those abnormal, often asymmetric forces (trunk and ground) that are most often responsible for the continued symptoms.

One relatively simple way to manage this condition during the initial phase of treatment is through use of a heel lift, which may help redistribute the weight line by altering the frontal plane position of the pelvis. This in itself may be considered a mechanism to unload any of the aforementioned tissues that may be symptomatic. The trunk and ground forces now converge into the lumbopelvic region in a more symmetric, less destructive manner. The injured tissue is slightly unloaded, which helps optimize the healing environment for the injured tissue. Redistributing the load in this manner is often a valuable adjunct during the initial phases of tissue healing, especially if the patient

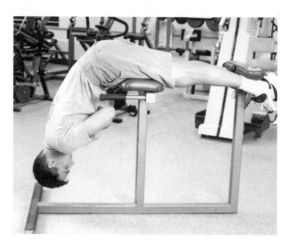

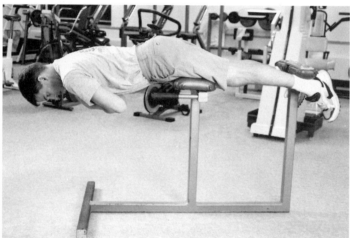

B

Figure 6–17. *continued*

responds favorably to the correction during the evaluation process.

These temporary lifts can be fabricated by using orthotic materials that do not "bottom out" as a result of compression. The lift is cut into the desired shape to fit the heel of the shoe, with the usual thickness being one-half of the discrepancy noted in the standing evaluation. Starting with this height gradually introduces the new forces into the axial skeleton, especially if the person is extremely active. A lift that is thicker than 3/8 inch often raises the heel out of the shoe's heelcounter and usually cannot be tolerated within the shoe. The heel lift can be incorporated into an orthotic.

Clinical Example 2

Pathoanatomic Diagnosis Correlated to Pathomechanics: Sacroiliac Joint Dysfunction

The various stresses to assess the pelvis were described in Chapter 5. Following is a treatment outline that matches the findings in the assessment to the objectives of treatment discussed above.

Sacroiliac joint involvement might be considered when the *history* suggests one of the following:

• History of fall? Force through ischial tuberosity?

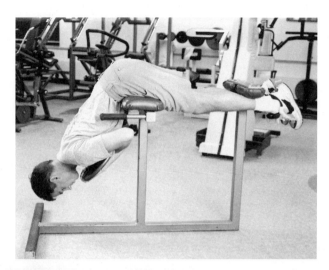

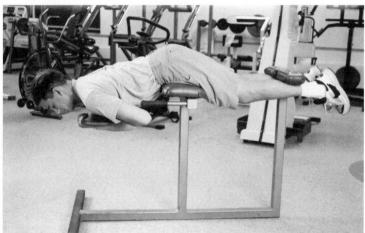

C

Figure 6–17. *continued*

- Pregnancy history—difficult delivery, multiparous, inability to decrease low back pain following pregnancy, even after a reasonable wait.
- "Lax" connective tissue framework of individual.
- Young individual—history of high kicks, abrupt step down.
- Referred pain into groin region, posterior thigh.

Sacroiliac joint involvement might be considered when the *physical assessment* suggests one of the following:

- Frontal plane asymmetry.
- Perception of unilateral asymmetry in the sagittal plane, i.e., one ilium appears rotated compared with the opposite. Consider the possibility that the pelvis is positioned to minimize anterior shear/compression at lumbosacral junction, rather than the ilium of the sacroiliac joint being rotated and "stuck."
- Inability to tolerate shear stresses at sacroiliac joint.
- Inability to tolerate torsional stresses. Care must be taken with this assessment because, in applying

Table 6–5. Training Focus: Muscles Related to Fascia Lata System

GLUTEUS MAXIMUS

Action: Resisted hip extension; returning to upright from forward bend

Goal: To increase tension-generating ability

Leg press
Squat (weight line anterior to hip)
Functional lift training (modified "deadlift," gluteus maximus/hamstring emphasis)
Walking lunge (with or without dumbbell resistance)
Step-ups
Hyperextensions over high bench (pelvis free to move)
Simulated skating

QUADRICEPS

Action: Control the rate of knee flexion in standing, knee extension

Goal: To increase hypertrophy

Squat (weight line posterior to knee joint)
Wall squat; hack squat
Lunge
Resistance cycling
Simulated skating

HAMSTRINGS

Action: Control the rate of hip flexion from standing; return pelvis to upright position from forward bend, knee flexion

Goal: To increase hypertrophy and tension-generating ability

Functional lift training—(modified "deadlift" gluteus maximus/hamstring emphasis)
Hyperextension over high bench (pelvis free to move)
Leg press
Resistance cycling

HIP ADDUCTORS

Action: Control pelvic motion on hip during gait

Goal: To increase hypertrophy

Freehand side lunge
Dumbbell side lunge
Simulated skating

Table 6–6. Raising and Lowering Body Weight Against Resistance: The Squat Exercise

GUIDELINES

- Keep the eyes forward and head up.
- Pinch scapula together—this assists facilitation of spinal extensors.
- Hips slightly externally rotated (usually about 30 degrees)
- Push through *heels* rather than toes during the move—this entails "sitting back" during the descent phase rather than shifting forward).
- During the descent, the patella should "track" over the second toe.
- If a bar is placed across the upper back, the weight line of the bar should fall through the midfoot.
- Begin with multiple repetitions without weight to encourage proper mechanics.

the treatment of sacroiliac joint dysfunction based on the objectives of treatment might be as follows:

Pain Modulation

- Consider use of iontophoresis or phonophoresis if subcutaneous fat is minimal over the region.
- Use of a nonsteroidal anti-inflammatory medication.
- Application of ice.

Application of Controlled Forces to Pelvis

- Muscle energy techniques in direction opposite manual stresses reproducing familiar pain
  Hip adductors
  Hip flexors
  Hip extensor
  Combined technique (contralateral hip flexion and hip extension)
- Joint mobilization techniques (torsional stresses to ilium)
- Sacroiliac orthosis—use of a support that increases the compressive force to the sacroiliac joint
- Crutches to control weight-bearing through lower extremity on the side of pain

Exercise Considerations

- Need for exceptionally strong hip extensors, but the training technique should not place hips into end-range positions.

torsion to the pelvis, it is very easy to generate a flexion force or extension/shear stress at the lumbosacral junction.

- Referred pain to groin, posterior thigh.

With the above findings in mind, and an understanding of the functional anatomy of the sacroiliac region considered (Chapters 3 and 4), a template for

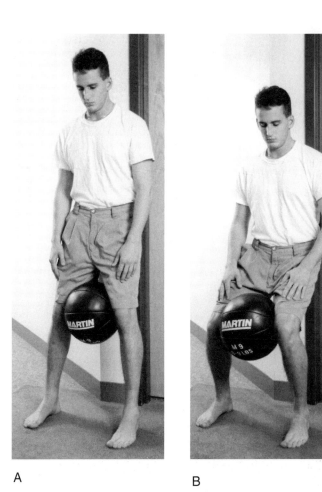
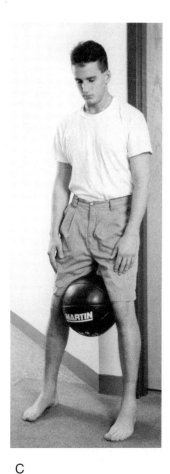

A   B   C

Figure 6–18. *A–C,* Use of a medicine or gymnastic ball during the squat exercise against a wall helps the patient track the patella over the second toe during the descent. The patient is also strongly recruiting the hip adductors and extensors, which helps control the position of the pelvis. The gymnastic ball is a safe way to begin learning the squat exercise.

- Avoid overload to hip muscles to such an extent that the resistance force of the exercise results in "isometric" muscle contraction.
- Train the latissimus dorsi muscles with resistance exercises.
- Train the erector spinae muscles with resistance exercises in invulnerable ranges.
- Train the abdominal mechanism.

Biomechanical Counseling

- Avoid deep squat.
- Avoid loading skeleton with lift from deep squat position.
- Avoid jumping.
- Avoid climbing stairs one leg over or two stairs at a time.

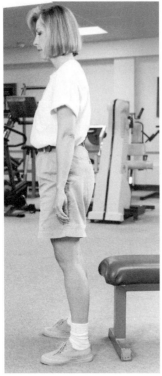

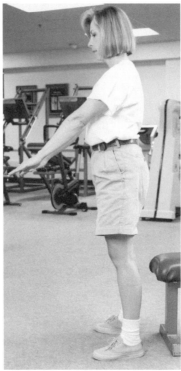

A

B

Figure 6–19. *A–D,* Slowly lowering to a bench is a safe way to begin teaching the patient how to strengthen and coordinate the hip extensors and thigh muscles. This sequence of four pictures shows the process. The emphasis is the slow speed of movement and the smooth transition between gently touching the bench and beginning the ascent. Use of the bench also provides the patient with the opportunity to learn to push through the heels during the ascent rather than leaning forward on the toes.

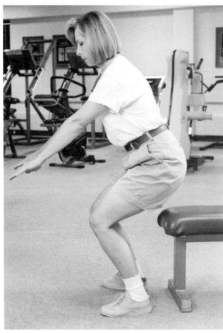

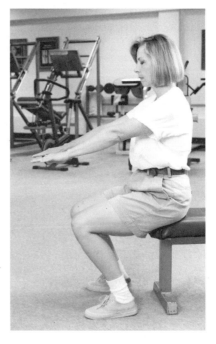

C

D

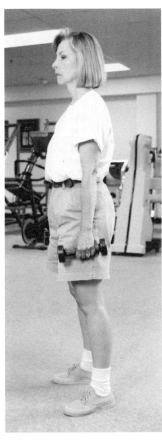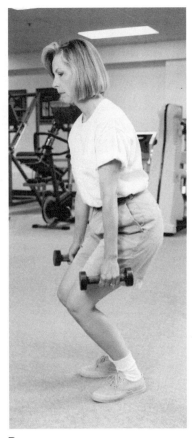

A   B

Figure 6–20. *A* and *B*, This sequence demonstrates resisted squatting using hand weights (dumbbells). Proper technique is the patella tracking over the second toe during the entire movement. Variations of this exercise might include the lunge and the step up, both of which can be performed with dumbbells for resistance.

- Understand the forces at sacroiliac joint and pubic symphysis with different sex positions, especially those positions in which hip is at end-range of motion or in Figure 4 position.
- Avoid sitting cross-legged.
- Avoid one-legged standing stresses.
- Recognize vulnerability of joint during menstrual cycle due to subtle increase in ligamentous laxity.

Although there are other means of assessing and treating suspected sacroiliac joint dysfunction, this template is provided because it illustrates an active approach toward rehabilitation designed around the objectives of treatment, with an emphasis on helping patients understand the mechanics of their problem.

Clinical Example 3

Pathoanatomical Diagnosis Correlated to Pathomechanics: Segmental Instability of the Lumbar Spine

In Chapter 3, instability of the lumbar spine was discussed in relation to a breakdown of the specialized connective tissues (due to injury or degenerative changes) resulting in aberrational motions between elements of the functional spinal unit due to applied physiologic stresses. It is a complex problem, and one without a universally accepted definition. What follows is a template for matching the pathomechanics found in the evaluation with a treatment process formulated around the objectives of treatment.

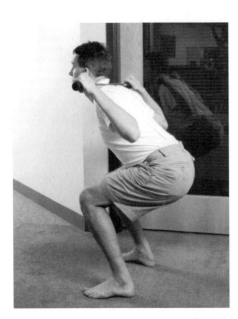

Figure 6–21. The squat exercise. Note that a plumb line dropped from the weight falls anterior to the hip and posterior to the knee. This ensures that the exercise challenges the hip extensors and the quadriceps muscles. The squat is one of the most important exercises that activates the main dynamic stabilizers of the lumbopelvic region.

Table 6–7. Functional Lift Training: The "Modified" Deadlift

HAMSTRING AND GLUTEAL EMPHASIS
- Individual fixes spine via abdominal and spine extensor co-contraction.
- Pelvis moves around the hips in both the controlled descent and the controlled ascent.
- Focus is on the ischial tuberosities going "upward" as one bends forward, and downward as one returns to the upright position.

SPINAL EXTENSOR FOCUS
- Pelvis is fixed via the hamstrings and the gluteals, i.e., the ischial tuberosities do not move during the descent or the ascent.
- Over the fixed pelvis, the lumbar spine gradually flexes in a controlled manner, and then returns to the upright position by extending the lumbar spine to restore the neutral lordosis. Range of movement in the lumbar spine is small and controlled.

Instability might be considered if findings during the functional assessment are suggestive of any of the following:

- Pain *during* forward-bend quadrants, but full forward-bending position with overpressure is tolerated reasonably well. End-range positions result in increased connective tissue tension which potentially augments segmental stability.
- Pain with standing extension quadrant with compression overpressure which increases lumbar shear stress.
- Pain with posterior–anterior shear stresses from prone position.
- Less pain with posterior–anterior shear stress from prone position when person is prone on elbows, which is an end-range, close-packed position for

the lumbar spine and allows less vertebral translation.
- Tenderness to palpation over PSIS. Pain over the region of the PSIS may be due to reflex muscle guarding by deep erector spinae muscle to minimize resultant shear force at lumbar spine due to instability.
- Greater stiffness and soreness in the morning on waking.

With the above findings on the exam, a treatment strategy and educational process for the patient might be matched to the objectives of treatment, emphasizing stability by utilizing trunk and abdominal muscles because the inert tissues have lost their stabilization capabilities. The patient must understand the effects of torsion and shear, which can occur during activities of daily living and work, because of their potential consequences over the lumbar spine. The patient must also begin to understand how the pain pattern is correlated to activities of daily living and work; the clinician provides this information in part by assessing those forces and movement patterns that reproduce familiar pain. Finally, a priority is developing power and strength in the hip and thigh muscles, as these are the primary "motors" for raising and lowering the body (squatting, stooping, lifting, etc.).

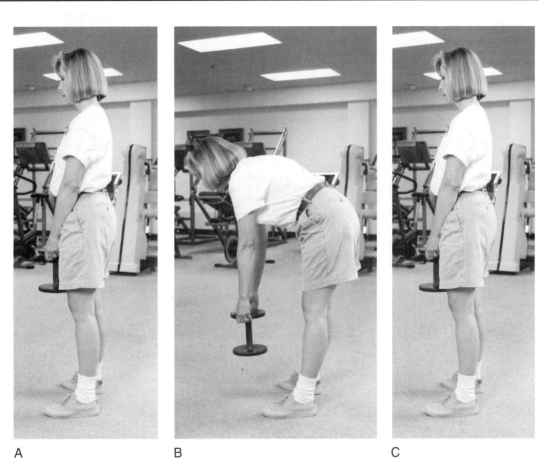

A   B   C

Figure 6–22. Functional lift training—the modified dead lift with emphasis on the hip extensor/hamstring or the spinal extensors. To focus on the hip extensor/hamstrings, the patient is instructed to slightly bend the knees, stabilize or fix the back, and concentrate the movement around the hip joints by placing the weight to an imaginary spot 4–8 inches in front of the toes *(A and B)*. The excercise should begin with a small range of motion and gradually reach the desired end range. Once this movement is completed to fatigue, it can be modified to place the emphasis to the lumbar extensors. The excercise can be described to the patient as follows: Keep the legs in the same position; start by flexing the neck and rounding the shoulders and back. Move the weight toward your toes. Slowly return to the starting position. The goal is a smooth, controlled, consistent movement until substitution or the slightest awareness of the provocation of symptoms.

Enhancing Neuromuscular Performance: Progression

Initially, the goal is to introduce exercises that begin conditioning and teach the patient vulnerable and invulnerable positions of low back. Start with stabilization exercises, but to make significant strength gains overload to the muscular system must be introduced, while avoiding reinjury. The patient should be made aware that morning stiffness is a key indicator of overtraining or reinjury.

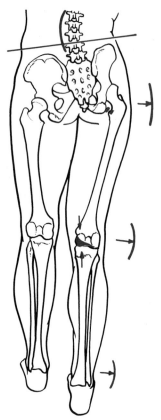

Figure 6–23. The frontal plane asymmetry results in increased compressive loading to the lumbosacral and lumbar joints on the long-leg side, increased shear loading on the long leg side, and different stresses to the soft tissues. The hip on the short-leg side is relatively abducted, which places the hip abductors in a shortened position while the hip abductors on the long-leg side are placed in a lengthened position. There is increased compressive loading to the trochanteric bursa on the long-leg side by the overlying gluteus maximus muscle. Note the forces to the long leg side as the pelvis drops in the frontal plane at heel strike.

Specific exercises to be performed are as follows:

• General conditioning exercises such as stationary cycling, because the lumbar spine is in a relatively flexed position.

Table 6–8. The Varus Condition

LUMBAR SPINE
↑ Compressive force to long-leg side
↑ Tensile force at short-leg side (HNP symptoms)

PELVIS
↑ Shear at the sacroiliac joint (long-leg side)

HIP
↑ Compressive force to hip joint and to tissues over greater trochanter on long-leg side (bursitis, tendinitis)

KNEE
↑ Tensile force at lateral compartment
↑ Compressive force at medial tibial plateau

ANKLE
↑ Tensile force to lateral compartment soft tissues
↑ Tensile force to the lateral talocrural joint

• Lumbar stabilization exercises.
• Abdominal set—pulling "stomach" away from belt line.
• Pulling exercises from the supine position, if very acute.
• Pulling exercises from the sitting position, but away from the quadrant that has been found to reproduce pain.
• Partial low back extension from the prone position (emphasize chin tuck scapular retraction during motions).
• Partial wall squats (emphasize scapular retraction during motion, and tracking of patella over second toe.
• De-emphasis on modalities, avoid joint mobilization or manipulation.

Specific exercises to be performed after the initial phase are as follows:

• General conditioning continued.
• Abdominal sets—pulling "stomach" away from belt line; progress to more aggressive abdominal muscle challenges such as standing pulleys.
• Pulling exercises from seated (toward but not into pain quadrant).
• Low back partial extensions—increases range (avoiding end range of extension) but still with emphasis on chin tuck and scapular retraction during motions.
• Squat exercises (lowering body center of gravity).

- Partial compound lift—gluteus maximus/hamstring emphasis with "stomach" pulled in.
- In the prone position, support the low back in a partially flexed position with pillows or gymnastic ball, and alternate arm raises.
- Standing alternate arm raises—emphasis on minimizing trunk torsion and lumbar postures that increase anterior shear.
- Leg pressing exercise.
- Modalities appropriate for pain relief following exercise.

Biomechanical Counseling

- Avoid torsion in back.
- Avoid ballistic "return to upright from bending" type of motions, as they have potential to increase anterior shear.
- Minimize times that heavy loads are lifted above head level.
- Minimize times of asymmetric lifts.
- Use of lumbar support in situations which can exacerbate the condition.

Clinical Example 4

Pathoanatomical Diagnosis Correlated to Pathomechanics: Inability of Posterior Joints to Tolerate Loading (Degenerative Joint Disease, Stenotic Spine)

The posterior joints are weight-bearing structures (Chapter 4) but begin to demonstrate degenerative changes resulting in their inability to tolerate loads. Findings in the evaluation that may be suggestive include:

- Frontal plane asymmetry with pain on the long leg side.
- Pain with extension quadrant overpressure (compression and shear), especially if this test reproduces familiar pain on same side as long-leg side.
- "Flattened buttocks" appearance due to tucking of pelvis; "loss" of abdominal wall.
- Pain with posterior-to-anterior stress directly over lumbar joints (compression–rotation stress).
- Pain increases in prone-on-elbows position, due to posterior-to-anterior overpressure. This position close-packs the joints, increasing joint compression.

- Adaptive changes in hips (cannot be changed with contract–relax techniques), such as asymmetrical (marked difference between right and left hips) FABERS test.

The rationale for treatment for abnormalities within the segment are exercise programs that offer stabilization of the range of motion by muscle activity and improved nutrition of the joint by mechanical activity. The treatment progression might be as follows:

Application of Controlled Forces to Promote Patient Function

- "Balance" frontal plane with heel lift if indicated.
- Stretch hip in Figure 4 position from sitting. Avoid stretching hamstrings; the hamstring force results in flexion at the lumbosacral junction, which decreases the compressive load to posterior lumbar joints.
- Physiologic mobilization—primarily sagittal plane and supplemented with techniques for frontal plane motion; begun passive but rapidly progressed to active. Progress to self-stretching of hips and low back; self-mobilization of back.
- Use of lumbar support in situations which can exacerbate the condition.

Enhance Neuromuscular Performance

- Pull "stomach" away from belt line—focus on abdomen below the umbilicus.
- General conditioning—seated cycling.
- Leg press exercises.
- Begin low back extension repetitions in range available—monitor where pain occurs in the range of motion to determine the safe range. Gradually work to increase range of low back extension exercises from increasingly flexed position.
- Walking, but with an emphasis on "pulling in" abdominal wall, squeezing buttocks, and working to maintain postural control.
- Supine-lying upper trunk lifts (scapula clear of table or floor) progressing to medicine ball or free-weight overhead; hips and knees flexed. When medicine ball or free weight is used, the rib cage must move toward the pelvis (true lumbar flexion motion). Contraction of the pectoralis major muscles should be part of the exercise.
- Alternate shoulder flexion–extension from sitting position with stomach away from belt line. Strong

emphasis on abdominal control during alternate shoulder flexions.
- Begin lowering of center-of-gravity exercises: squat, compound lift, lift with gluteus and hamstring focus.

Biomechanical Counseling

- The patient must understand the concept of the vulnerable and invulnerable range of motion.
- Provide rest posture instructions that focus on positions that decompress apophyseal joints, such as side lying with painful side up and top hip crossed over the opposite (pelvis rolled slightly forward).
- Patient should minimize overhead pushing activities as much as possible, as this increases lumbar extension and loading.

Clinical Example 5

Pathoanatomical Diagnosis Correlated to Pathomechanics: Sprain and Strain

Many activity-related disorders of the low back are often classified as "sprain and strain" injuries," because their time course to resolution often mimics the healing of muscle–connective tissue structures. Sprain–strain injuries might be considered when results of the functional assessment suggest the following:

- The history is "intensive"—onset does not appear to be insidious or gradual but more likely related to an injury mechanism such as lifting or bending to pick up heavy object.
- Pain is worse in any of forward-bending quadrants and is easily made worse with tensile overpressure.
- Tenderness to palpation lateral to spinous processes, above or below pelvis.
- Disproportionate referral into extremities with forward-bending assessment.

The rationale for the treatment strategy is to promote functional healing while at the same time recognizing the limits of soft tissue repair capabilities. Treatment progression might be as follows:

Application of Controlled Forces to Promote Patient Movement

- Active mobilization—prone hyperextension, press-ups (especially if pain is reproduced or peripheralizes with forward-bending tests).

- Active flexion and extension of lumbar spine from "all fours" position.
- Avoid stretching anterior hip structures initially, as this helps minimize the flexion force at the lumbosacral junction.
- Soft tissue/joint mobilization.
- Use of lumbar support if needed.

Enhancing Neuromuscular Performance

- Isometric low back extension progressing to unresisted low back hyperextension.
- Overhead pressing activities against light resistance from sitting or standing (medicine ball or free weight).
- Active PNF (nonresisted) diagonals for lower extremities.
- Overhead pressing activities against moderate resistance from standing.
- Seated rowing exercises with caution to avoid end-range forward-bending quadrants.
- One-arm rowing exercises from semiquadruped position.
- Controlled lumbar range of motion compound lifting with gluteus maximus and hamstring emphasis. During such training, the lumbar spine should be isometrically maintained in neutral lumbar spine position, avoiding end-range lumbar flexion.
- Leg press activities.
- Lumbar hyperextension exercises.

Biomechanical Counseling

- Instruct the patient in postural positioning for rest, such as prone on elbows, if this is an acute injury (first 7 days following injury)—patient must understand the concept of active and passive rest.
- Instruct the patient in tissue healing, especially the time constraints and the favorable natural course of healing events
- Instruct the patient in lifting, especially keeping loads close to center of gravity.
- Avoid pulling, jerking motions.

SUMMARY

The purpose of this chapter was to examine the different treatment techniques for low back pain and evaluate them as a means to meet the four basic objectives of treatment. An emphasis on exercise, considered for its effect on enhancing neuromuscular performance, is suggested as being highly indicated for most activity-related low back disorders, especially for the exacerbation of previous injury and chronic pain groupings. The rehabilitation process emphasizes the restoration of function by means of early activity and education for self-management. The treatment goal in all cases is to assist patients in maximizing their potential for functional healing and enhancing their ability to attenuate stresses in the lumbopelvic region. The musculoskeletal system responds favorably to the stimuli of exercise, and the health, fitness level, and understanding of the problem contribute greatly to the ability to manage low back pain of mechanical origin.

REFERENCES

1. Biering-Sorenson F: Physical measurements as risk indicators for low back trouble over a one year period. Spine 9:106, 1984.
2. Bigos S, Battie MC: Acute care to prevent back disability. Ten years of progress. Clin Orthop 221:121, 1987.
3. Bogduk N, Macintosh JE: The applied anatomy of the thoracolumbar fascia. Spine 9:164, 1984.
4. Conroy BP, Earle RW: Bone, Muscle, and Connective Tissue Adaptations to Physical Activity. In Baechle TR (ed): Essentials of Strength Training and Conditioning, Champaign, IL Human Kinetics, 1994, p. 51.
5. Deyo RA, Diehl AK, Rosenthal M: How many days bed rest for acute low back pain? A randomized clinical study. N Engl J Med 315:1064, 1986.
6. DeRosa C: Physical Therapy in the Management of Mechanical Spinal Disorders. J Musculoskel Med July:60, 1994.
7. DeRosa C, Porterfield JA: A physical therapy model for the treatment of low back pain. Phys Ther 72:261, 1992.
8. Dudley GA, Harris RT: Neuromuscular Adaptation to Conditioning. In Baechle TR (ed): Essentials of Strength Training and Conditioning, Champaigne, IL Human Kinetics, 1994, p. 12.
9. Farfan HF: Mechanical Disorders of the Low Back. Philadelphia: Lea & Febiger, 1973.
10. Guyton AC: The microcirculation and the lymphatic system: Capillary fluid exchange, interstitial fluid, and lymph flow. In: Textbook of Medical Physiology, 8th ed. Philadelphia: WB Saunders, 1991, p. 170.
11. Hansson T, Sandstrom J, Roos B, et al: The bone mineral content of the lumbar spine in patients with chronic low back pain. Spine 10:158, 1985.
12. Hakkinen KM, Alen M, Komi PV: Changes in isometric force and relaxation time, electromyographic and muscle fiber characteristics of human muscle during strength training and detraining. Acta Physiol Scand 125:573, 1985.
13. Hides JA, Stokes MJ, Saide M, Jull GA, Cooper DH: Evidence of lumbar multifidus muscle wasting ipsilateral to symptoms in patients with acute/subacute low back pain. Spine 19:165, 1994.
14. Kahanovitz N, Nordin M, Verdame R, et al: Normal trunk muscle strength and endurance in women and the effect of exercises and electrical stimulation and exercises to increase trunk muscle strength and endurance. Spine 12:112, 1987.
15. Komi PV: Training of muscle strength and power: Interaction of neuromotoric, hypertrophic, and mechanical factors. Int J Sports Med 7(Suppl):10, 1986.
16. Kraemer WJ: Neuroendocrine Responses to Resistance Exercise. In Baechle (ed): Essentials of Strength Training and Conditioning, 1994, p. 86.
17. Mooney V: Where is the pain coming from? Presidential address, International Society for the Study of the Lumbar Spine. Spine 12:754, 1987.
18. Porterfield JA, DeRosa C: Mechanical Low Back Pain: Perspectives in Functional Anatomy. Philadelphia: WB Saunders, 1991.
19. Rantanen J, Hurme M, Falck B: The lumbar multifidus muscle five years after surgery for a lumbar intervertebral disc herniation. Spine 18:568, 1993.
20. Saal JA, Saal JS: Nonoperative treatment of herniated lumbar intervertebral disc with radiculopathy: An outcome study. Spine 14:431, 1989.
21. Staron RS, Leonardi MJ, Karapondo DL, et al: Strength and skeletal muscle adaptation in heavy resistance trained women after detraining and retraining. J Appl Physiol 70:631, 1991.
22. Stone MH: Implications for connective tissue and bone alterations resulting from resistance exercise training. Med Sci Sports Exerc 20(Suppl):162, 1988.
23. Tesch PA: Acute and long term metabolic changes consequent to heavy resistance training. Med Sports Sci 26:67, 1987.
24. Tesh KM, Dunn JS, Evans JH: The abdominal muscles and vertebral stability. Spine 12:501, 1987.
25. Tipton CM, Vailas AC, Matthes RD: Experimental studies on the influences of physical activity on ligaments, tendons, and joints: A brief review. Acta Med Scand 711(Suppl):157, 1985.
26. Trafimow JH, Schipplein OD, Novak GJ, Andersson GBJ: The effect of quadriceps fatigue on the technique of lifting. Spine 18:3647, 1993.
27. van der Muelen JCH: Present state of knowledge on processes of healing in collagen structures. Int J Sports Med 3:4, 1982.
28. Videman T: Connective tissue and immobilization. Key factors in musculoskeletal degeneration? Clin Orthop 221:26, 1987.
29. Vleeming A, Pool-Goudzwaard AL, Stoeckart R, et al: The posterior layer of thoracolumbar fascia: Its function in load transfer from spine to legs. Spine 20:753, 1995.
30. Vleeming A., VanWindergarden JP, Snijders LJ, et al: Load application of the sacrotuberous ligament: Influences on sacroiliac joint mechanics. Clin Biomech 4:203, 1989.
31. Woolf CJ: Generation of acute pain: Central mechanisms. Br Med Bull 47:523, 1991.

INDEX

Note: Page numbers in italics indicate figures; those with a *t* indicate tables.

A

Abdomen, fascia of, 62t, 89, *90, 91*
    tension to, 96–98
    muscles of, 89–101, *90–101*
        actions of, 62t
        exercises for, 244–245, 245t, *246–251*
        lumbar shear and, 131t
        pubic symphysis and, *162*
    pendulous, *87,* 87–88
Abdominal oblique muscles, 89–91, *91–95*
    actions of, 62t
    attachments of, 89–90, *91, 95, 96*
    cross section of, *64*
    exercises for, 244–245, 245t, *246–251*
    sacroiliac joint and, 157, *160*
Abdominal wall, 89
    functions of, 62t, 95–100, *98, 100, 101*
    lumbar lordosis and, 96
    pelvis rotation and, *136*
    thorax and, 99, *100*
Actin, 53, *54*
Adaptive change, loading zone and, 19, *19*
Afferent-efferent pathways, anatomy of, 31, *31*
    imbalance of, 25
    nociceptors and, *47,* 47–49
Age, intervertebral discs and, 138
    optimal loading zone and, 18, *19*
Analgesia, 227
Angiotensin, 27t
Annulus fibrosus, *138, 140,* 140–141. *See also* Intervertebral discs.
    buckle in, *145*
    compressive force of, *142,* 142–143

Annulus fibrosus, (*continued*)
    during forward bending, 140–141, *141*
    nociceptors in, 139
Anterior superior iliac spine (ASIS), *151,* 180–182, *185*
Apophyseal joint, *122*
    nociceptors in, 28
Arthrosis, hip, 164
ASIS (anterior superior iliac spine), *151,* 180–182, *185*
Assessment, functional, 169–171, 170t
    gait, 188–189
    of leg length discrepancies, 185–188, *187*
    of low back pain, 169–171, 170t
        care pathways for, 254–255
    working, 171–172, 172t
Asymmetry, frontal plane, 159–161, *160*
    assessment of, 182–188, *187*
    compressive loading in, *266*
    exercises for, 255–258, *266,* 266t
    functional spinal unit and, *123*
    sacroiliac joint and, 159–161, *160*
Axoplasmic transport, *37,* 38–40

B

Back, locked, 136
Back pain. *See* Low back pain.
Bending. *See also* Lifting.
    annulus fibrosus in, 140–141, *141*
    mechanics of, 149
Body types, 15–17, *16*
Bursitis, trochanteric, 116

C

Calcitonin gene-related peptide, 27, 27t, 33
Capsules, joint, 12
    zygapophyseal, 128–130
Care pathways, for functional assessment, 254–255

ISBN 0-7216-6837-2